Bayesian Applications in Environmental and Ecological Studies with R and Stan

Modern ecological and environmental sciences are dominated by observational data. As a result, traditional statistical training often leaves scientists ill-prepared for the data analysis tasks they encounter in their work. Bayesian methods provide a more robust and flexible tool for data analysis, as they enable information from different sources to be brought into the modelling process. This book provides a Bayesian framework for model formulation, parameter estimation, and model evaluation in the context of analyzing environmental and ecological data.

Features:

- An accessible overview of Bayesian methods in environmental and ecological studies

- Emphasizes the hypothetical deductive process, particularly model formulation

- Necessary background material on Bayesian inference and Monte Carlo simulation

- Detailed case studies, covering water quality monitoring and assessment, ecosystem response to urbanization, fisheries ecology, and more

- Advanced chapter on Bayesian applications, including Bayesian networks and a change point model

- Complete code for all examples, along with the data used in the book, are available via GitHub

The book is primarily aimed at graduate students and researchers in the environmental and ecological sciences, as well as environmental management professionals. This is a group of people representing diverse subject matter fields, which could benefit from the potential power and flexibility of Bayesian methods.

Chapman & Hall/CRC

Applied Environmental Series

Series Editors

Douglas Nychka, *Colorado School of Mines*
Alexandra Schmidt, *Universidade Federal do Rio de Janero*
Richard L. Smith, *University of North Carolina*
Lance A. Waller, *Emory University*

Recently Published Titles

Statistical Geoinformatics for Human Environment Interface
Wayne L. Myers, Ganapati P. Patil

Introduction to Hierarchical Bayesian Modeling for Ecological Data
Eric Parent, Etienne Rivot

Handbook of Spatial Point-Pattern Analysis in Ecology
Thorsten Wiegand, Kirk A. Moloney

Introduction to Ecological Sampling
Bryan F.J. Manly, Jorge A. Navarro Alberto

Future Sustainable Ecosystems: Complexity, Risk, and Uncertainty
Nathaniel K Newlands

Environmental and Ecological Statistics with R
Second Edition
Song S. Qian

Statistical Methods for Field and Laboratory Studies in Behavioral Ecology
Scott Pardo, Michael Pardo

Biometry for Forestry and Environmental Data with Examples in R
Lauri Mehtätalo, Juha Lappi

Bayesian Applications in Environmental and Ecological Studies with R and Stan
Song S. Qian, Mark R. DuFour, Ibrahim Alameddine

For more information about this series, please visit: https://www.crcpress.com/
Chapman--HallCRC-Applied-Environmental-Statistics/book-series/ CRCAPPENVSTA

Bayesian Applications in Environmental and Ecological Studies with R and Stan

Song S. Qian
Mark R. DuFour
Ibrahim Alameddine

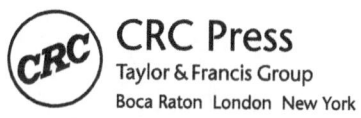

CRC Press
Taylor & Francis Group
Boca Raton London New York

CRC Press is an imprint of the
Taylor & Francis Group, an **informa** business
A CHAPMAN & HALL BOOK

First edition published 2023
by CRC Press
6000 Broken Sound Parkway NW, Suite 300, Boca Raton, FL 33487-2742

and by CRC Press
4 Park Square, Milton Park, Abingdon, Oxon, OX14 4RN

© 2023 Taylor & Francis Group, LLC

CRC Press is an imprint of Taylor & Francis Group, LLC

LCCN: 2022941760

ISBN: 9781138497399 (hbk)
ISBN: 9781032290072 (pbk)
ISBN: 9781351018784 (ebk)

DOI: 10.1201/9781351018784

Typeset in CMR10
by KnowledgeWorks Global Ltd.

Publisher's note: This book has been prepared from camera-ready copy provided by the authors.

To the Reckhow Lab

Contents

Foreword   **xi**

Preface   **xv**

Acknowledgments   **xvii**

1   Overview   **1**

    1.1   Two Modes of Reasoning: Deduction vs. Induction   1
        1.1.1   Testing for Snake Fungal Disease   6
    1.2   Bayesian versus Classical Statistics   10
    1.3   Guiding Principles   13
    1.4   Examples   15
        1.4.1   Gill-net Monitoring Data   15
        1.4.2   Effects of Urbanization on Stream Ecosystems   16
        1.4.3   Everglades Studies   18
        1.4.4   Compliance Assessment under the U.S. Clean Water Act   21
    1.5   Summary   22

2   Bayesian Inference and Monte Carlo Simulation   **25**

    2.1   The Role of Simulation in Statistics   25
    2.2   Bayesian Monte Carlo   26
    2.3   Sampling from Known Distributions   28
        2.3.1   Inverse-CDF Methods   28
        2.3.2   Acceptance-Rejection Methods   30
        2.3.3   Relationships Method   32
        2.3.4   Numeric Integration   33
        2.3.5   A Statistical Estimation Example   36
    2.4   Markov Chain Monte Carlo Simulation   41
        2.4.1   Metropolis-Hastings Algorithm   42
        2.4.2   Gibbs Sampler   45
            2.4.2.1   Examples   46
    2.5   Bayesian Inference Using Markov Chain Monte Carlo   54
        2.5.1   Metropolis-Hastings within a Gibbs Sampler   55

2.6   MCMC Software   57
      2.6.1 Stan   58
2.7   Summary   61

3 An Overview of Bayesian Inference   63

3.1   The General Approach   65
3.2   Example: Assessing Water Quality Standard Compliance in the
      Neuse River Estuary   66
      3.2.1 Background   66
      3.2.2 Study Area and Data   67
      3.2.3 The Problem of Specification   68
      3.2.4 The Problem of Estimation and Distribution . . .   68
             3.2.4.1   Likelihood Function and Prior Distribution .   68
             3.2.4.2   Deriving the Posterior Distribution . . .   71
             3.2.4.3   Predictive Distribution   72
      3.2.5 Application in the Neuse River Estuary   73
3.3   Specifying Prior Distributions   76
3.4   Summary   80

**4 Environmental Monitoring and Assessment – Normal
    Response Models   83**

4.1   A Simulation-Based Inference   84
      4.1.1 Using Stan through R Package `rstan`   85
4.2   Examples of Analysis of Variance   91
      4.2.1 The Seaweed Grazer Example   93
      4.2.2 The Gulf of Mexico Hypoxia Example 100
             4.2.2.1   Study Background 101
             4.2.2.2   Prior Analysis 102
             4.2.2.3   Implementation in Stan and Alternative
                       Models 103
4.3   Regression Models 108
      4.3.1 Linear Regression Example 109
      4.3.2 Nonlinear Regression Models 117
             4.3.2.1   Calibration-Curve Methods 117
             4.3.2.2   The Toledo Water Crisis of 2014 119
             4.3.2.3   ELISA Test Data 119
             4.3.2.4   Alternative Parameterization 123
4.4   Fitting a Hierarchical Model Sequentially 126
4.5   A Mixture of Two Normal Distributions 131
      4.5.1 Estimating Background Contaminant Concentrations . 132
4.6   Summary 139

5 Population and Community: Count Variables   141

5.1   Poisson and Negative Binomial Distributions   142
5.2   Analysis of Variance/Deviance   146
    5.2.1   The Liverpool Moth Example   148
    5.2.2   The Seedling Recruitment Example   156
       5.2.2.1   The Classical Generalized Linear Models . .   157
       5.2.2.2   Bayesian Implementation of GLM   158
       5.2.2.3   Over-dispersion   162
       5.2.2.4   Spatial Auto-correlation   165
5.3   Imperfect Detection   168
    5.3.1   The Data Augmentation Algorithm   170
    5.3.2   Example: COVID-19 Testing in Ohio, USA   177
       5.3.2.1   Initial Testing   178
       5.3.2.2   Shelter in Place and Reopening   179
       5.3.2.3   Programming Notes   181
    5.3.3   Zero-Inflation   183
       5.3.3.1   Example: Simulated Data and ZIP Model . .   186
       5.3.3.2   Example: Seabird By-Catch Data   188
       5.3.3.3   Example: Estimating Sturgeon Population Trends   191
       5.3.3.4   Example: Effects of Urbanization on Stream Ecosystems   196
5.4   Multinomial Count Data   206
    5.4.1   The Insect Oviposition Example   210
    5.4.2   The EUSE Example – Multinomial Logistic Regression   215
    5.4.3   The Everglades Example – A Missing Data Problem .   217
5.5   Summary   222

6 Hierarchical Modeling and Aggregation   225

6.1   Aggregation in Science and Management   226
6.2   Subjective Ignorance and Objective Knowledge   228
6.3   Stein's Paradox and Bayesian Hierarchical Model   232
6.4   Examples   236
    6.4.1   Example 1: Setting Environmental Standards in the Everglades   237
    6.4.2   Example 2: Environmental Standard Compliance . . .   243
    6.4.3   Example 3: Multilevel Modeling with Group-Level Predictors   250
    6.4.4   Example 4: Multilevel Modeling for Evaluating Fisheries Sampling Methods   261
       6.4.4.1   Regional Differences in Gill-net Catchability   262
       6.4.4.2   Species-length relationships   268
    6.4.5   Censored Data and Imperfect Detection   271

6.4.5.1   Example 5: Drinking Water Safety Review in
            the US   273
6.4.5.2   Example 6: Water Quality Survey of China's
            Drinking Water Sources   276
6.4.5.3   Example 7: Developing a Drinking Water
            Regulatory Standard in the U.S.   278
6.5   When Data from Nonexchangeable Units Are Mixed   288
6.5.1   Example 8: Are Small Wetlands More Effective in
            Nutrient Retention?   289
6.6   Summary   293

7   Bayesian Applications   297

7.1   Bayesian Networks   298
7.1.1   Model Structure and Conditional Probability Tables .   299
7.1.1.1   Building a BN Model   300
7.1.1.2   Populating the CPTs   309
7.1.1.3   Discretization and Its Impacts on a BN . . .   311
7.1.2   Model Diagnostics and Sensitivity Analysis for Bayesian
            Networks   320
7.1.2.1   Sensitivity to Findings   320
7.1.2.2   Model Validation   323
7.1.3   Spatio-temporal BN   324
7.2   Bayesian Change Point and Threshold Models   326
7.2.1   Hierarchical Change Point Model   335
7.2.2   Modeling Temporal Changes in the Flow-Concentration
            Relationship   338

8   Concluding Remarks   343

8.1   Model Formulation   344
8.2   Estimation   349
8.3   Model Evaluation   351
8.4   Statistical Significance and Bayesian Posterior Distribution .   355
8.5   Formulating a Prior Distribution Based on Hyper-distribution   360
8.5.1   Example: Forecasting the Likelihood of High Cyanobacterial
            Toxin Concentration Events in Western Lake Erie . .   363

Bibliography   367

Index   391

Foreword

I arrived at Duke University in 1980, eager to begin a research program focusing on statistical analysis and uncertainty analysis based on lake water quality data. I had learned about Bayesian analysis in my PhD program at Harvard, but I had yet to apply Bayesian techniques in my research. As a water quality modeler focused on statistical methods, I began to realize that Bayes' Theorem provided a logical framework for learning with new information. So, why not utilize the expert knowledge of water quality scientists to augment the information in water quality data? This expert judgment could become an informative prior probability to be updated with a likelihood function based on data. Ironically, at this time in the mid-1980s, Bayesian analysis was dominated by noninformative priors. This emphasis was gradually changing. So, in the mid-1980s I began research work with informative priors. An article in *Science* magazine [Malakoff, 1999] describes the emergence of applied Bayesian statistics, beginning with a brief description of my experiences attempting to apply Bayesian analysis to a water quality modeling problem in the mid-1980s.

Over the next 30+ years, I was fortunate to work with exceptional Ph.D. students who became my colleagues and friends. Beginning with Bill Warren-Hicks in the late 1980s, I established a significant intellectual collaboration with Robert Wolpert, a Bayesian statistician who successfully endeavored to understand the water quality modeling issues as he worked with us on Bayesian methods. That work with Bill and Robert was followed by Craig Stow's dissertation, which was the first of several addressing water quality in the Florida Everglades region. At the same time, Robert and I worked with Laura Steinberg, my Ph.D. advisee from Civil and Environmental Engineering, on a Bayesian model for PCB transport in the Hudson River. During this time, I continued to learn from my Ph.D. students and my Duke colleagues. Yet it was so much more than a rich learning experience. These students became my friends, and they became friends and colleagues with each other. Song Qian was with our group in the mid-1990s, and he helped me understand nonparametric Bayes. Song, Laura Steinberg, Robert Wolpert, and Michael Lavine increased my depth of understanding of Bayesian methods during those years. Beginning with this work, Song became the most adept Bayesian statistical modeler in my research lab. From 1996 to 2004, on a part-time basis, I became Director of the University of North Carolina Water Resources Research Institute. During that time, Craig Stow assumed some of my Duke teaching responsibilities, as well as advising my grad students. In this position, Craig developed into an excellent scholar and mentor, producing several outstanding Bayesian water quality modeling papers. In the late 1990s, I became interested in Bayesian networks. Mark Borsuk was a member of our grad student group at that time, and in his dissertation research, Mark demonstrated the merits of Bayesian networks applied to a water quality modeling problem. Mark is a terrific communicator and scholar, as confirmed by his academic position at Duke. Thanks to Bill, Craig, Laura, Song, and Mark, our program at Duke became the academic center for Bayesian water quality modeling. At that same time, our lab group included several Ph.D. students who contributed to the sharing of knowledge and camaraderie through their own research; these students/colleagues were Conrad Lamon, Barbara Van Harn Adams, Pauline Vaas, and Tom Stockton. Prior to their Ph.D. research, Pauline and Tom were professional master's students with me in the 1980s. Tom and I were distance running companions, competing in local 5/10 Ks and training/running in the Boston Marathon! Also during that time, we were fortunate to have George Arhonditsis as a post-doc in my lab. George's intellect and engaging personality were great assets to our lab. Ph.D. student Melissa Kenney provided a similar energy and leadership in my lab, particularly with my professional master's students. During that time, Song and I worked with my Ph.D. student Roxalana Kashuba along with USGS scientists on Bayesian Methods to assess the effect of urbanization on aquatic ecosystems using the USGS NAWQA data. Also during that time, Farnaz Nojavan Asghari added intellectually and internationally to our lab; aside from US researchers in the Reckhow lab, students/colleagues in our group were from China, Lebanon, Iran, Greece, and South Korea. Around that time, Drew Gronewold and Ibrahim Alameddine joined our lab group. Drew and Ibrahim continued to expand the application of Bayesian statistics in water quality modeling. They were not only great scholars; they were great mentors, as evidenced by each assuming academic positions following completion of the Ph.D. As I moved toward academic retirement in 2010, my group included two Ph.D. students from South Korea, Boknam Lee and Yoonkyung Cha. Boknam did some terrific work on Bayes nets focused on pollutant export from the hundreds of high-intensity hog operations in coastal North Carolina. Yoonkyung collaborated with Craig Stow at NOAA, modeling the *spirogyra* and *cladafora* that accumulated on the shores and beaches of Saginaw Bay. This work brought back distant memories; in the mid-1960s as a high school student, I would go with my classmates to Lake Erie beaches in Canada where we would have to wade through shoreline accumulations of *cladafora* to get to clear swimming water! I am delighted and humbled that Song and Ibrahim have dedicated their book to our lab group. As with many of life's endeavors, I ventured on an academic career that was fraught with uncertainty, least of which was the uncertainty in the water quality modeling that was the focus of my career! Without doubt, the most gratifying outcome of my academic career is to have worked with the wonderful scholars and friends who were

part of the "Reckhow lab." This honor that Song, Mark, and Ibrahim have bestowed on our research group is something that I will cherish forever.
  – Kenneth H. Reckhow

In my final year of graduate school at Duke University, we had a new student from China enter the program. We came from very different backgrounds and had very different life experiences, but we had something in common – we were both excited. He was excited to be starting and I was excited to be finishing. Another thing we had in common was a shared recognition of the potential to contribute to environmental decision-making by immersing ourselves in learning more about quantitative approaches. Although we overlapped in graduate school, what we learned there was very different. During my tenure, Bayesian statistics was fairly controversial and, for most applied problems, not very practical. By the time Song enrolled, fast, cheap computing and the coevolution of modern software resulted in an explosion of new possibilities and applications. I learned about Bayesian statistics; Song learned how to really make it work. Those complementary experiences served us well as we became friends, colleagues, and frequent collaborators (and PhDs). Song has become an ace programmer who dives deeply into statistical theory for use in environmental applications and typically offers-up novel approaches to problems I've been pondering. Our collaborations often work something like this – I approach him with data from a particular system (often a lake) and ask: "what if we did this?" He'll think it over and reply: "here's a better approach." And it usually is. Song's (or rather Dr. Qian's) updated book captures his interest in both statistics and environmental science and reflects what is now 25+ years of experience. Along with our respected colleagues Drs. DuFour and Alameddine, he presents a range of applied problems, a bit of statistical theory for context, and code to reveal the stories lurking in the data. I've learned a lot from working with Song over the years and I know readers will learn a lot from this book.
  – Craig A. Stow

Preface

We wrote this book to summarize our journey of learning and using statistics in our careers as environmental scientists. Statistics is a tool for inductive reasoning, using hypothetical deduction as the main inference method. The hypothetical deductive nature of statistical inference often dictates how statistics is taught and learned: we learn the deductive part of statistics and largely ignore the hypothetical nature of the deductive process. The statistical curriculum in a typical environmental sciences, biology, or ecology graduate program remains strongly influenced by biostatistics – a sub-field of statistics that focuses on statistical models developed to assess experimental data. Because proper experimental design can ensure that the resulting data meet the intended models, we learn which statistical model is suitable for each type of experiment.

The modern ecological and environmental sciences are, however, dominated by observational data. As a result, our traditional statistical training often leaves us ill-prepared for the data analysis tasks in our professional work. The three of us worked for a few years after college before going back to graduate school. A common motive for pursuing a graduate degree was the need to be better educated in statistics. In different ways, we were attracted by the potential of Bayesian statistics, although we initially had no idea what it was. Through our graduate studies and, more importantly, our professional work, we gradually learned the art of applying statistics and honed our abilities to use Bayesian statistics. We decided to write this book to summarize what we learned and re-learned in our combined approximately 45 years of professional life. In the process of writing the book, we revisited many of our published papers and reviewed them with critical eyes. We want to present the process of statistical application in our field, with an emphasis on how to propose and justify the model – the hypothetical part of the statistical inference. The deductive part is quite straightforward under a Bayesian framework – through Bayes' theorem to derive the posterior distribution, combining the prior (summarizing what we already know) and the likelihood (the support of the proposed model from data). By organizing our work based on the type of response variable data, we hope to provide our colleagues with a collection of case studies that can help them avoid some of the detours we encountered.

Chapter 1 is an overview of the book, including a summary of our understanding of applied statistics, an overview of the general principles in application, and a summary of some of the examples used in the book. Chapter 2 documents some of the most commonly used methods for generating random numbers from a probability distribution. Chapter 3 introduces the general process of the Bayesian inference, including our understanding of where and how to start when proposing a proper informative prior. These three chapters form the methodological basis of the rest of the book. The methods discussed in Chapter 2 are largely incorporated in most modern computer software for Monte Carlo simulation. They are unlikely to be directly used by a practitioner. A summary of our experience in writing Stan code is included in this chapter. Chapter 4 summarizes a number of examples with response variables approximated by the normal distribution. Examples in Chapter 4 are mostly related to environmental monitoring and assessment. Chapter 5 describes some commonly used models for modeling count data. The focus of Chapter 5 is on imperfect detection – a common feature in many ecological data sets. Chapter 6 is a collection of examples to illustrate the Bayesian hierarchical model (BHM). We see BHM as a tool for properly analyzing "big data" – data collected from multiple sources. We argue that properly modeling the hierarchical structure of the data is the key to resolving Simpson's paradox. Chapter 7 includes two relatively independent topics – the Bayesian network model and the Bayesian change point/threshold model. The book ends with a number of concluding remarks in Chapter 8, where we revisit the general themes of statistical inference with references to some of the examples covered in the book, as well as a discussion of the connection between classical hypothesis testing and Bayesian statistics. Our approach to the subject is application oriented, which may be justifiably criticized by both classical and Bayesian statisticians.

A casual reader can start the book with Chapter 1, Chapter 3, and Sections 2.5–2.6, then go to a chapter (Chapters 4–7) of choice (e.g., matches the application in hand), and finish with Chapter 8.

The R and Stan code printed in the book are not complete by themselves. They should be used as a reference. Complete code for all examples, along with the data used in the book, are available at the book's GitHub repository (`github.com/songsqian/beesrstan`). The GitHub repository is regularly updated.

Song S. Qian   Mark R. DuFour   Ibrahim Alameddine
Sylvania, Ohio   Sandusky, Ohio   Beirut
USA   USA   Lebanon

Acknowledgments

This book is possible due largely to the support and mentoring we had from Professor Kenneth H. Reckhow. Ken fostered a warm and collegiate environment in his lab. Ken's conviction and enthusiasm for adopting Bayesian statistics as a means to better understand modern environmental problems was and continues to be irresistible. Ken is serious about two things in life: Bayesian statistics and his support for the Blue Devils. His pioneering work in the use of Bayesian statistics in environmental modeling and management was seminal and remains inspiring. His lab attracted researchers from different backgrounds and varied prior experiences. His dedication to simplifying complex problems, ensuring that the forest is not missed for the trees, and his curiosity to explore topics at the fringe of his expertise have helped us become productive researchers and educators, each with a unique trajectory and a different focus area. In our years with Ken, we were given the freedom and encouraged to explore. Our dissertation research often established novel linkages between surface water quality modeling and research questions raised by policy makers, city planners, ecologists, toxicologists, and engineers. Ken always found a way to build on the individual strength of each of his students and was always open to exploring a new avenue as long as we could justify the approach to him. The process of developing a research topic, rather than being handed one, and the focus on being able to convincingly defend the adopted rationale made us all better researchers. The only mandatory task that Ken ever assigned to his students was to sit for Robert L. Winkler's class in Bayesian statistics and decision theory. While we all struggled through the class and, in the process, developed a habit of working with our fellow lab mates to work through hard problems, we all came out of that class with a better appreciation of Ken's commitment to Bayesian statistics as a means for environmental modeling and decision making. Over the years, the Reckhow lab has become a big family that now spans the globe with colleagues and collaborators who continue to work together. Many of us can trace many of the most important events that shaped our development journey to the time we spent at Ken's lab. For the first author (SSQ), the most memorable quote from Ken was "if a regression model has an R^2 value of more than 0.9, you should check to see if there is anything wrong with it." Reading Efron and Morris [1977] (a group activity organized by Laura J. Steinberg) in Spring 1991 is another important event in his tenure as a graduate student. Although the content of the paper was beyond his comprehension at the time, the paper was the initial inspiration for his pursuit of the Bayesian hierarchical modeling approach. The paper led to numerous discussions with Ken, and later with Craig A. Stow in the years after graduate school (sometimes over a shot of bourbon), and these discussions inspired many exciting ideas. For the third author (IA), Ken's summer book club that was dedicated to exploring the inner workings of Bayesian networks and SSQ's unwavering diligence to adopt the hierarchical Bayesian modeling framework as a means to tease out the signal from the noise, when data are collected at different spatial scales, are two landmark moments. Over the years, we had chances to collaborate with many of Ken's students, including E. Conrad Lamon, Mark E. Borsuk, Yoonkyung Cha, Andrew D. Gronewold, Farnaz Nojavan Asghari, and George B. Arhonditsis.

Ken's lab was open and inclusive. Each of us had committee members from statistics and other departments. Professors Michael L. Lavine and Robert L. Wolpert were popular committee members among Ken's students. We owe them gratitude for their tutelage of the fine points of applied statistics.

For the second author (MRD), his journey in contributing to this book began with an opportunity to join Professor Christine M. Mayer's lab and explore the use of Bayesian statistical applications in fisheries. The appeal of Bayesian methods was great while the struggle was real. As luck would have it, SSQ soon joined the department and immediately became a mentor and friend. Ken's emphasis on thought-provoking discussion, freedom to intellectually explore, development of coherent research topics, and culminating in statically rigorous applications continues to generate a learning and working environment that allows each of our students to grow as a researcher and person, and future students will continue to benefit from this influence.

Outside the extended "Reckhow family," we owe gratitude to many colleagues. Curt J. Richardson helped to clarify many questions we had regarding wetland nutrient retention in the Everglades examples. Boping Han and Dengsheng Lu discussed many potential applications of Bayesian statistics in limnology and remote sensing. Thomas F. Cuffney, Jonathan G. Kennen, Mary C. Freeman, Jason May, and Gerald McMahon were instrumental in shaping up the EUSE example. Michael J. Messner and Jonathon Koplos introduced us to the world of drinking water safety assessment. The idea of imperfect detection and the snake fungal disease example were given to us by Jennifer A. Moore. Christine M. Mayer, who mentored MRD, gave us fisheries insight to make the discussions of walleye examples less fishy.

We are indebted to Freya E. Rowland, Patrick M. Kočovský, Jason C. Doll, Jean Adams, and Robin White who read an early version of the book. They corrected many errors and provided helpful comments and suggestions. Our editors Rob Calver and Vaishali Singh oversaw the entire process, the book proposal, the writing, and the manuscript review. Without them, the book would have been impossible.

All errors remaining in the book are ours. A live errata is on the book's GitHub repository (`https://github.com/songsqian/BeesRStan`).

Any use of trade, product, or firm names is for descriptive purposes only and does not imply endorsement by the U.S. Government.

Chapter 1

Overview

This is a book for practitioners. Our goal is to introduce the procedure of using Bayesian statistics in environmental and ecological studies. As a practical application-oriented book, we use examples from the literature, most of them our work, to illustrate our approach to an applied statistics problem. In this chapter, we outline the inductive nature of statistical inference, the three basic questions in statistical inference, our guiding principles, and examples we use in multiple chapters. Our guiding principles are further summarized in Chapter 8, with an emphasis on the iterative nature of using Bayesian statistics in a problem (Figure 1.5).

1.1 Two Modes of Reasoning: Deduction vs. Induction

Bayesian statistics is named after the British Presbyterian minister Thomas Bayes (1702–1761), whose posthumously published paper entitled "An essay towards solving a problem in the doctrine of chances" appeared in the *Philosophical Transactions of the Royal Society of London* in 1763. In the paper, Bayes presented a solution to a problem of inverse probability regarding the quantification of a binomial distribution probability. Some speculated that the motivation of the paper was to respond to David Hume's essay in which Hume questioned the validity of inductive reasoning. Inference from cause to effect is an example of deductive reasoning, while the inverse problem, inference about the cause based on observed effects, is inductive reasoning. Although the differences are philosophical, the validity of induction brings into question all empirical claims, including science and religion (e.g., miracles as evidence supporting the existence of God). At the time, the concept of probability was only explored in the context of gambling. Although methods for calculating the probability of an effect (e.g., the chance of having a hand with four aces in a poker game) from a cause (e.g., dealt from a fair deck of cards) was well understood, the inverse problem (e.g., what is the chance that the deck is loaded if a poker player receives four aces in four consecutive hands) was hardly obvious at the time. The statistical question answered in Bayes' essay is related to a binomial problem. A deduction in this problem is to calculate the probability of observing x positives (or successes) in n trials when the probability of success is known, a question long answered by Bernoulli. Bayes' paper is about how to calculate the probability of success after observing x successes in n trials. This problem is actually very hard. The solution Bayes provided requires an initial guess of what the likely probability (p) would be. For example, we may limit the likely value to be one of the five values: $p_1 = 0.1, p_2 = 0.2, p_3 = 0.3, p_4 = 0.4$, and $p_5 = 0.5$. Then we can use Bayes' theorem to calculate the probability of each of the five possible values to be the true probability of success provided we also know, a priori, how likely each of the five probabilities are to be true.

Suppose we don't know how likely each of the five values are to be true. One way to express this ignorance is to assume that the five values are equally likely. In other words, we set $\Pr(p = p_i) = 0.2$ for $i = 1, \cdots, 5$. For a binomial process with probability of success p_i, the number of successes X is a random variable and its distribution is described by the binomial distribution. The probability of observing x successes in n trial is $\Pr(Y = y, n|p_i) = \binom{n}{y}p_i^y(1-p_i)^{n-y}$. Using Bayes' theorem, we can update the probability of being the true probability of success (p_i) after observing $data = \{y, n\}$:

$$\Pr(p = p_i|data) = \frac{\Pr(p_i)\Pr(data|p_i)}{\sum_{j=1}^5 \Pr(p_i)\Pr(data|p = p_j)}. \tag{1.1}$$

If we suppose that we conducted a study and obtained $x = 3$ successes in $n = 10$ trials, then equation (1.1) can be tabulated (Table 1.1).

TABLE 1.1: A discrete binomial distribution problem – tabulated for easy calculation and accuracy check.

	$p = 0.1$	$p = 0.2$	$p = 0.3$	$p = 0.4$	$p = 0.5$	sum
$\Pr(p_i)$	0.2	0.2	0.2	0.2	0.2	
$\Pr(data|p_i)$	0.0574	0.2013	0.2668	0.2150	0.1172	
$\Pr(p_i) \times \Pr(data|p_i)$	0.0115	0.0403	0.0534	0.0430	0.0234	0.1715
$\Pr(p_i|data)$	0.0669	0.2347	0.3111	0.2506	0.1366	

This tabulated method was initially used by Pierre-Simon Laplace, who was responsible for the general form of Bayes' theorem we use now. Using the general form of equation (1.1), we can tabulate the calculation, so that the tedious arithmetic is organized and easy to check for accuracy. Although we now can easily automate the calculation process using an R function, Table (1.1) is conceptually appealing.

```
#### R code ####
y <- 3
n <- 10
pri <- (1:5)/10
```

```
prior <- rep(0.2,5)
likelihood <- dbinom(y,n, pri)
post <- likelihood*prior/sum(likelihood*prior)

## in a function ##
bayes_binom <- function(y, n, p_i=pri, prior=NULL){
  k <- length(p_i)
  if (is.null(prior)) prior <- rep(1/k, k)
  likelihood <- dbinom(y, n, p_i)
  return(likelihood * prior / (sum(likelihood * prior)))
}
### End ###
```

The posterior probabilities $\Pr(p_i|y)$ show that, upon observing $y = 3$ successes in $n = 10$ trials, we believe that the probability of success is most likely to be $p = 0.3$, with a "posterior" probability of 0.3111.

Let's suppose that we carried out another study with a result of $y_2 = 2$ successes in $n_2 = 12$ trials. Because of the previous study, we have a better understanding the relative likelihood of the five possible values. Our interpretation of the new data should be based on the most recent information. That is, we should use the estimated posterior probabilities as the prior probabilities:

```
#### R code ###
> bayes_binom(y=2, n=12, prior=post)
[1] 0.10108542 0.43676278 0.34264060 0.10505992 0.01445127
>
### End ###
```

The information contained in the two batches of data should be the same with or without our two successive applications of Bayes' theorem. That is, our posterior probabilities should be the same if we use the flat prior (0.2) and the combined data of $\{y = 5, n = 22\}$:

```
#### R code ###
> bayes_binom(y=5, n=22)
[1] 0.10108542 0.43676278 0.34264060 0.10505992 0.01445127
>
### End ###
```

The above example illustrates the difference between deductive and inductive reasoning. Using deductive reasoning, we start from what we know to predict the outcome. As long as what we know is correct, the prediction will be correct. If we know the probability of success is $p = 0.3$, we can easily calculate the likelihood of observing $x = 3$ successes in $n = 10$ trials (dbinom(x=3, n=10, p=0.3)). Induction is the inverse process of figuring out the likely value of the probability of success when observing the data. In the binomial example, we start the process by providing an initial guess (the prior) and Bayes' theorem updates the prior with data. The updating process can be iterative.

The updating process is straightforward, but often tedious. In the above example, we limited the estimation accuracy of p_i to one decimal point (increment of 0.1). If we reduce the incremental increase to 0.05, we have nine potential values.

```
#### R code ####
pi <- seq(0.1,0.5,0.05)
post <- bayes_binom(y=5, n=22, p_i=pi)

print(cbind(pi, post))
print(pi_gvn_y <- pi[post==max(post)])
### End ###
```

Using this method we can achieve an arbitrary level of accuracy; by decreasing the increments thus increasing the number of potential values of p_i. This approach was used in the 1990s and is often known as Bayesian Monte Carlo (BMC), where thousands of potential values are used. When the number of potential values increases, equation (1.1) can be expressed in a continuous form:

$$\pi(p|y) = \frac{\pi(p)L(y|p)}{\int_p \pi(p)L(y|p)dp} \qquad (1.2)$$

where $\pi(\cdot)$ represents a probability density function. For example, $\pi(p)$ is now the prior probability density function of the binomial distribution parameter p. $L(\cdot)$ is the likelihood function. Because the observed data are discrete integers (e.g., $\{y = 5, n = 22\}$), the likelihood is a function proportional to the probability of observing y. In this case, $L(y|p) \propto p^y(1 - p)^{n-y}$. Now all we need is a probability density function of p (the prior probability) to describe our uncertainty on the value.

In practice, we often use a beta distribution to describe the uncertainty in a probability variable. The beta distribution has two shape parameters, α and β: $p \sim beta(\alpha, \beta)$ with a probability density function $\pi(p|\alpha, \beta) = \frac{\Gamma(\alpha+\beta)}{\Gamma(\alpha)\Gamma(\beta)}p^{\alpha-1}(1 - p)^{\beta-1}$, where $\Gamma(\cdot)$ is the gamma function. The mean of the distribution is $\alpha/(\alpha + \beta)$, the mode is $(\alpha - 1)/(\alpha + \beta - 2)$ (for $\alpha > 1$ and $\beta > 1$), and the variance is $\alpha\beta/((\alpha + \beta)^2(\alpha + \beta + 1))$. By using a properly selected combination of the two parameters, we can use a beta distribution to approximate our uncertainty about p. For example, if we are entirely ignorant about the probability, we can assume that any given value of p is equally likely as any other value, or $\pi(p) = 1$ (the flat prior), which is $beta(1, 1)$. Sometimes based on the available information, we may believe that the probability is more likely to be either 0 or 1 than any other value. A beta distribution with $\alpha = \beta < 1$ can be used (Figure 1.1).

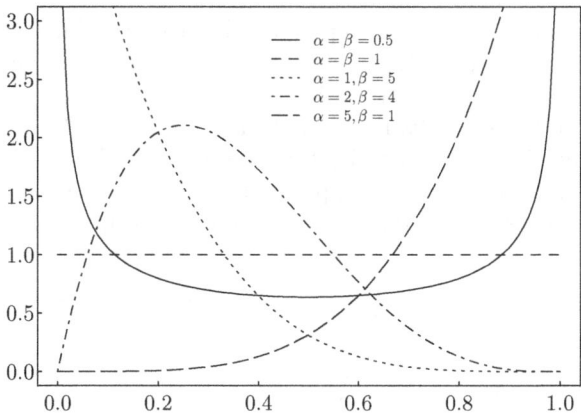

FIGURE 1.1: The beta distribution – commonly used to represent uncertainty in a variable bounded by 0 and 1.

Combining the prior $beta(\alpha, \beta)$ and the likelihood function, we derive the posterior distribution:

$$\pi(p|y) = \frac{p^{\alpha-1}(1-p)^{\beta-1}p^y(1-p)^{n-y}}{\int_{p=1}^{1} p^{\alpha-1}(1-p)^{\beta-1}p^y(1-p)^{n-y}dp}$$
$$= \frac{p^{y+\alpha-1}(1-p)^{n-y+\beta-1}}{\int_p p^{y+\alpha-1}(1-p)^{n-y+\beta-1}dp}.$$

Recognizing that the numerator is proportional to the density function of the beta distribution with parameters $y+\alpha$ and $n-y+\beta$ and the denominator is a constant, we can deduce that the posterior distribution is a beta distribution with parameters $y+\alpha$ and $n-y+\beta$. A quick shortcut for solving the integral in the denominator is to multiply both the denominator and the numerator by the beta distribution constant $\frac{\Gamma(y+\alpha+n-y+\beta)}{\Gamma(y+\alpha)\Gamma(n-y+\beta)}$ such that the denominator is an integral of a beta distribution density, which is 1. Using the data $\{y = 5, n = 22\}$ and a flat prior $beta(1,1)$, the posterior of p is $beta(6,18)$. This distribution has a mean of $6/(6+18) = 0.25$, a mode of $(6-1)/(24-2) = 0.2273$, and the 90% credible interval of the posterior distribution is $(0.1202, 0.4039)$ (Figure 1.2).

This binomial example illustrates a general framework of the Bayesian inductive inference. In any applied problem, the first step is always the identification of the response variable. In the binomial example, the response is the number of successes in a given number of trials. A probability distribution model is then applied to the response variable to summarize the data-generating process. A probability distribution model is defined through one or more unknown parameters. The unknown parameter(s) is the target of the inference once observations of the response variable are available.

Characterizing the data generating process is what Fisher called the problem of model formulation, the first step of a statistical modeling problem [Fisher, 1922]. The second step is Fisher's problem of parameter estimation – quantifying the unknown parameter(s) using observed data. The Bayesian approach is to derive the posterior distribution of the parameter, which is proportional to the product of the prior density function and the likelihood function. The difficulties of using the Bayesian approach are (1) finding the appropriate prior distribution and (2) computation (potentially high-dimensional integration).

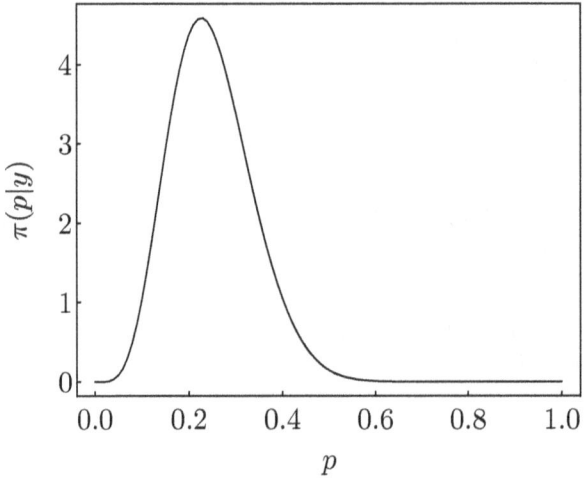

FIGURE 1.2: The posterior distribution of the binomial parameter is a beta distribution.

Many methods can be found in the literature for deriving an appropriate prior distribution. Frequently, researchers choose a class of priors that represents little or no information. The flat prior $beta(1, 1)$ is an example of a "non-informative" prior. In our work, we often find that these non-informative priors are worrisome, especially for parameters without a theoretical upper or lower bound. In the rest of the book we will discuss our understanding of the prior and how to derive a relevant prior in an application whenever appropriate.

1.1.1   Testing for Snake Fungal Disease

We use an example to explain the use of the Bayesian framework and show the difference between deduction and induction. When we have the model parameters, we often want to know the likelihood of an outcome (deduction). Conversely, when we have the outcome, we may want to infer the model parameter values (induction). This example is typical of many applied problems.

Snake fungal disease (SFD), caused by the fungus *Ophidiomyces ophiodi-icola*, is an emergent pathogen known to affect at least 30 snake species from 6 families in eastern North America and Europe [Allender et al., 2015, Lorch et al., 2016]. SFD was detected in eastern massasaugas (*Sistrurus catenatus*), a small, federally threatened rattlesnake species in Michigan, USA in 2013 [Tetzlaff et al., 2015]. The estimated SFD prevalence ranges from 3–17% in three Michigan populations [Hileman et al., 2017].

A commonly used method for detecting SFD is quantitative polymerase chain reaction (qPCR) to identify the fungal DNA using a skin swab. The method often leads to a false negative because swabbing can miss the disease agent. Hileman et al. [2017] show that a single swab of an eastern massasauga with clinical signs of SFD (skin lesions) can often result in a false negative; a positive result (detecting fungal DNA on an individual snake) does not always indicate that the individual has SFD (false positive). In other words, the test is imperfect and we are uncertain of the snake's true state regardless of the test result. Such uncertainty is quantified using probabilities, specifically, conditional probabilities.

For the purpose of discussion, we used a sample of 20 snakes, 5 of which tested positive for SFD. As the effectiveness of using qPCR for testing SFD is still under study, we use optimistic hypothetical rates of false positive (7%) and false negative (5%). With these facts, how we carry out further analysis depends on the objective of the study. If we are interested in the 20 individual snakes, the question is likely whether the five positive snakes are truly infected and whether the 15 negative snakes are truly free of the fungal disease. If the objective is to learn about the status of the disease in the snake population, the question is likely, "what is the prevalence of the disease in the population?"

To simplify the presentation, we use "+" to represent a positive test result and "−" to represent a negative test result. Likewise, we use *pr* and *ab* to denote the presence and absence of the fungus, respectively. That is, the unknown true state of the world is represented by *pr* or *ab* and the observed test results are + or −. Once we observe a + or − from a snake, we want to know the likelihood that the snake is infected or not. Using a probability symbol, we want to learn $\Pr(pr|+)$ (and $\Pr(ab|-)$).

Deduction: The following calculation shows that the disease prevalence is necessary in the deductive process. To summarize, we know the following quantities:

$$\Pr(pr) = 0.03, \Pr(+|ab) = 0.07, \text{ and } \Pr(-|pr) = 0.05$$

and observed a positive test result (+, data). If the objective is specifically the disease status of the 20 individual snakes, we have a deductive problem. There are two possible true states of the world: each snake is either infected (*pr*) or not infected (*ab*). From the known quantities and the data, we want to learn $\Pr(pr|+)$, the probability that *pr* is the true state of the world.

Before a formal statistical analysis, let us consider a hypothetical population of 10,000 snakes. Suppose that we can test all 10,000 snakes. The known prevalence of the disease (3%) tells us that 300 snakes are infected. These 300 infected snakes (and a 5% false negative rate) will result in 15 false negatives and 285 true positives. The 9,700 healthy snakes (and a 7% false positive rate) will result in 679 false positives and 9,021 true negatives. After testing all 10,000 snakes, there will be a total of 964 (679+285) positives and 9,036 (9,021+15) negatives. Among the 964 positives, 285 are truly infected. As a result, the likelihood of a positive snake being truly infected is 285/964 = 0.2956. This calculation is a deductive reasoning process. That is, we start from the known causes of a positive result to infer the probability of a positive snake being truly infected.

Bayes' theorem can be interpreted by this deductive calculation:

$$\Pr(pr|+) = \frac{\Pr(pr)\Pr(+|pr)}{\Pr(pr)\Pr(+|pr) + \Pr(ab)\Pr(+|ab)}. \tag{1.3}$$

When we know the prevalence $\Pr(pr)$ (3%), we can see that Bayes' theorem represents the same deductive calculation as illustrated in the previous paragraph. Before a snake is tested, we don't know whether the snake is infected or not. The prevalence of SFD allows us to make a probabilistic statement about the snake's status. Once the snake is tested, the snake population is now divided into two virtual populations: those would-be positive snakes and those would-be negative snakes. Bayes' theorem updates the prevalence in these two virtual populations. In the would-be positive population, the prevalence is now 0.2956. In other words, we can update the probability statement with regard to the positive snake.

Induction: If the prevalence $\Pr(pr)$ is unknown, and the goal of testing snakes is to estimate the prevalence, we then have an induction problem. That is, we infer the cause (the prevalence) from the effects (observing five positives in 20 snakes). Bayes' theorem of equation (1.3) cannot be used directly because the population prevalence ($\Pr(pr)$) is unknown; therefore, testing just one snake is no longer a viable option. Let us now return to the original data of 5 positives from a sample of 20 snakes.

To simplify the discussion, we will first assume that the test is perfect with $\Pr(+|ab) = 0$ and $\Pr(-|pr) = 0$, which brings us back to the binomial problem. As before, we can simplify the problem by limiting the prevalence value to one decimal point, that is, $\Pr(pr) = \theta = 0.0, 0.1, 0.2, \cdots, 0.9, 1.0$. More generally, $\theta = \theta_1, \cdots, \theta_k$. Alternatively, we can use a beta distribution (e.g., $beta(1,1)$) to represent the prior distribution of the prevalence. The posterior distribution of the prevalence is also a beta distribution ($beta(1 + 5, 1 + 20 - 5)$).

The problem is considerably more complicated because the test is imperfect. With an imperfect test, the probability of observing a positive result is no longer the prevalence. Using the Bayesian notation, we use θ to represent the unknown parameter of interest. In this case, it is the prevalence $\theta = \Pr(pr)$. Also, we use $f_p = \Pr(+|ab)$ to represent the false positive probability and $f_n = \Pr(-|pr)$ to represent the false negative probability. The data we obtain from testing a number of snakes are a binomial variable. The probability of observing a positive result is $p_+ = \theta(1 - f_n) + (1 - \theta)f_p$. The probability of observing $y = 5$ positive in $n = 20$ trials is:

$$L(y = 5, n = 20|p_+) = \binom{20}{5}p_+^y(1 - p_+)^{n-y}.$$

Using Bayes' theorem (equation (1.2), the posterior distribution of θ is:

$$
\begin{aligned}
\pi(\theta|y) &= \frac{\theta^{1-1}(1-\theta)^{1-1} \times p_+^y(1-p_+)^{(n-y)}}{\int_\theta \theta^{1-1}(1-\theta)^{1-1} \times p_+^y(1-p_+)^{n-y}d\theta} \\
&= \frac{(\theta(1-f_n)+(1-\theta)f_p)^y(1-\theta(1-f_n)-(1-\theta)f_p)^{n-y}}{\int_\theta (\theta(1-f_n)+(1-\theta)f_p)^y(1-\theta(1-f_n)-(1-\theta)f_p)^{n-y}d\theta}.
\end{aligned}
\tag{1.4}
$$

The integral in the denominator is no longer simple. However, we can derive numerical solutions using the characteristics of a probability density function, namely, the density function integrates to unity: $\int_0^1 \pi(\theta|y)d\theta = 1$, or the area under the density curve is 1. We can approximate the area under the curve by summing the numerator values on the right-hand side of equation (1.4) evaluated over an evenly spaced grid of θ between 0 and 1 and multiplying the sum by the width of the grid. Dividing these same numerator values by the approximate area under the curve, we have the estimated posterior density function, both numerically and graphically (Figure 1.3).

```
post_impft <- function(y=5, n=20, fp=0.07, fn=0.05, k=100){
    theta <- seq(0, 1,, k)
    fpst <- theta*(1-fn) + (1-theta)*fp
    post <- y*log(fpst) + (n-y)*log(1-fpst)
    return(exp(post)/(theta[2]*sum(exp(post))))
}

plot(seq(0, 1, , 100), (post2 <- post_impft()), type="l",
    xlab="$\\theta$", ylab="$\\pi(\\theta|y)$")
### End ###
```

With these two examples, we show the difference between deduction and induction. The most important difference is the target of the inference. When we know the prevalence, we want to know the likelihood of infection of an individual snake (deduction). Consequently, Bayes' theorem calculated $Pr(pr|+) = 0.2956$ is specific to individual snakes. The flow of information goes from the cause and data to the quantity of interest. When the prevalence is unknown, our goal becomes the estimation of the prevalence based on the test result (induction). The flow of information goes from data back to the cause (Figure 1.4). While the deductive calculation is definite, the inductive process requires additional information about the quantity of interest.

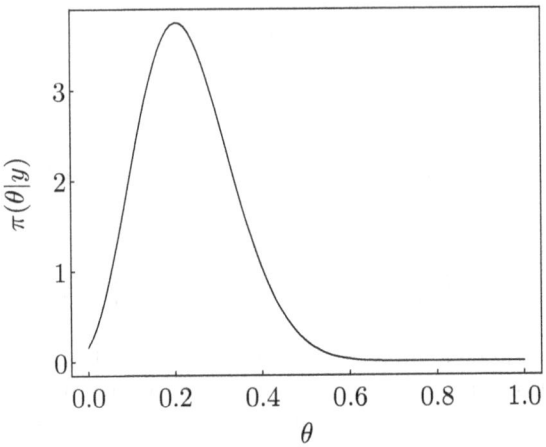

FIGURE 1.3: The posterior distribution of the unknown prevalence of snake fungal disease is graphically displayed.

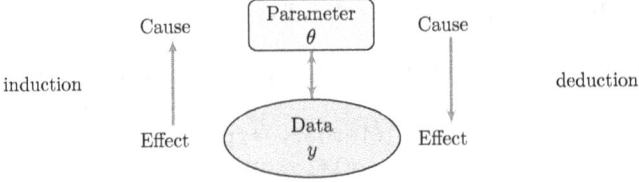

FIGURE 1.4: Deduction reasoning goes from cause to effect, whereas induction goes from effect to cause.

1.2   Bayesian versus Classical Statistics

Neyman and Pearson started their 1933 paper that developed the classical statistical hypothesis testing theory (the Neyman-Pearson lemma) with a review of existing methods for testing statistical hypothesis. They cited Bayes as the first to develop a test to learn about a causal relationship – what are the probabilities that the observed data (e.g., $y = 5, n = 20$) are caused by several likely events (e.g., p_j)? They quickly declared that their work was about a different kind of hypothesis testing – a procedure for discovering a "characteristic" of the data, upon which one can determine whether to reject the hypothesis of interest. The procedure ensures that the hypothesis will be rejected only infrequently when it is correct, and rejected when it is wrong with a high probability. This is the classical null hypothesis testing, where a null hypothesis (e.g., $p = 0.3$) is set against an alternative hypothesis ($p \neq 0.3$). A test statistic, for example, number of successes (y) in n trials, a binomial random variable with $p = 0.3$ under the null hypothesis, is compared to a set of criteria. In this case, if $2 \leq y \leq 10$, we do not reject the null hypothesis and otherwise we do. This procedure ensures that when the null hypothesis is true (i.e., $p = 0.3$) the probability of rejecting the null is approximately $\alpha = 0.05$. Neyman and Pearson [1933] showed that when the null is not true, this procedure will reject the null hypothesis with the highest probability among any other kind of tests. In the introduction section of their paper, Neyman and Pearson stated that the objective of such procedure is not to determine how likely it is taht the null hypothesis is true. Rather, the procedure provides a rational "rule of behavior:"

> Without hoping to know whether each separate hypothesis is true or false, we may search for rules to govern our behaviour with regard to them, in following which we insure that, in the long run of experience, we shall not be too often wrong. Here, for example, would be such a "rule of behaviour": to decide whether a hypothesis, H, of a given type be rejected or not, calculate a specified character, x, of the observed facts; if $x > x_0$ reject H, if $x < x_0$ accept H. Such a rule tells us nothing as to whether in a particular case H is true when $x \leq x_0$ or false when $x > x_0$. But it may often be proved that if we behave according to such a rule, then in the long run we shall reject H when it is true not more, say, than once in a hundred times, and in addition we may have evidence that we shall reject H sufficiently often when it is false.

This long-run frequency interpretation of statistics is the foundation of all classical statistics. For example, confidence intervals are used to measure the uncertainty in almost all estimated parameters. The interpretation of a confidence interval is not about the likely range of the parameter, rather a rule of behavior. That is, the parameter of interest is a fixed number and the confidence interval is random. The probabilistic statement of being 95% confident is about the confidence interval, not about the parameter of interest – if we repeat the same estimation process and construct the confidence interval each time, 95% of the intervals will include the true parameter value. But for the specific confidence interval at hand, there is no hope to determine whether the true parameter value is inside or outside of the confidence interval. This is a rule of behavior, in that, if we use the confidence interval as a guide to make decisions about the parameter of interest, we will be correct 95% of the time. This rule of behavior may be fine in some situations, but is often confusing when used in scientific research.

In scientific research, we are interested in the underlying causal relationship, that is, we want to know the value of the SFD prevalence θ. Any specific value of the prevalence (e.g., $\theta = 0.3$) is unlikely to be exactly true. As a result, a long-run frequency approach (e.g., testing whether $\theta = 0.3$) is simply unsatisfactory. The Bayesian approach is focused on the understanding of the causal relationship. As a result, the Bayesian approach is more focused on the problem of estimation. Although the core component of the Bayesian framework, the likelihood function, is the same used in the classical statistics, the Bayesian view of the role of data in our quest for the truth is fundamentally different from the long-run frequency perspective. However, scientists are often naturally Bayesian, in that, we rarely interpret statistical results in terms of long-run frequency. Because graduate-level statistics instruction in scientific disciplines is nearly inevitably based on classical statistics, we are accustomed to the standardized classical statistical models, from t-test, to linear regression and generalized linear models, and sometimes multilevel models (most likely referred to as the mixed effect models). When Bayesian statistics is introduced, we often use non-informative priors on familiar models, which leads to posterior distributions of parameters of interest similar to the classical statistical estimates (most likely using the maximum likelihood estimator). As a result, some question the need for Bayesian statistics, especially with the added computational burden.

Because of the shared likelihood function in both classical and Bayesian statistics, they also share some basic principles as we discussed earlier. We would start a statistical inference problem with the problem of model formulation and likely arrive at the same probabilistic model, regardless of our statistical denomination. Suppose that the Bayesian statistician has no prior knowledge for the parameter of interest; both the classical statistician and the Bayesian statistician summarize information in the data using the same likelihood function. The difference between the two lies in how they present the information represented in the likelihood function. The classical statistician would present the parameter value that maximizes the likelihood function as the best estimate of the unknown parameter (i.e., developing the maximum likelihood estimator). Finding the value is a mathematical optimization process, mainly through derivative operation. The Bayesian statistician would normalize the likelihood function and present the unknown parameter as a probability distribution. The Bayesian computation is mostly solving integrals. For example, in the snake fungal disease example, the likelihood function of the problem in equation (1.4) is

$$L = (\theta(1 - f_n) + (1 - \theta)f_p)^y (1 - \theta(1 - f_n) - (1 - \theta)f_p)^{n-y}.$$

The maximum likelihood estimator (MLE) of θ is often derived by setting the first derivative of the likelihood function to 0. Because the log transformation is a monotonic transformation, we can find the MLE using the log-likelihood, which often simplifies the operation. In this case,

$$\frac{d\log(L)}{d\theta} = \frac{y(1 - f_n - f_p)}{\theta(1 - f_n - f_p) + f_p} - \frac{(n - y)(1 - f_n - f_p)}{1 - \theta(1 - f_n - f_p) - f_p}.$$

Setting the right-hand side to be 0, the MLE of θ is

$$\theta_{MLE} = \frac{y - nf_p}{n(1 - f_n - f_p)}.$$

The posterior distribution function, on the other hand, requires the integration of the likelihood function. In many cases, the integral may not have an analytic solution. As a result, numerical approximation is necessary.

Classical statistics has a tradition of emphasizing easy access, for example, the early effort of tabulating commonly used probability distributions. As a result, efficient and fast analytic/numeric algorithms for a large number of standard problems, including linear, nonlinear, and the generalized linear models, were developed and implemented long before the advent of powerful personal computers, making classical statistics methods readily available for scientific applications. The same did not happen in Bayesian statistics.

However, routine applications of classical statistics are limited to a number of standard models. These methods limit the choices of models in an applied problem. As a result, practitioners are advised to design their experiment with the intended statistical methods in mind. In ecology, the institutionalized approach of randomized experimental design for causal inference and the concerns of "pseudo-replication" are examples of this influence. The lack of computer algorithms for standard models in Bayesian statistics, however, has required us to formulate a model, which is perhaps why we have perceived it as more difficult. A purposely formulated model is often more realistic, hence more relevant.

Because of the commonality of the classical and Bayesian statistics, especially the inductive nature of both, applications of statistics should not be limited to one or the other. A more effective data analysis approach often combines elements of both. In this book, we often use classical algorithms to explore potential models for a problem. If a standard classical model fits the data, we can either directly use the output for inference (e.g., interpreting the 95% confidence interval as the range of the middle 95% of the respective posterior distribution, or the credible interval) or use Monte Carlo simulation based on classical sampling distribution theory to approximate the posterior distribution. In most applications, standard models in classical statistics are often inadequate. Nevertheless, using these standard models as a starting point can often lead to better model specification for subsequent Bayesian analysis.

1.3 Guiding Principles

Throughout the book, we describe the Bayesian analysis as part of the inference process of a specific environmental and ecological problem. As such, when we use the term "Bayesian analysis," we imply that it is part of the larger scientific problem, of which we aim to understand the underlying environmental/ecological processes and develop models to describe them. This emphasis takes the Bayesian analysis beyond the simple application of Bayes' theorem to derive the posterior distribution. In this process, we need to develop a procedure of inquiry of the most appropriate model in a study, and this should be guided by the three basic problems of statistics: specification, estimation, and distribution [Fisher, 1922]. Both classical and Bayesian statistics must address these three problems; however, classical biostatistic studies typically address these problems in a linear fashion. In contrast, many environmental and ecological studies require feedback among these three basic problems, which we refer to moving forward as model formulation, parameter estimation, and model evaluation (Figure 1.5). At each step, we have feedback on the model itself, which we argue is particularly suited for a Bayesian approach.

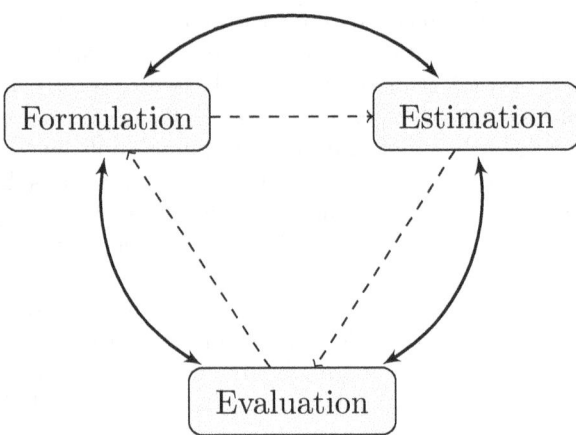

FIGURE 1.5: Bayesian analysis is an iterative process among the three problems of a statistical analysis (solid arrows), while the classical statistics inference is largely a linear process (dashed arrows).

To find the appropriate model for a study requires a process of proposing and evaluating alternative models. Comparing multiple alternative models was recognized long ago as an effective method to guard against personal and professional bias. In Chamberlin's words, proposing only a single model can "menace the integrity of the intellectual processes" because the single model quickly instills "parental affections" in the mind of the researcher [Chamberlin, 1890]. Chamberlin advocated the method of "multiple working hypotheses." The disadvantage of this approach is the burden of proposing alternative models, especially when the first model that springs into our mind is always the preferred model. In Chamberlin's words: "we cannot put into words more than a single line of thought at the same time; and even in that the order of expression must be conformed to the idiosyncrasies of the language, and the rate must be relatively slow." We emphasize that proposing the right model cannot be isolated from addressing the questions of parameter estimation and model evaluation. As a result, a Bayesian analysis is characterized by the iterative interactions among the three questions, rather than the linear process of moving from model formulation to parameter estimation to model evaluation. Throughout the book, we use examples to emphasize the steps of finding the most appropriate model.

1.4 Examples

In this book, we emphasize practical applications of Bayesian statistics with examples from several large studies. In this section, we introduce some of the examples that appear in multiple chapters. We used materials from these studies in multiple chapters because of the complicated nature of these problems. In this section, we summarize the scientific background of these examples.

1.4.1 Gill-net Monitoring Data

Three of the focal studies in this book involve fisheries-related research, including from studies of populations of Lake Erie walleye (*Sander vitreus*) [DuFour et al., 2019, 2021] and Hudson River Atlantic sturgeon (*Acipenser oxyrinchus*). A common feature of these studies is the use of gill nets as sampling gear to collect target fish in study areas. Gill nets are passive sampling gear, as they are placed in a designated location underwater and capture fish that swim into them. Panels of the net are attached on the top to floaters and on the bottom to weights so that the net fishes vertically, and can be set on the bottom or suspended in the water column. A gill net is set in a straight line and is characterized by its mesh size. A gill net is typically set (or soaked) in water for a predetermined period of time. The net is then retrieved and the number of fish caught in the net is counted, identified to the species level, and fish length and weight are measured. The number of fish caught in the net divided by the time the net was deployed is called the catch per unit effort (CPUE). In many fisheries studies, CPUE is used as an index of the population abundance. Fisheries management agencies carry out standard surveys to routinely monitor fish population. Standardized surveys use consistent sampling protocols to allow comparison of survey results through time. As a result, changes in CPUE over time are assumed to indicate changes in fish population.

In many fisheries studies, CPUE is usually treated as a continuous response variable in analysis, implying that the population is proportional to CPUE.

Because our interests are typically in the population, the process linking the population to CPUE (the data-generating process) can invalidate this implicit assumption, due to circumstances of data collection, spatial and temporal scales represented by the data, uneven fish distribution, and environmental influences. Specifically, we are interested in quantifying the proportionality of CPUE and the underlying population, and how the proportion constant changes spatially and under different environmental conditions. To accomplish the goal, the Lake Erie walleye project used a paired hydroacoustic survey to better quantify the number of fish in the vicinity of each gill net. We used the hydroacoustic estimated number of walleyes as a surrogate of the population of fish available to the passive gill net. In doing so, DuFour et al. [2019] showed that the gill net's catchability (measured as the ratio of CPUE and the underlying population size) varies among three distinct regions of Lake Erie. By sharing information across regional boundaries to improve region-specific estimates of survey gear efficiency (Chapter 6), we can improve the overall accuracy of the estimated population trends. In addition, the Lake Erie walleye example also demonstrates the advantage of using the Bayesian approach for quantifying uncertainty and its propagation in estimating intermediate variables (Chapter 2). We use the Atlantic sturgeon example to explicitly account for the processes of resulting in a zero count in the model to better estimate the relative abundance indices (Chapter 5).

1.4.2   Effects of Urbanization on Stream Ecosystems

The topical study on the Effects of Urbanization on Stream Ecosystems (EUSE) was part of U.S. Geological Survey's (USGS) National Water Quality Assessment Program (NAWQA). The study was designed to mimic a typical ecological experiment to study the effect of a dose-response effect of a treatment, which is the level of urbanization. As the levels of urbanization cannot be manipulated and applied to selected watersheds, the EUSE study selected nine metropolitan areas (or regions) across the continental U.S. These metropolitan regions (Atlanta, Georgia (ATL); Boston, Massachusetts (BOS); Birmingham, Alabama (BIR); Denver, Colorado (DEN); Dallas-Fort Worth, Texas (DFW); Milwaukee-Green Bay, Wisconsin (MGB); Portland, Oregon (POR); Raleigh, North Carolina (RAL); and Salt Lake City, Utah (SLC)) represent different environmental settings.

Within each region, 30 watersheds were identified based on a multimetric national urban intensity index (NUII) to represent gradients of urbanization within relatively homogeneous environmental settings [McMahon and Cuffney, 2000, Cuffney and Falcone, 2008]. These watersheds are similar in all other aspects except their levels of urbanization and data from these watersheds were collected using the same sampling protocol. The sampling design was guided by the principle of a randomized experiment for causal inference, even though the treatment (levels of urbanization) cannot be randomly assigned.

The intended analysis method was regression: modeling of various watershed-level indicators calculated based on observed biological data as functions of the watershed urbanization level. The biological data are counts of individuals of various species representing aquatic biota (fish, invertebrates, and algae) in samples collected using the same sampling protocol throughout the EUSE studies. For example, benthic macroinvertebrate communities are widely used to represent stream ecological conditions. Species in these communities are relatively long-lived (compared to algae), to integrate the temporal changes in water quality, and are of limited mobility (compared to fish), to reflect the impact of activities in the immediate upstream watershed.

Ecologists often use univariate metrics, instead of the counts of each species, to describe a community [Barbour and Paul, 2010, Barbour et al., 1999, e.g.]. For macroinvertebrates and algae, the total number of individuals counted is typically limited to a manageable value (e.g., 300 or 500 individuals). As a result, many of the metrics are based on the relative abundances of individual species. These univariate metrics are often used as response variables in regression analysis, with predictors represented by various water chemistry variables and physical habitat variables.

Many authors have examined metrics representing the rate and form of biological responses. Through regression analysis, researchers with the EUSE project identified watershed characteristics most strongly associated with biological responses and compared responses among urban areas [Coles et al., 2004, Cuffney et al., 2005, Brown et al., 2009, Cuffney et al., 2010]. As mentioned above, the biological responses used in these studies were univariate biological metrics calculated based on the observed counts of individual species of the target ecological community. For example, the metric Cuffney et al. [2005] used for measuring the level of pollution in an aquatic environment is the average tolerance level of benthic macroinvertebrates, a richness-weighted average of individual taxa tolerance values (RichTOL). Later, RichTOL was used in Qian et al. [2010] to illustrate the multilevel modeling approach to quantify the region-specific effects of the main treatment (watershed-level urbanization), as well as to explore the regional-level factors (e.g., annual average temperature and precipitation) that influence the urbanization effect (the regression slope). The multilevel modeling approach was further detailed in Qian [2016].

The basic form of the macroinvertebrate community data is counts of various species (taxa) from stream segments near the outlets of respective watersheds. These taxa counts are commonly used to derive univariate indicators or metrics to represent different features of the community. We use univariate indicators (in Chapter 6) to discuss the multilevel model, especially the multivariate normal priors for a Bayesian hierarchical model. We also directly use the observed count data to discuss two types of models: (1) the zero-inflated Poisson model and how such models can be used in a hierarchical model and (2) the multinomial regression model. Through these applications, we hope to show the multi-faceted nature of the study.

Although the EUSE studies were designed to mimic a randomized experiment, the data collected from these studies are largely observational. For example, there were differences in land use patterns and weather conditions among the nine metropolitan regions, which make the comparisons across the regions tentative. In all metropolitan areas except RAL and SLC, the distribution of levels of urbanization in sampling watersheds was skewed toward the lower end of the urban gradient because the number of streams available for study dropped precipitously at higher levels of urbanization (Figure 1.6). DEN, DFW, and MGB have high levels of antecedent agricultural land use compared with the other six metropolitan areas and are known to respond to urban development differently [Qian et al., 2010]. SLC differs from the other metropolitan areas by having development that has progressed from the valley floor up the Wasatch Mountains to the east of Salt Lake City. The upper limit of development is determined by the water supply infrastructure resulting in a sudden jump in urban intensity (i.e., ca. 0 to 20% developed land) as the water supply boundary is crossed. As a result, averages of % developed land in RAL and SLC are higher than the averages in the other four low antecedent agriculture regions [Qian and Cuffney, 2014].

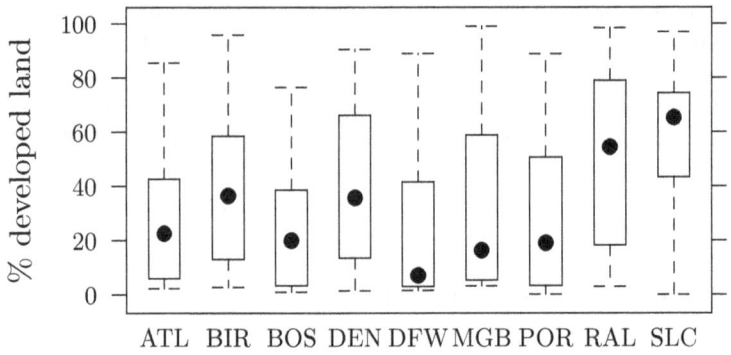

FIGURE 1.6: Watershed level % developed land distribution in the nine metropolitan regions.

1.4.3 Everglades Studies

Data from various aspects of the Everglades research are used in this book. These research activities were prompted, in large part, by a series of legal actions focused on the protection of the Everglades ecosystem in south Florida. Qian and Lavine [2003] summarize these legal actions and the subsequent research activities supporting the establishment of an environmental standard for phosphorus in the Everglades. In this section, we summarize some of these studies.

Legal actions related to the Everglades environmental protection started in the late 1980s. The current Everglades is largely represented by the Everglades National Park in the southern tip of the Florida peninsula. Over one hundred years ago, the Everglades was nearly one million hectares, covering almost the entire area south of Lake Okeechobee [Davis, 1943]. In the 1940s, settlers drained a small portion of the land for agriculture. Through the U.S. federal project Central and Southern Project for Flood Control and Other Purposes of 1948, the Everglades was systematically drained through the establishment of a system of canals, pumping stations, water storage areas, and levees [Light and Dineen, 1994]. As a result, large agricultural tracts were established within the Everglades, south of Lake Okeechobee, leading to the increased input of nutrient enriched agriculture runoff to the remaining Everglades [Snyder and Davidson, 1994]. The Everglades is a historically phosphorus-limited freshwater wetland ecosystem [Steward and Ornes, 1975b,a, Swift and Nicholas, 1987, Flora et al., 1988, Richardson et al., 1997]. The intense agriculture activity in the area resulted in an increased supply of phosphorus to the wetlands causing changes to its ecosystem, including major alterations in the water chemistry and elevated phosphorus concentrations in soils, extensive shifts in algal species, and altered community structure in areas with high and moderate phosphorus enrichment.

In a legal action brought by the federal government in 1988, the U.S. Department of Justice accused the state of Florida (represented by the South Florida Water Management District and the then Florida Department of Environmental Regulation) of violations of state water quality standards, particularly phosphorus, in the Loxahatchee National Wildlife Refuge and the Everglades National Park. In the settlement reached in 1991, the state of Florida recognized the severe harm to the Everglades National Park to the south and the Loxahatchee Wildlife Refuge to the east of the Everglades Agriculture Area. The 1992 consent decree of the settlement commits all parties to achieve the water quality and quantity needed to preserve and restore the unique flora and fauna of the Park and Refuge and to require agricultural growers to use best management practices to control and cleanse discharges from the Everglades Agricultural Area.

The 1991 settlement agreement was superseded by the 1994 Everglades Forever Act (EFA), requiring compliance with all water quality standards in the entire Everglades by December 31, 2006. The EFA authorized the Everglades Construction Project, including schedules for construction and operation of six storm water treatment areas to remove phosphorus from the EAA runoff. The EFA created a research program to understand phosphorus impacts on the Everglades and to develop additional treatment technologies. Finally, the EFA required the Florida Department of Environmental Protection (FDEP) to establish a numeric criterion for phosphorus.

To accomplish the task of setting environmental criterion for phosphorus, several studies focused on how the Everglades ecosystem responded to the elevated phosphorus input through both observational and experimental studies. A prominent mesocosm experimental study was carried out by the Duke University Wetland Center (DUWC) in the interior of a large water conservation area (the Water Conservation Area – 2A, or WCA2A), where the remaining wetland ecosystem is known not to be impacted by the agricultural runoff. In this experiment, six experimental flumes (10m × 2m channels) were constructed. At the upstream end, an automatic feeding machine pumped a continuous stream of water into the flume. Five of the channels were dosed with different levels of phosphorus, the sixth was a control. The purpose of the channels was to create phosphorus concentration gradients. Total phosphorus (TP) concentrations were measured biweekly at each meter mark along each channel for six years (1992–1998). The mean TP concentrations in those channels ranged from 10 to 75 μg/L. After the system stabilized, biological samples were collected regularly from 1995 to 1998. These biological samples were used to derive attributes representing biological responses at several trophic levels. Finally, an analysis was done to see what level of TP resulted in significant ecological change.

Data from DUWC's mesocosm study (known as the dosing study) were used to estimate the Everglades ecosystem's TP thresholds. The concept of an ecological threshold is based on the ecological concept of ecosystem resilience and alternative stable states. An ecosystem and its functions are resilient to disturbance when such disturbance is within certain limits. Because of the resilience, indicators of the ecosystem are often stable even when the disturbance increases. In ecological studies, we can observe the behavior of several similar ecosystems with different levels of disturbances (observational study), or create small replicas of the target ecosystems and apply different levels of disturbance (experimental study). The varying levels of disturbance (in this case, the disturbance is TP) is often known as the disturbance gradient. A threshold is a point along a disturbance gradient across which an ecosystem (or certain aspects of the ecosystem) changes abruptly from one stable state to another. The six experimental flumes created a TP gradient both within and among the flumes. In the DUWC's Bayesian analysis, the sequence of the observed ecological response variable is ordered along the TP gradient. In Chapter 7 we use data from the dosing study as part of the change point model examples. In Chapter 6, the separately estimated ecological thresholds for several ecological indicators are combined to derive an ecosystem-level threshold.

The task of establishing treatment wetlands for removing phosphorus requires an understanding of the effectiveness of a constructed wetland in removing phosphorus. Observation data from WCA2A were used in several studies to study the effectiveness of WCA2A as a treatment wetland. Because only a portion of WCA2A was affected by the agricultural runoff, historical soil TP in the wetland was of interest. Knowing the historical (or background)

TP levels, we can estimate the size of WCA2A that is impacted by agricultural runoff [Qian, 1997, e.g.,]. Using the changes in algal species (diatom) composition along the TP gradient in present-day Everglades, we illustrate the multinomial missing data problem in Chapter 5. Qian and Richardson [1997] used the ecological threshold concept to propose a separate model for estimating a wetland's phosphorus retention capacity. We used the data from Qian and Richardson [1997] as an example of the Gibbs sampler in Chapter 2.

1.4.4 Compliance Assessment under the U.S. Clean Water Act

The U.S. Clean Water Act (CWA, 33 U.S.C. §1251 et seq. (1972)) requires that states in the U.S. periodically submit a list of impaired waters, that is, waters that are "too polluted or otherwise degraded to meet water quality standards." This requirement is part of Section 303(d) of CWA, and the process of compiling the list is known as 303(d) listing. Once a water is listed, CWA further requires that the state develop total maximum daily load (TMDL) programs for mitigating the impairment. With a TMDL program implemented, monitoring is usually the basis for assessing compliance and determining if any management modifications are needed. The U.S. Environmental Protection Agency is responsible for developing rules and regulations to implement the law including setting specific standards for compliance assessment. Enforcement actions will take effect once a noncompliance is identified. Consequently, compliance assessment is often the important first step of environmental management.

As inference based on monitoring data is associated with errors because of, for example, measurement uncertainty, sampling error, seasonal and other periodicity caused auto-correlation, statistical analysis is inevitably an important consideration in compliance assessment based on monitoring data. In the U.S., most states developed procedures of standard compliance assessment based on statistical null hypothesis testing, mostly comparing an upper percentile (e.g., 80–90%) to the established environmental standard [Keller and Cavallaro, 2008]. Qian and Miltner [2018] discussed legal and management background of the environmental standard compliance assessment in the U.S., including the legal definition of a water quality standard as the mean concentration of a pollutant, the varying practices among states, and the "magnitude, duration, and frequency (MDF)" components of a water quality standard. They concluded that the practice of using hypothesis testing, common in nearly all states, was designed to address statistical uncertainty (sampling and measurement error). The MDF components of a water quality standard define (1) the harmful level of a pollutant (magnitude) determined by a toxicity study for toxic pollutants and by reference conditions for non-toxic pollutants such as nutrients, (2) the assessment period (duration) for which the mean concentration is estimated (e.g., annual mean concentration), and

(3) a recurring probability (frequency) which defines how to address the estimation uncertainty in the estimated annual mean [Qian, 2015]. The frequency component is the most confusing aspect of the MDF components. Qian [2015] suggested that the frequency component defines an upper quantile of the sampling distribution of the estimated mean. In subsequent chapters, we use the topic to discuss the advantage of a Bayesian estimation-oriented approach in compliance assessment.

1.5   Summary

Although we emphasize the two modes of inference in Bayesian and classical statistics, both follow the hypothetical deduction approach as described by Fisher [Fisher, 1922]. The common starting point of statistical inference is a probability distribution assumption on the response variable. The assumed probability distribution includes parameter(s) that are potentially function(s) of predictor variable(s). This step establishes the hypothesis in the hypothetical deduction process. In classical statistics, model parameters are estimated using the maximum likelihood method, while the estimation uncertainty is represented by the sampling distributions of these parameters. In Bayesian statistics, model parameters are estimated via Bayes' theorem producing posterior distributions which simultaneously characterize estimation uncertainty. The oft-neglected third step of the hypothetical deduction process is model evaluation. In classical statistics, this step is based on various hypothesis testing procedures. In classical statistics, a model parameter is a fixed (but unknown) constant and the estimate is a random variable. Model evaluation relies on the sampling distribution of the estimated parameter – a probability distribution of all potential estimates based on random sampling of the same population. As such, the classical statistical inference relies on not just the estimated parameter, but all unrealized potential estimates. When using Bayesian statistics, a probability is not necessarily representing a long-run frequency. As a result, we can use a probability distribution to represent our uncertainty about a parameter. The prior and posterior distributions represent what we know and do not know before and after observing data, respectively. Instead of using hypothesis testing, we use predictive distribution in Bayesian statistics for model evaluation.

We emphasize the iterative nature of model development – model formulation, parameter estimation, and model evaluation are inter-dependent in an applied problem.

This is a book for practitioners. Consequently, we want to emphasize applications, especially the thought-process behind the examples we used throughout the book. Because there is only one equation in Bayesian statistics, the process of applying Bayesian statistics is inevitably centered around two questions. First, "What is the statistical model describing the response variable?"

A model is parameterized with one or more parameters. Once these parameters are identified, the second question is, "Do we have any prior knowledge about these parameters?" If we do, how can our knowledge be quantified in terms of a probability distribution of these parameters? Once we have the answers to these two questions, the remaining tasks of a Bayesian application are mostly related to computation – calculating the posterior distribution and making inference (e.g., through posterior predictive inference).

Chapter 2

Bayesian Inference and Monte Carlo Simulation

This chapter discusses the now dominant computational tool in Bayesian analysis – Monte Carlo simulation. Although this topic requires knowledge of advanced mathematical subjects, a simulation-based method is often relatively simple to use. We start with the use of Monte Carlo simulation (a process of generating independent random numbers) for numeric integration and for statistical inference. In most Bayesian applications, however, we use Markov chain Monte Carlo simulation that will result in correlated random numbers. The Markov chain Monte Carlo method is rooted in mathematical features of Markov chains. These Markov chain features are highly technical. Although mathematical theories of a Markov chain are important in ensuring the resulting Markov chain converges to the target probability distribution, only fairly mild conditions are needed for most practical problems. In most cases, we can directly use these Markov chain methods with little risk of violating these conditions. As a result, we document the algorithmic details of two of the most commonly used Markov chain Monte Carlo methods: the Metropolis-Hastings algorithm and the Gibbs sampler. The algorithmic details are no longer needed as these algorithms are written into computer programming languages. As such, this chapter serves as a record. Readers may choose to skip the last three sections of this chapter for now and come back to them later.

2.1 The Role of Simulation in Statistics

We assume that most of our readers are familiar with classical statistics, especially with concepts of long-run frequency-based probability and sampling distributions. This familiarity is convenient because simulation uses a large (but finite) number of iterations to approximate the "long-run" frequency.

Monte Carlo simulation has been part of statistical inference since before computers were widely available [Metropolis and Ulam, 1949, e.g.,]. The work of Metropolis and Ulam proposed the Monte Carlo simulation as a statistical approach to the study of integro-differential equations. In most modern applications, we use simulation to replicate the behavior of a random process. Early simulation examples were focused on demonstrating certain features of a concept or a statistical process. For example, the multiple comparison problem can be demonstrated with a simulation where random numbers of multiple random variables were drawn from the same probability distribution repeatedly and each time a t-test is carried out between the group with the smallest mean and the group with the largest mean. The frequency of rejecting the null hypothesis is the probability of a family-wise type I error. Similarly, Box [1976] used a simulation to demonstrate the robustness of a t-test with respect to the normality assumption. These simulations are easy to understand and easy to replicate without getting into complicated mathematics. Simulation is especially effective as a model evaluation tool as illustrated in Qian [2016, Chapter 11] and Qian and Cuffney [2018]. In many cases, Monte Carlo simulation is often a practical means for solving a problem. We describe two main uses of Monte Carlo simulations: as a numerical algorithm for complex integrals and as a tool for drawing random variates from complex probability distributions.

2.2   Bayesian Monte Carlo

We mentioned Bayesian Monte Carlo in Chapter 1. At the center of this method is the use of computer simulation to obtain an approximation of the posterior distribution, thereby avoiding the evaluation of the potentially difficult integral in the denominator of the Bayes' theorem. We will explain this method by showing its potential to estimate the posterior distribution of a binomial problem. In the binomial example, this method is unnecessary because we have the analytical result of the posterior distribution; yet this example will allow us to compare between the simulation results and the analytic solution. In many moderately complicated problems, the need for a computational short-cut is real. The Bayesian Monte Carlo (BMC) was a classic example of how computer simulation can be used to solve complicated computation tasks. It is a brute force approximation of the posterior distribution. We start by using a simple example, where simulation is unnecessary, to explain the process.

In the snake fungal disease example (Section 1.1.1 on page 6), the posterior distribution can be expressed as a function that is proportional to the prior density times the likelihood:

$$\pi(\theta|y) \propto \pi(\theta) \times (\theta(1 - f_-) + (1 - \theta)f_+)^x (1 - (\theta(1 - f_-) + (1 - \theta)f_+))^{n-x}$$

We used a numerical method to approximate the posterior distribution of the parameter of interest (Figure 1.3), assuming that we have a flat prior ($\theta \sim beta(1, 1)$). In using the Bayesian Monte Carlo method, we first draw a number of random samples of the parameter θ from its prior distribution.

We consider these random samples are equally likely under the prior distribution. Now let us assume that n is large enough and these n random samples represent all possible values of θ. In other words, we approximate the infinite population of possible values of θ using a finite number of n values $p_1, \cdots, p_n$. The discrete version of the Bayes' theorem can be used in this case. For each value p_i, we can calculate the likelihood of the data given p_i and multiply the likelihood by $1/n$, the prior probability of an individual value in the sample. Each product is then divided by the sum of all the n products to obtain the posterior probability of the respective value of p_i. These posterior probabilities can be directly used to derive the cumulative density function (CDF) of the posterior probability distribution. The cumulative distribution is often used in risk assessment. Examples of BMC application can be found in Qian et al. [2003b]. The determination of the posterior distribution probability density function (PDF) of θ, however, requires a few additional steps. The most direct method uses a "histogram" method: divide the range of θ (0, 1) into a number of bins and then the histogram heights for these bins are calculated as the sum of the posterior probabilities for those p_i's within the range of each bin. If the number of data points n is large enough, we can make the size of the bins small enough to approximate the posterior distribution. Alternatively, we can use the CDF to derive the PDF.

```r
#### R code ####
## BMC of the SFD example
n_sims <- 100000

bmc_sfd_post <- function(prior = sort(runif(n_sims)),
                         x=5, n=20, fp=0.07, fn=0.05,
                         pdfgrid=seq(0,1,0.01)){
    log_likelihood <- x * log(prior*(1-fn) + (1-prior)*fp) +
        (n-x) * log(1-prior*(1-fn)-(1-prior)*fp)
    post <- exp(log_likelihood)/sum(exp(log_likelihood))
    post_cdf <- cumsum(post)
    pdf_interval <- findInterval(prior, pdfgrid)
    post_pdf <- unlist(by(post, pdf_interval, sum))
    return(list(p=prior, cdf=post_cdf, pdf=post_pdf,
                grid=pdfgrid[-1]))
}
sfdbmc <- bmc_sfd_post()
plot(sfdbmc$cdf ~ sfdbmc$p, type="l", ylab="cdf", xlab="p")
plot(sfdbmc$pdf ~ sfdbmc$grid, type="l", ylab="pdf", xlab="p")
### End ###
```

BMC illustrates two points. First, simulation can be used to simplify computation, specifically, simplify the task of solving difficult integrals. With BMC, estimating the posterior CDF is as simple as applying the R function `cumsum()`. The second point is that a simulation algorithm is designed with a specific purpose in mind. If the objective is to present the density function of parameter distributions, BMC is not effective. In general, a simulation algorithm is most effective when it is designed to draw random samples from the target probability distribution directly. In Chapter 1, Figure 1.3 was obtained by evaluating the numerator of the Bayes' theorem (which is proportional to the posterior density function) at 100 evenly spaced grid points. Using BMC, a simulation with 10,000 iterations resulted in a jagged PDF. The posterior PDF is reasonably smooth only when the number of iterations increased to above 250,000. This is a large overhead for simplifying computation.

2.3   Sampling from Known Distributions

The basic operation of a simulation is drawing random numbers from random variables with known probability distributions. This operation is now a routine task that can be easily accomplished using modern statistical software such as R. We will take full advantage of these existing computer programs (the family of `rDist` functions in R, such as `rnorm, rbinom`). In some cases, we may have to develop purpose-built algorithms to generate random numbers from some difficult distributions. In this section, we summarize some of the most generic methods that can be used in conjunction with functions for generating uniform random numbers to generate random samples from random variables with non-standard distributions.

2.3.1   Inverse-CDF Methods

Almost all random number generators rely on the availability of uniformly distributed random variates. The process of generating random variates of a random variable with a known (cumulative) probability distribution $F(X)$ can be quite simple if its inverse function $F^{-1}(U)$ is known. When considering a value u between 0 and 1 as a cumulative probability from the distribution $F(X)$, we can find the X variable value with $\Pr(X \leq x) = u$ using the inverse CDF: $x = F^{-1}(u)$. In other words, we can draw random variates from the distribution $F(X)$ by drawing random variates, $u^{(1)}, \cdots, u^{(m)}$, from the uniform distribution between 0 and 1 and substitute the resulting values into the inverse CDF to obtain random variates of $X : x^{(1)}, \cdots, x^{(m)}$ (Figure 2.1). We can write a simple function to draw random variates from a normal distribution $X \sim N(\mu, \sigma^2)$ in R and compare it to the function `rnorm()`:

```
### R Code ###
set.seed(101)
mu <- 2
sigma <- 1.25
```

```
u <- runif(10000)
x <- qnorm(u, mu, sigma)
summary(x)

y <- rnorm(10000, mu, sigma)
summary(y)

hist(x, col=rgb(0.1,0.1,0.1,0.5), xlim=c(-3,6), ylim=c(0, 1800),
    nclass=20, main="")
hist(y, col=rgb(0.8,0.8,0.8,0.5), nclass=20, add=T)
box()
### End ###
```

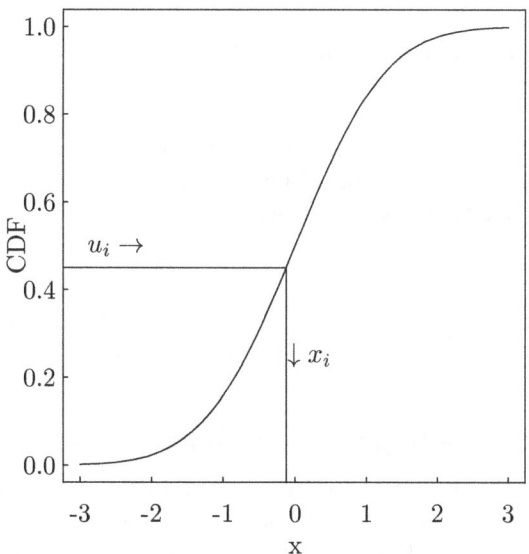

FIGURE 2.1: Inverse cumulative density fuction (CDF) method: random variate x_i is drawn as the inverse CDF of a random variate u_i from the uniform distribution between 0 and 1.

In general, numerical approximation is possible as long as a probability distribution is specified up to a proportional constant. Fortunately, in Bayesian statistics, the posterior probability density function is proportional to the product of the prior density and the likelihood function. As a result, we can use the inverse CDF method in many problems. In the snake fungal disease example, the posterior density function in equation (1.4) is numerically approximated because we want to avoid the integration of the denominator. The numerical approximation process requires only the function of the numerator.

The posterior density can be evaluated over a number of evenly spaced θ values.

These numerically evaluated density values can be converted into cumulative densities:

```
### R Code ###
post_impft_cdf <- function(x=5, n=20, fp=0.07, fn=0.05, k=100){
    theta <- seq(0, 1,, k)
    fpst <- theta*(1-fn) + (1-theta)*fp
    post <- x*log(fpst) + (n-x)*log(1-fpst)
    return(cumsum(exp(post)/sum(exp(post))))
}
n <- 1000 ## draw 1000 random numbers
post_cdf <- data.frame(theta=seq(0,1,,1000),
                    cdf=post_impft_cdf(k=1000))
u <- runif(n)
tmp <- apply(post_cdf, 1, function(x, unf)
    return(x[2]-unf), unf=u)

theta <- apply(tmp, 1, function(x, theta)
    return(theta[abs(x)==min(abs(x))]),
            theta=post_cdf$theta)
hist(theta)
### End ###
```

Using numerical approximation, we now limit the posterior probability distribution to be represented by 1000 evenly spaced values between 0 and 1.

2.3.2   Acceptance-Rejection Methods

The basis of the acceptance-rejection method is a theorem [Robert and Casella, 1999], which states that if generating random variates from a probability distribution with a PDF of $\pi(x)$ is difficult, but a random variate from an alternative distribution $g(x)$ can be easily obtained, then random variates from $\pi(x)$ can be obtained by using the following algorithm.

1. Determine a constant M such that $\pi(x) \leq Mg(x)$.

2. Generate $x \sim g$ and U from the uniform distribution between 0 and 1.

3. Accept x as a random variate from $\pi(x)$ if $U \leq \pi(x)/Mg(x)$.

4. Return to 1, otherwise.

We call this alternative distribution, $g(x)$, a candidate-generating (or instrumental) distribution.

The most commonly used example of this algorithm is to generate normal (the target distribution) random variates from an exponential distribution (the instrumental distribution). First, random variates from an exponential distribution with a cumulative density of $\Pr(X \leq x) = 1 - e^{-x}$ can be easily generated as the negative natural log of random variates from a uniform distribution between 0 and 1 [Robert and Casella, 1999, Example 2.2.1]. That is, if $U \sim U(0,1)$, $X = -\log(U)$ is a random variable from an exponential distribution with the rate parameter of 1. In general, $X = -\log(U/\lambda)$ is distributed from the exponential with a rate parameter of λ. The density function of the exponential distribution is $\lambda e^{-\lambda x}$. For our alternative ($g(x)$) distribution, we will choose the exponential density with a rate of 1. Thus, $g(x) = e^{-x}, x \geq 0$. The density function of the standard normal distribution ($N(0,1)$) is $\frac{1}{2\pi}e^{-\frac{x^2}{2}}$. As the exponential distribution is defined for $X > 0$, the exponential random variates are positive. Because the standard normal distribution is symmetric, we can consider that the target distribution is the distribution of the absolute value of a stadard normal random variable, which has a density of $\sqrt{2/\pi}e^{-\frac{x^2}{2}}$. The ratio of the two density functions $\pi(x)/g(x) = \sqrt{2/\pi}e^{1-x^2/2}$. The maximum of the ratio is $\sqrt{2e/\pi}$ (reached at $x = 0$). As a result, we can set $M = \sqrt{2e/\pi}$. That is, $\pi(X)/Mg(x) = e^{-\frac{(1-x)^2}{2}}$. The acceptance-rejection algorithm is as follows:

1. Generate $U_1 \sim U(0,1)$ and calculate $x = -\log(U_1)$.

2. Generate $U_2 \sim U(0,1)$ and calculate $r = e^{-\frac{(1-x)^2}{2}}$.

3. If $U_2 \leq r$, accept x as a random variate from the standard normal distribution.

4. Otherwise, go back to 1.

5. Generate $u_3 \sim U(0,1)$, if $u_3 < 0.5$, $x = -x$.

Because a normal random variate $X \sim N(\mu, \sigma^2)$ can be expressed as $X = \mu + \sigma Z$, only the algorithm for $Z \sim N(0,1)$ is necessary. This algorithm can be implemented in R using a nested function:

```
my.rnorm <- function(n, mu=0, sigma=1){
    x <- -log(runif(n))
    r <- exp(-0.5*(1-x)^2)
    x <- x[r>=runif(n)]
    m <- length(x)
    if (m < n)
        x <- c(x, my.rnorm(n-m, mu, sigma))
    return (mu + sigma*x*ifelse(runif(n) < 0.5, -1, 1))
}
### End ###
```

The acceptance-rejection method is a basic building block of the Markov chain Monte Carlo simulation. As a result, it is probably the most widely used algorithm in Bayesian computation. We will discuss this method further in Section 2.4.

2.3.3   Relationships Method

When a random variable (variable of interest) can be expressed as a function of one or more other random variables, we can exploit the relationship if random variates from these other variables can be easily obtained. Specifically, we can draw random variates of the one or more other random variables and use the relationship to derive a random variate of the variable of interest. For example, a random variable with a binomial distribution $(Bin(x; p, n))$ is the sum of n Bernoulli random variables $(bern(p))$. If we are limited to using runif() only, we can draw a binomial random variate in two steps:

1. Draw $u_j \sim unif(0, 1)$ and set $J_j = 1$ if $u_j \leq p$.

2. Return $x = \sum_j J_j$.

```
### R Code ###
my.rbinom <- function(m, p, n)
return(unlist(apply(matrix(as.numeric(runif(n*m)<p),
                    nrow=n), 2, sum)))
### End ###
```

In general, the probability distribution function of a random variable $y = f(x)$ can be derived directly from the probability distribution of x through the inverse function $x = g^{-1}(y)$:

$$\pi_y(y) = \pi_x \left(f^{-1}(y) \right) \left| \frac{d}{dy} g^{-1}(y) \right| \tag{2.1}$$

where $\pi_y(\cdot)$ is the density function of y, $\pi_x(\cdot)$ is the density function of x, and $g^{-1}(y)$ is the inverse function. Using random samples of $x^i \sim \pi(x)$, we directly derive random samples of $y^i = f(x^i)$, thereby avoiding the derivative computation in equation (2.1).

We can use this method to greatly simplify computation, especially in propagating estimation uncertainty from one or more variables to the variable of interest. For example, log transformation is commonly used in analyzing environmental and ecological data as many commonly used variables (e.g., concentration variables) can be approximated by the log-normal distribution. As such, log transformation can often linearize the relationship between the response and the predictor variable and stabilize the model error variance. However, we are typically interested in making prediction and interpretation in the natural metric. For example, when a log-log linear regression model is used:

$$\log(y) = \alpha + \beta \log(X) + \epsilon$$

we typically report the retransformed relationship:

$$y = e^{\hat{\alpha}} x^{\hat{\beta}}.$$

While $\hat{\alpha} + \hat{\beta} \log(\tilde{x})$ is the estimated mean of $\log(y|\tilde{x})$, the exponential of the same ($e^{\hat{\alpha}+\hat{\beta}\log(\tilde{x})}$) is not the mean of $y|\tilde{x}$. Using the log-normal distribution results, the mean of $y|\tilde{x}$ should be $e^{\hat{\alpha}+\hat{\beta}\log(\tilde{x})+\sigma^2/2}$, where σ^2 is the residual variance. Because both the regression coefficients (α, β) and the residual variance (σ^2) are estimated with uncertainty, the retransformation correction is not simply a multiplicative factor of $e^{\hat{\sigma}^2/2}$. Using simulation, we can draw random samples of the regression coefficient and the residual variance to derive random samples of the predicted mean. Stow et al. [2006] used Bayesian regression implemented in WinBUGS [Lunn et al., 2000] where random samples of α, β, and σ^2 are drawn from their joint posterior distribution (see Chapter 4). Random samples of these model coefficients are used to derive random samples of $y \mid \tilde{x}$ (which are used to estimate the desired mean). Qian [2016, Chapter 9] approximated the joint posterior distributions of linear and nonlinear regression coefficients using their classical sampling distributions.

2.3.4 Numeric Integration

Using Monte Carlo simulation to numerically approximate an integral is based on the definition of the expected value of a random variable, that is, $E(x) = \int_x x \cdot \pi(x)dx$, where $\pi(x)$ is the density function. We can approximate the integral using the average of a large number of random variates from the distribution of x. If random variates from the distribution can be efficiently drawn, the simulation can be an effective method. In fact, this method can be applied to any integral $I = \int_x g(x)dx$, as long as $g(x)$ can be partitioned into a product $g(x) = h(x)\pi(x)$, where $\pi(x)$ is a probability density function. The integral can be approximated by first drawing $x^{(1)}, \cdots, x^{(k)}$ random numbers from the probability distribution defined by $\pi(x)$, and

$$I \approx \frac{1}{k} \sum_j h(x^{(j)}).$$

By increasing k, we can make the approximation as accurate as we desire. In both Bayesian and classical statistics, integration can quickly become complicated even for a simple model. For example, Qian [2016] used an example of establishing an environmental standard in the Everglades National Park, where the water quality standard of total phosphorus (TP) concentration is defined in terms of the 75th percentile of the concentration distribution in reference areas (areas that are not impacted by human activities). When setting the standard, we use data (TP concentrations from a reference area) to estimate the reference TP concentration distribution. In studying water quality, we often assume that a concentration variable can be modeled by a log-normal distribution. This assumption is widely used and Ott [1995] justified the assumption based on the central limit theorem. As a result, a rule of thumb in analyzing environmental data is to log transform a concentration variable and estimate the log-mean and log-variance. That is, the log-concentration variable y is assumed to follow a normal distribution:

$$y \sim N(\mu, \sigma^2).$$

The density function of y is

$$\pi(y|\mu, \sigma^2) = \frac{1}{\sqrt{2\pi}\sigma} e^{-\frac{(y-\mu)^2}{2\sigma^2}}.$$

If the parameters μ and σ are known, the 75th percentile of the distribution can be directly estimated (in R, qnorm(0.75, mu, sigma)). Let us first assume that σ^2 is known but μ is unknown. The uncertainty of the estimated mean $\hat{\mu}$ in classical statistics is described by a normal distribution defined by the central limit theorem (i.e., $\hat{\mu} \sim N(\mu, \sigma^2/n)$). In Bayesian statistics, the posterior distribution of μ is similar to the sampling distribution when a non-informative prior is used:

$$\mu|y \sim N(\hat{\mu}, \sigma^2/n).$$

With the posterior distribution of μ, the predictive distribution of y is

$$\pi(\tilde{y}|y) = \int_\mu \pi(\tilde{y}|\mu, \sigma^2)\pi(\mu|y)d\mu.$$

Although an analytic result of this integral can be derived with little effort, we use it to illustrate the use of Monte Carlo simulation for numerically evaluating the integral. As $\pi(\mu|y)$ is a probability density function, the integral can be approximated by the average of $\pi(\tilde{y}|\mu^{(i)}, \sigma^2)$, where $\mu^{(i)}$ for $i = 1, \cdots, k$ are random variates drawn from the posterior distribution of μ. We can numerically present the marginal density of $\tilde{y}$ by estimating the density over a grid of $\tilde{y}$ values $\tilde{y}_j$ with $j = 1, \cdots, n$.

$$\pi(\tilde{y}_j) \approx \frac{1}{k}\sum_i \pi(\tilde{y}_j|\mu^{(i)}, \sigma^2)$$

```
### R Code ###
nsims <- 10000
## simulated data
### predictive distribution with known sigma
set.seed(2)
sigma <- 2
n <- 25
y <- rnorm(n, 3, sigma)
hat_mu <- mean(y)
```

```
rhat_mu <- rnorm(nsims, hat_mu, sigma/sqrt(n))
y_grid <- matrix(seq(1,6,length=500), ncol=1)

pi_yj <- apply(y_grid, 1,
    function(x)dnorm(x, rhat_mu, sigma/sqrt(25)))
pi_y1 <- apply(pi_yj, 2, mean)

plot(pi_y1~y_grid[,1], type="l")
### End ###
```

When σ^2 is unknown, the predictive distribution is estimated by a double integral:

$$\pi(\tilde{y}|y) = \int_{\hat{\mu}} \int_{\hat{\sigma}^2} \pi(\tilde{y}|\mu, \sigma^2)\pi(\mu, \sigma^2|y)d\hat{\mu}d\hat{\sigma}^2.$$

The joint distribution $\pi(\mu, \sigma^2|y) = \pi(\mu|\sigma^2, y)\pi(\sigma^2|y)$ can be sampled by first drawing σ^2 from its posterior distribution (a re-scaled inverse-χ^2 distribution), then sampling μ from its conditional posterior.

```
### R Code ###
### predictive distribution with unknown sigma
hat_s <- sd(y)
rhat_sig <- sqrt((n-1)*hat_s^2/rchisq(nsims, n-1))
rhat_mu <- rnorm(nsims, hat_mu, rhat_sig/sqrt(n))

pi_yj <- apply(y_grid, 1,
            function(x)dnorm(x, rhat_mu, rhat_sig/sqrt(25)))
pi_y2 <- apply(pi_yj, 2, mean)

lines(pi_y2 ~ y_grid[,1], lty=2, type="l")
### End ###
```

The goal of this problem is, however, not to derive the marginal distribution of y, but rather to estimate the 75th percentile of the distribution of y. The 75th percentile of a normal distribution can be calculated by $q_{0.75} = \mu + \sigma\Phi(0.75)$, where $\Phi(\cdot)$ is the inverse cumulative density function of the standard normal distribution ($N(0, 1)$), which allows us to quickly draw random samples of $q_{0.75}$ using random samples of μ and σ we already have, using the relationships method (Section 2.3.3):

```
### R Code ###
### random samples of q75
q75 <- rhat_mu+rhat_sig * qnorm(0.75)
hist(q75)
### End ###
```

2.3.5   A Statistical Estimation Example

In this example, we illustrate how simulation can be used in a more complicated problem. The basic idea is the process of (1) using random samples of a quantity to represent the uncertainty and (2) propagate the uncertainty from one parameter to the other through empirical or mechanistic models using Monte Carlo simulation to carry out the necessary differential and integral calculus. The example is from DuFour et al. [2019], who explored the use of hydroacoustic survey data to estimate the abundance of walleye, a large fish species in Lake Erie - a Laurentian Great Lake. The basic premise of the study is as follows: in hydroacoustic data, each fish detected is recorded with a "target strength," which can be used to infer the fish's size (length). Given that walleye is one of the largest predator fish in Lake Erie, the target strength inferred fish size can then be used to estimate the likelihood of the detected fish being a walleye. In the process, we used a Bayesian method to quantify the uncertainty in the mean target strength and a logistic regression model to estimate the probability of a given-length fish being a walleye. Uncertainty in the estimated coefficients included using integration. Data and R code can be found in our GitHub repository.

Lake Erie walleye is an ecologically and economically important fish. The U.S. and Canadian governments maintain a long-term walleye population-monitoring program including a fishery independent gill-net survey. The monitoring in Ohio is conducted by the Ohio Department of Natural Resources, Division of Wildlife (ODNR-DOW). The survey provides measures of relative abundance, and species- and size-compositions of the fish community. Catches of fish in gill nets are affected by vulnerability of fish to the gear and selectivity of the net for certain species and sizes of fish. These shortcomings prompted researchers to consider the use of hydroacoustic surveys in conjunction with the existing gill net survey to improve data used in population models that guide harvest quota decisions. A hydroacoustic device mounted on a moving boat transmits a sound pulse into the water. When the pulse encounters a fish, part of the sound energy is reflected, and the strength of the reflected sound pulse (known as target strength or TS) is related to a fish's size. The reflected sound pulse is referred to as backscatter or an echo. The number and strength of returns, along with the volume of sampled water, can be used to estimate fish density and abundance. As a result, using hydroacoustic surveys, we can estimate both the abundance and the size composition of the fish population. Studies have shown that TS is a good indicator of fish size and empirical models have been developed to link TS and fish total length (TL). The widely cited model used here was developed by Love [1971].

Although we can use hydroacoustic data to estimate abundance and size composition of the fish community, fish species information is not available. In Ohio waters of Lake Erie, walleye are the most common large fish. Consequently, fish size is used as an indicator; the longer the fish, the more likely it is a walleye. Using data from gill-net surveys, DuFour et al. [2019] derived a logistic regression model for estimating the probability that a fish is a wall-eye using fish length as a predictor. Combining this logistic model and Love's equation allows us to estimate the probability that a detected fish is a walleye.

Specifically, when a sound pulse encounters a fish, it returns a distribution of backscattered echoes as the fish moves through the acoustic beam, each echo with various strength (TS) due to measurement uncertainty and the fish's orientation with respect to the survey boat. Love's equation is a regression model with TS as the response variable and $\log_{10}(TL)$ as the predictor. Unfortunately, Love [1971] did not report the regression model uncertainty statistics. As a result, the regression model was used as a deterministic formula without considering the associated uncertainty. Love's equation $(E(TS) = 19.2 \times \log_{10}(TL) + 0.9 \times \log_{10}(\lambda) - 62.3)$ computes the expected target strength $E(TS)$ based on the known fish length (TL) and the wavelength of the transmitted sound (λ), which is also known. In this example, $E(TS)$ is estimated by fitting a log-normal distribution using the measured TS values from multiple echoes. Log-normality of the TS measurement is a standard assumption. Using a Bayesian estimation method (see Chapter 3 for details), we can estimate the posterior probability distribution of the log mean $\mu_{TS,i}$ $(\pi(\mu_{TS,j[i]}|y)$ and log variance $(\pi(\sigma^2|y))$ using equation (2.2).

$$y_i \sim N(\mu_{TS,j[i]}, \sigma^2) \tag{2.2}$$

Using the log-normal distribution formula for the expected value, we transform the model estimated parameters (log-mean and log-variance) to the expected target strength: $E(TS) = e^{\mu_{TS,j} + \sigma^2/2}$. Using the Markov chain Monte Carlo simulation (see Section 2.4), we draw random samples of $\mu_{TS,j}$ from its posterior distribution. Each random sample of $\mu_{TS,j}$ is then used to calculate a random sample of $E(TS)$. Given that we are using Love's equation as a deterministic formula, the posterior distribution of fish length can be determined by using the inverse formula:

$$TL = g(TS) = 10^{\frac{E(TS) - 0.9 \times \log_{10}(\lambda) + 62.3}{19.2}}. \tag{2.3}$$

Using equation (2.3), we derive random samples of TL for each fish from their respective random samples of the expected target strength.

When estimating the probability of a detected fish being a walleye, we use the logistic regression model. The logit transformed probability is a linear function of TL.

$$\text{logit}(p) = \alpha_0 + \alpha_1 TL. \tag{2.4}$$

Just as we did in the step of drawing random samples of TL, we can use equation (2.4) to convert random samples of TL to samples of p. The random samples of p represent random variates from the probability distribution of p. When we have the estimated p for each fish in the sampling region, the sum of these probabilities across all fish is an estimate of the total number of the target fish (walleye). Because there are multiple samples of p for each fish, we have multiple estimates of the total number of fish to summarize the estimation uncertainty.

We now examine the details of each of the three steps focusing on targets detected in one location. For each target j, we estimate the $E(TS)$ from multiple target strength returns. The $E(TS)$ is then used to estimate the distribution of the target length. Through the logistic regression, the estimated length is used to estimate the probability that the target is a walleye.

1. Estimating the distribution of the expected TS based on multiple observations.

   The distribution of TS_{ij} is a log-normal distribution:

   $$\log(TS_{ij}) \sim N(\mu_{TS,j}, \sigma_{TS}^2) \tag{2.5}$$

   where ij represents the ith measurement for the jth target. For simplicity, we will drop the subscript j when doing so will not lead to confusion. Based on the central limit theorem, we know that the estimated mean $\hat{\mu}_{TS}$ has a normal distribution. We have multiple fish in the hydroacoustic data and we estimated them together by imposing a relatively vague prior on the mean target strength for individual fish μ_{TS}:

   $$\mu_{TS} \sim N(0, \sigma_\mu^2). \tag{2.6}$$

   After passing TS return data through a data quality filter, some individual fish had only one while others have multiple associated TS measurement. These associate TS measurements can be grouped together into a fish track. We impose a reasonable prior for σ_μ (half normal with mean 0 and standard deviation 25) to make the estimation of σ_μ possible. For now, we will borrow the results from Gelman and Hill [2007] and simply state that the mean of the distribution is the sample average of observed log TS and the variance is the sample variance divided by the sample size (n_i). The sample variance itself has an inverse χ^2 distribution with degrees of freedom $n_i - 1$. In other words, the distribution of $\hat{\mu}_{TS}$ is a conditional normal distribution. The density function of the marginal distribution of $\hat{\mu}_{TS}$ is

   $$\pi(\hat{\mu}_{TS}) = \int_{\hat{\sigma}^2} \pi(\hat{\mu}_{TS}|\hat{\sigma}^2) \times \pi(\hat{\sigma}^2) d\hat{\sigma}^2.$$

   We will see later in Chapter 3 that the marginal distribution is a Student-t distribution. Hence, we can draw random samples of $\hat{\mu}_{TS}$ directly. In this example, we directly implement the model (equations (2.5) and (2.6)) in Stan and using the resulting random samples of μ_{TS} and σ_{TS}^2 to obtain a random sample of the expected value of TS: $E(TS) = e^{\hat{\mu}_{TS} + \hat{\sigma}_{TS}^2/2}$ (Figure 2.2, left column).

2. Estimating the distribution of TL conditional on knowing the distribution of the expected value of TS.

Although directly estimating the density function is possible, we can use the inverse Love's equation to draw a random sample of TL by substituting the random sample from the previous step (step 1) into equation (2.3) (Figure 2.2, right column).

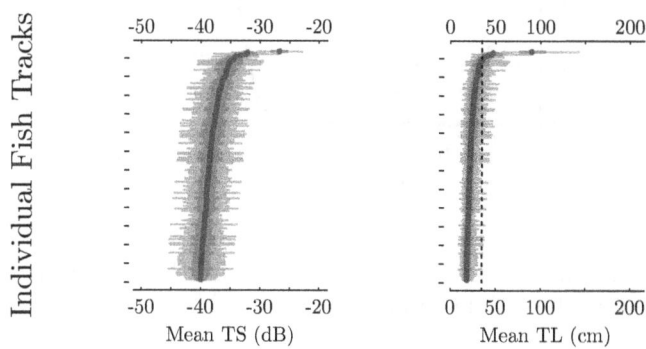

FIGURE 2.2: The estimated mean hydroacoustic target strength distributions (left column) and the corresponding mean fish length distributions (right column) are shown using the simplified boxplots. The solid dots are the means, the thick shaded lines are the middle 50% credible intervals, and the thin shaded lines are the 95% credible intervals.

3. Estimating the probability of a given length fish is a walleye (*Sander vitreus*) using a logistic regression. From equation (2.4), the probability is

$$p = \frac{1}{1 + e^{-(\alpha_0 + \alpha_1 TL)}}. \qquad (2.7)$$

Again, the parameter of interest p is a function of three random variables: logistic regression model coefficients (α_0 and α_1) and the estimated fish length TL. Using the relationships method (Section 2.3.3) we can directly convert random variates of α_0, α_1, and TL to random variates of p.

These steps lead to random variates of p for one fish track, from which we can approximate the distribution of p as a summary of the uncertainty we have on whether the observed target is a walleye or not. This process is carried out for each target.

In our R code, we estimated the 5087 fish tracks in one survey grid simultaneously. Using the estimated mean length for each fish, the estimated probability of each fish being a walleye ranges between 0 and 1 (Figure 2.3). The vast majority of the fish (5065) were unlikely to be walleye (probability less than 0.2).

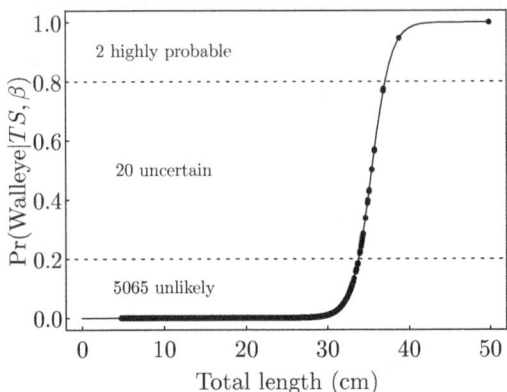

FIGURE 2.3: The estimated probability of a fish being a walleye (*Sander vitreus*) based on the estimated mean length.

The objective of this hydroacoustic survey is to estimate the abundance of walleye in Lake Erie. Each target is a Bernoulli random variable: the detected fish is either a walleye or some other fish. (For the moment, we ignore the possibility that a moving signal is a non-fish object.) The total number of fish is then the sum of the 5087 random variables. As we discussed in Section 2.3.3, we can draw random variates of the total number of fish in two steps:

- For each fish with the probability of being a walleye p_{ij}, draw a random variate from the Bernoulli distribution with the probability of success of p_{ij}, where the subscript ij represents the ith random sample of p from fish j obtained from step 3 of the simulation process discussed previously.

- Sum the Bernoulli random samples for all fish as a random sample of the total number of fish.

Random samples of the total number of walleye (Figure 2.4) can be used to estimate the mean total and its standard deviation (or other measures of uncertainty).

This example is a frequently seen practical problem. There is estimation uncertainty associated with each step, and the outcome is represented using a (conditional) probability distribution. From the observed target strength values of an individual fish, we estimate the probability distribution of the expected target strength. Given a target strength, we estimate a probability distribution of the fish's length. Conditional on the fish's length, we estimate the probability distribution of the probability of the fish being a walleye.

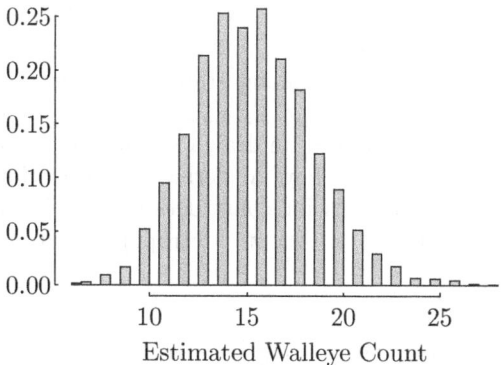

FIGURE 2.4: The estimated probability distribution of total number of walleye in the sampled water encountered by the survey vessel is presented in a histogram.

2.4 Markov Chain Monte Carlo Simulation

We have seen methods for generating random variates from mostly univariate random variables with known probability distributions. When we want to generate random variates from multivariate random variables, a more general method is needed. The various Markov chain Monte Carlo algorithms are such methods.

In mathematics, a Markov chain refers to a system that hops from one state (e.g., a set of values) to another. The list of all (finite) states is known as the state space. A Markov chain defines the state space, as well as the probability of transitioning from one state to the other. In a finite state space $S = \{1, \cdots, N\}$, a Markov chain is a sequence of random variables, where the probability of being in a particular state at step $k + 1$ only depends on the state at step k. For a time-homogeneous Markov chain (transition probability independent of k) we can define a transition matrix $P = \{p_{ij}\}$, where p_{ij} is the probability of transitioning from state i to state j (and $\sum_{j=1}^{N} p_{ij} = 1$). When a Markov chain is ergodic, that is, a state does not recur in a regular pattern (aperiodic) and the chance of a state occurring is larger than 0 (positive recurrent), any state can be reached from any other state in a finite number of steps.

Furthermore, an ergodic Markov chain has a unique stable distribution $\pi = (\pi_1, \pi_2, \cdots, \pi_N)$ on the state space (π_i = the probability of state i) with the property that $\pi = \pi P$ (or $\pi_j = \sum_i \pi_i p_{ij}$). The Markov chain Monte Carlo simulation (MCMC) methods are based on this stable distribution [Richey,

2010]. To obtain a sample from π, we can take a sample s_1 from any position of the Markov chain. If $s_1 = i$ we select $s_2 = j$ with probability p_{ij}, if $s_2 = k$ we select $s_3 = l$ with probability p_{kl}, and so forth. In the resulting series $s_1, s_2, \cdots, s_M$, the fraction of s's taking state j is π_j when $M \to \infty$. For any large number m, the sequence $s_{m+1}, s_{m+2}, \cdots, s_{m+n}$ is an approximate sample of π. Using this feature, we can draw random samples from the stable distribution as long as we know how to derive the transition probabilities. Surprisingly, there exist methods for constructing such "transition kernels" that are valid for almost any density π. Metropolis et al. [1953] presented such a method.

2.4.1   Metropolis-Hastings Algorithm

The Metropolis-Hastings algorithm is based on a version of the acceptance-rejection method. In the algorithm, we know the target density $\pi(x)$ and an easy-to-sample-from candidate-generating density $q(y \mid x)$. The candidate-generating density is a conditional probability density. If it is the transition kernel, it should satisfy the condition $\pi(x)q(y \mid x) = \pi(y)q(x \mid y)$. That is, $q(y \mid x)$ is reversible. In most cases, q is not reversible. If we found a q that for some x, y,

$$\pi(x)q(y \mid x) > \pi(y)q(x \mid y),$$

the transition moves x to y too frequently and needs to be slowed down. One way to slow the process is to introduce a probability $\alpha(x, y) < 1$ so that the move does not happen every time (i.e., $\pi(x)q(y \mid x)\alpha(x, y) = \pi(y)q(x \mid y)$). The algorithm developed in Metropolis et al. [1953] and generalized by Hastings [1970] defines this probability of move as

$$\alpha(x, y) = min \left[\frac{\pi(y)q(y \mid x)}{\pi(x)q(x \mid y)}, 1 \right].$$

The algorithm starts with an arbitrary value $x^{(0)}$, and repeats for $j = 1, \cdots, N$:

1. Generate y from $q(y \mid x^{(j)})$ and u from $U(0, 1)$.

2. If $u \leq \alpha(x^{(j)}, y)$, set $x^{(j+1)} = y$.

3. Else, set $x^{(j+1)} = x^{(j)}$.

The distinct advantage of the Metropolis-Hastings algorithm is that the full analytic form of the target density is not needed. The algorithm draws samples from $q(y|x)$ and decides whether to accept the sample based on the ratio $r = \frac{\pi(y)q(y|x)}{\pi(x)q(x|y)}$. As a result, in a Bayesian analysis, when the posterior density is hard to derive because of the integral in the denominator, we can simply define the posterior as proportional to the prior times the likelihood and still be able to draw random samples from the posterior.

The Metropolis-Hastings algorithm is generic. It applies to any target distribution π. It can be easily implemented in R for any generic q.

```
### R Code ###
## rq(n, x) is a generic function for generating
##           random numbers from q
x <- rep(0, n_sims) # initial values
for (j in 1:n_sims){
  y <- rq (1, x[j])
  alpha <- (pi(y)/pi(x[j]))*(q(y, x[j])/(q(x[j], y)))
  if (runif(1) < alpha) x[j+1] <- y
  else x[j+1] <- x[j]
}
### End ###
```

As an example, we modify this generic program to generate random variables from a beta distribution. We can use a uniform distribution between 0 and 1 as q. As a result, the density $q(x \mid y) = q(y \mid x) = 1$.

```
### R Code ###
set.seed(10)
n_sims<-4000
x <- numeric()
x[1] <- rbeta(1,1,1) # initial value
a <- 2
b <- 5
for (j in 1:n_sims){
  y <- runif(1)
  alpha <- dbeta(y, a, b)/dbeta(x[j], a, b)
  if (runif(1) < alpha) x[j+1] <- y
  else x[j+1] <- x[j]
}

x <- x[round(1+n_sims/2):n_sims]
hist(x, prob=T, main="Metropolis-Hastings Algorithm")
curve(dbeta(x, a, b), add=T)
### End ###
```

Discarding the first 2000 iterations (burn-in), the histogram of the second 2000 random samples matches the target distribution ($beta(2,5)$) and the random samples appear "random" (Figure 2.5).

In practice, the target density is often more complicated than the beta distribution density. In Bayesian analysis, the target distribution is most likely the posterior distribution derived by the product of the prior density and the likelihood function. In the snake fungal disease example (Section 1.1.1 on page 6), the posterior distribution (equation (1.4) on page 9) is numerically

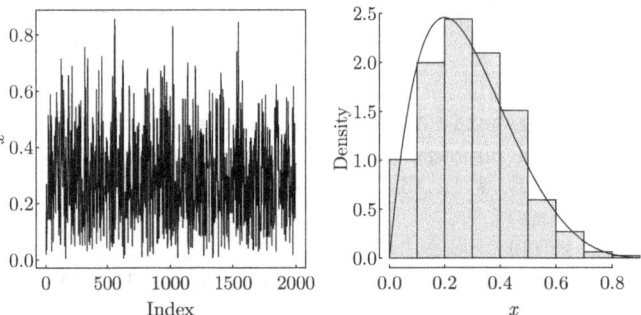

FIGURE 2.5: The Metropolis-Hastings algorithm generated random samples from the beta distribution with parameters 2 and 5. The left panel shows the trajectory of the second 2000 samples. The right panel show the histogram of the second 2000 random samples, compared to the density function of $beta(x \mid \alpha = 2, \beta = 5)$.

evaluated. Using the Metropolis-Hastings algorithm, we can directly draw random variates from equation (1.4) using only the numerator:

```
### R Code ###
## Snake fungal disease example
log_lk <- function(theta, x=5, n=20, fp=0.07, fn=0.05){
         ## log-likelihood function
    pp <- theta*(1-fn)+(1-theta)*fp
    llk <- x*log(pp)+(n-x)*log(1-pp)
    return(llk)
}

for (j in 1:n_sims){
  y <- runif(1)
  alpha <- exp(log_lk(y)-log_lk(theta[j]))
  if (runif(1) < alpha) theta[j+1] <- y
  else theta[j+1] <- theta[j]
}
### End ###
```

The results from the Metropolis-Hastings algorithm is comparable to the same posterior distribution numerically evaluated based on equation (1.4) on page 9 (Figure 2.6).

A properly selected candidate distribution is often the key to the performance of the Metropolis-Hastings algorithm. Most of the considerations in selecting a candidate density is out of the scope of this book and can be found in Robert and Casella [2010].

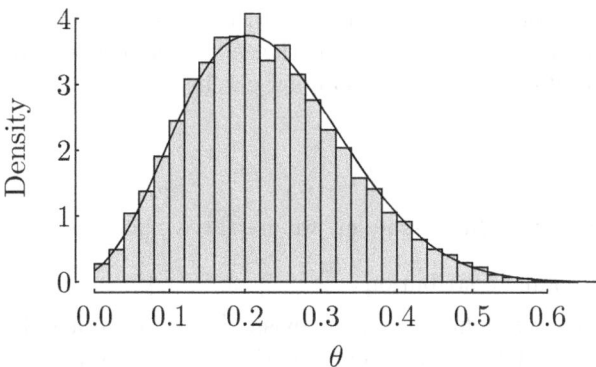

FIGURE 2.6: The Metropolis-Hastings algorithm generated random samples from the posterior distribution of the snake fungal disease prevalence θ (equation (1.4)) are shown in the histogram. The numerically evaluated same posterior (Figure 1.3) is superposed (the thin black line).

2.4.2 Gibbs Sampler

A special case of the Metropolis-Hastings algorithm is the Gibbs sampler for sampling from a multivariate density. The Gibbs sampler became a popular tool of choice after Gelfand and Smith [1990] illustrated its use in Bayesian inference. We describe the Gibbs sampler using the process for generating random samples from a joint distribution of Z_1, Z_2, and Z_3. Suppose the analytic form of the joint distribution is difficult to evaluate. However, it is often true that the conditional distributions of $(Z_1|Z_2, Z_3)$, $(Z_2|Z_1, Z_3)$, and $(Z_3|Z_1, Z_2)$ are relatively easy to define. Drawing random variates from a univariate probability distribution is often possible even when we do not know the density function exactly. Starting from a set of arbitrary initial values of Z_1^0, Z_2^0, and Z_3^0, the Gibbs sampler generates a set of random variates from their corresponding conditional distributions, that is, $Z_1^1 \sim (Z_1|Z_2^0, Z_3^0)$, $Z_2^1 \sim (Z_2|Z_1^1, Z_3^0)$, and $Z_3^1 \sim (Z_3|Z_1^1, Z_2^1)$. Replacing the initial values with newly generated random variates, we can generate a second set of random variates. Continuing to generate successively for k times, we have k sets of random variates of Z_1, Z_2, and Z_3. Geman and Geman [1984] showed that when k is large enough, (Z_1^k, Z_2^k, Z_3^k) can be considered as a sample from the joint distribution. In other words, the conditional densities are the candidate-generating densities that are also reversible in the Metropolis-Hastings algorithm. As a result, if we continue to generate random variates, we can take $Z_i^k, Z_i^{k+1}, \cdots$ as samples from the marginal distribution of Z_i (here $i = 1, 2, 3$). Since the marginal and/or joint densities are estimated from random variates, only procedures that can be used to generate these random variates from their respective conditional distributions are needed, the conditional probability densities themselves do not have to be fully described. Details of the Gibbs sampler can be found in the earlier cited references, and a simple and intuitive exposition of the Gibbs sampler can be found in Casella and George [1992].

2.4.2.1   Examples

To illustrate the Gibbs sampler, we use three examples.

1. Beta-binomial distribution

    We go back to Chapter 1 and revisit the problem of estimating the binomial distribution parameter p (Figure 1.2). Suppose that before we observe data, we want to have a better understanding of what to expect. That is, we would like to know how many positives we should expect under different p and the likely range of p if we observe x. The posterior distribution of p is proportional to the product of the prior of p ($beta(\alpha, \beta)$) and the likelihood

    $$\pi(p \mid n, x) \propto \frac{\Gamma(\alpha)\Gamma(\beta)}{\Gamma(\alpha + \beta)} p^{\alpha-1}(1-p)^{\beta-1} \times \binom{n}{x} p^x (1-p)^{n-x}.$$

    It is a conditional distribution of p given x. Likewise, if p is known, the data x have a binomial distribution, another conditional distribution. That is, we have

    $$\begin{aligned} p \mid x, n &\sim beta(\alpha + x, \beta + n - x) \\ x \mid p, n &\sim bin(p, n). \end{aligned}$$

    To draw random numbers from the joint distribution, we can start with an initial value for p (e.g., a random draw from $beta(1, 1)$), followed by a random draw of x from a binomial distribution.

```
### R Code ###
alpha <- 2
beta <- 2
n <- 20
x <- numeric()
p <- numeric()
p[1] <- rbeta(1, 1, 1)
x[1] <- rbinom(1, n, p[1])
for (j in 2:n_sims){
  p[j] <- rbeta(1, alpha+x[j-1], beta+n-x[j-1])
  x[j] <- rbinom(1, n, p[j])
}
plot(p, x)
### End ###
```

2. The change point model

Qian and Richardson [1997] proposed a model for estimating a wetland's long-term total phosphorus retention capacity as part of the Everglades study (Section 1.4.3). They reasoned that the long-term fate of phosphorus in a wetland is either dissolved in water or buried in the sediment because phosphorus does not have a gaseous phase. Phosphorus used by microorganisms, algae, and plants is transient. Once these organisms die, a large portion of the incorporated phosphorus will be released either to the water column or be buried in the sediment. As sediment buildup increases, part of the phosphorus buried in the sediment will be out of the reach of rooted plants and can be considered permanently removed. Each wetland has its rate of sediment buildup, hence a capacity for removing phosphorus. If a wetland receives phosphorous-enriched input from surface runoff or sewage treatment effluent, some of the phosphorus can be permanently stored in the wetland. If the input phosphorus loading rate is below the wetland's retention capacity, we expect that phosphorus concentrations in the outflow of the wetland would be low and stable. When the input loading rate exceeds the wetland's retention capacity, the excess amount will eventually be in the water column and the outflow phosphorus concentration will increase and fluctuate. If we plot the effluent phosphorus concentrations against the input loading, we expect to see a pattern that can be modeled by a piecewise linear function. A piecewise linear model is a statistical change point problem, where the linear model's slope changes at the change point.

$$y_i = \begin{cases} \alpha_0 + \alpha_1 x_i + \epsilon_i & \text{if } x \leq \gamma \\ \beta_0 + \beta_1 x_i + \epsilon_i & \text{if } x > \gamma \end{cases} \tag{2.8}$$

The model has six parameters (two slopes (α_1, β_1), two intercepts (α_0, β_0), a change point (γ), and the residual variance (ϵ_i)). The two lines intercept at the change point. That is,

$$\alpha_0 + \alpha_1 \gamma = \beta_0 + \beta_1 \gamma,$$

reducing the number of free parameters to five $(\theta = \{\alpha_0, \alpha_1, \beta_1, \gamma, \sigma^2\})$. The piecewise linear model used to be computationally challenging. The likelihood function is potentially discontinuous:

$$L = \frac{1}{\sigma^n} e^{-\frac{1}{2\sigma^2}(L_1 + L_2)} \tag{2.9}$$

where $L_1 = \sum_{x \leq \gamma} (y_i - \alpha_0 - \alpha_1 x_i)^2$ and $L_2 = \sum_{x > \gamma} (y_i - \alpha_0 - \beta_1 x_i - (\alpha_1 - \beta_1)\gamma)^2$. The joint posterior distribution of the five free parameters is proportional to the product of the priors and the likelihood. We can use the standard non-informative priors $\pi(\alpha_0, \alpha_1, \beta_1, \gamma, \sigma^2) \propto 1/\sigma^2$.

To use the Gibbs sampler for this problem, we need to find the full set of conditional posterior distribution functions. To shorten the expression, we use $\pi(\alpha_0 \mid \theta_{-\alpha_0})$ to represent the conditional probability of α_0 given all other parameters: $\pi(\alpha_0 \mid \theta_{-\alpha_0}, Y) = \pi(\alpha_0 \mid \alpha_1, \beta_1, \gamma, \sigma^2, Y)$. To further shorten the notation, we omit Y from the expression here as we are discussing the posterior conditionals. As a result, the full set of conditional probabilities is $\pi(\alpha_0 \mid \theta_{-\alpha_0}), \pi(\alpha_1 \mid \theta_{-\alpha_1}), \pi(\beta_1 \mid \theta_{-\beta_1}), \pi(\sigma^2 \mid \theta_{-\sigma^2})$, and $\pi(\gamma \mid \theta_{-\gamma})$. Although the joint distribution (the product of the prior ($\propto 1/\sigma^2$) and the likelihood function (equation (2.9)) is perhaps intractable because of the discontinuity from the two summations, the conditional posteriors can be derived relatively easily through straightforward (but tedious) algebraic manipulation. For example, the conditional posterior density of β_1 can be expressed as follows:

$$\pi(\beta_1 \mid \theta_{-\beta_1}) \propto \frac{1}{\sigma^{n+2}} e^{-\frac{L_1+L_2}{2\sigma^2}}.$$

The core part of the conditional probability density is the second summation term (L_2) because the rest of the conditional posterior density function is a constant multiplicative factor. As a result, the conditional posterior of β_1 can be simplified to

$$\pi(\beta_1 \mid \theta_{-\beta_1}) \propto e^{-\frac{1}{2\sigma^2} \sum_{x>\gamma} (y_i - \alpha_0 - \beta_1 x_i - (\alpha_1 - \beta_1)\gamma)^2}.$$

Regrouping the sum of squares term to express it as a quadratic function of β_1, that is,

$$
\begin{aligned}
L_2 &= \sum_{x>\gamma} (y_i - \alpha_0 - \beta_1 x_i - (\alpha_1 - \beta_1)\gamma)^2 \\
&= \sum_{x>\gamma} (y_i - \alpha_0 - \alpha_1\gamma)^2 - 2\beta_0 \sum_{x>\gamma} (x_i - \gamma)(y_i - \alpha_0 - \alpha_1\gamma) \\
&\quad + \beta_1^2 \sum_{x>\gamma} (x_i - \gamma)^2 \\
&= \sum_{x>\gamma} (x_i - \gamma)^2 \left(\beta_1 - \frac{\sum_{x>\gamma}(x_i-\gamma)(y_i-\alpha_0-\alpha_1\gamma)}{\sum_{x>\gamma}(x_i-\gamma)^2} \right)^2.
\end{aligned}
$$

The posterior is then proportional to

$$e^{-\frac{1}{2\sigma^2} \left(\sum_{x>\gamma}(x_i-\gamma)^2 \left(\beta_1 - \frac{\sum_{x>\gamma}[(x_i-\gamma)(y_i-\alpha_0-\alpha_1\gamma)]}{\sum_{x>\gamma}(x_i-\gamma)^2} \right)^2 \right)},$$

which is proportional to the normal density function with mean

$$\mu_{\beta_1} = \frac{\sum_{x>\gamma}[(x_i-\gamma)(y_i-\alpha_0-\alpha_1\gamma)]}{\sum_{x>\gamma}(x_i-\gamma)^2}$$

and variance

$$\tau_{\beta_1}^2 = \sigma^2 / \left(\sum_{x>\gamma}(x_i-\gamma)^2 \right).$$

As a result, the conditional distribution of β_1 is $\beta_1 \mid \theta_{-\beta_1} \sim N(\mu_{\beta_1}, \tau_{\beta_1}^2)$.

Likewise, we can show that the conditional posterior distribution function of $\alpha_0 \mid \theta_{-\alpha_0}$ is also a normal distribution with mean

$$\mu_{\alpha_0} = \frac{A_0 + B_0}{n_1 + n_2}$$

where $A_0 = \sum_{x \leq \gamma}(y_i - \alpha_1 x_i)$, $B_0 = \sum_{x > \gamma}(y_i - \beta_1 x_i - (\alpha_1 - \beta_1)\gamma)$, n_1 is the number of observations with $x \leq \gamma$, and n_2 is the number of observations with $x > \gamma$, and variance

$$\tau_{\alpha_0}^2 = \frac{\sigma^2}{n_1 + n_2}.$$

The conditional posterior of $\alpha_1 \mid \theta_{-\alpha_1}$ is a normal with mean

$$\mu_{\alpha_1} = \frac{A_1 + B_1}{n_2 \gamma^2 + \sum_{x \leq \gamma} x_i^2}$$

where $A_1 = \sum_{x \leq \gamma} x_i(y_i - \alpha_0)$ and $B_1 = \gamma \sum_{x > \gamma}(y_i - \alpha_0 + \beta_1(x_i - \gamma))$, and variance

$$\tau_{\alpha_1}^2 = \frac{\sigma^2}{n_2 \gamma^2 + \sum_{x \leq \gamma} x_i^2}.$$

The conditional posterior of $\sigma^2 \mid \theta_{-\sigma^2}$ is an inverse gamma distribution:

$$1/\sigma^2 \sim gamma\left(\frac{n}{2} + 2, \frac{L_1 + L_2}{2}\right).$$

Finally, the conditional posterior distribution of γ is not of any standard distribution we know:

$$\pi(\gamma \mid \theta_{-\gamma}) \propto e^{\frac{1}{2\sigma^2}(L_1 + L2)}.$$

However, we can use the acceptance-rejection method to draw random variates from the conditional posterior distribution. The strategy is to first draw a candidate random number from an instrumental distribution (e.g., uniform within the observed range of x), and then estimate the maximum value of the conditional density to calculate the acceptance probability. Specifically,

- Draw $\gamma^* \sim U(x_{min}, x_{max})$.
- Once γ^* is selected, L_1 is no longer a function of γ and L_2 reaches its minimum when

$$\gamma = \gamma^{min} = \frac{\sum_{x > \gamma^*}(y_i - \alpha_0 - \beta_1 x_i)}{n_2(\alpha_1 - \beta_1)}.$$

- Hence, we accept γ^* as a random variate from the conditional posterior of $\gamma \mid \theta_{-\gamma}$ with probability $p_a = e^{\frac{L_2(\gamma^{min}) - L_2(\gamma^*)}{2\sigma^2}}$, where $L_2(\gamma^{min})$ and $L_2(\gamma^*)$ are L_2 evaluated at γ^{min} and γ^*, respectively.

The Gibbs sampler program is included in the GitHub companion of the book. The computer code of a Gibbs sampler is often impossible to verify because, unlike a program for a maximum likelihood estimator, we cannot check the accuracy of the code using standard testing data with known results. The outcome from a Gibbs sampler consists of random numbers. In this example, the tedious algebraic derivation can be difficult to check as well. For this reason, we used a different formulation of the model as a comparison. The change point model in equation (2.8) can be rewritten as

$$y_i = b_0 + (b_1 + \delta I(x - \gamma))(x - \gamma) + \epsilon_i \qquad (2.10)$$

where $I(a) = \begin{cases} 0 & \text{if } a \leq 0 \\ 1 & \text{if } a > 0 \end{cases}$ is a unit step function. With this formulation, $b_0 = \alpha_0 + \alpha_1 \gamma$, $b_1 = \alpha_1$, and $\delta = \beta_1 - \alpha_1$. We can compare the simulation results to ensure coding accuracy.

The likelihood function is

$$L = \frac{1}{\sigma^n} e^{\frac{L_1^\delta + L_2^\delta}{2\sigma^2}}$$

where

$$L_1^\delta = \sum_{x_i \leq \gamma} (y_i - b_0 - b_1(x_i - \gamma))^2$$

and

$$L_2^\delta = \sum_{x_i > \gamma} (y_i - b_0 - (b_1 + \delta)(x_i - \gamma))^2.$$

The conditional posterior distributions for this formulation are:

- $b_0 \mid \theta_{-b_0} \sim N\left(\frac{S_1 + S_2}{n_1 + n_2}, \frac{\sigma^2}{n_1 + n_2}\right)$,
  where $S_1 = \sum_{x_i \leq \gamma}(y_i - b_1(x_i - \gamma))$ and $S_2 = \sum_{x > \gamma}(y_i - (b_1 + \delta)(x_i - \gamma))$.

- $b_1 \mid \theta_{-b_1} \sim N\left(\frac{S_3 + S_4}{\sum_{i=1}^n (x_i - \gamma)^2}, \frac{\sigma^2}{\sum_{i=1}^n (x_i - \gamma)^2}\right)$,
  where $S_3 = \sum_{x_i \leq \gamma}(x_i - \gamma)(y_i - b_0)$ and $S_4 = \sum_{x_i > \gamma}(x_i - \gamma)(y_i - b_0 - \delta(x_i - \gamma))$.

- $\delta \mid \theta_{-\delta} \sim N\left(\frac{S_5}{\sum_{x > \gamma}(x_i - \gamma)}, \frac{\sigma^2}{\sum_{x > \gamma}(x_i - \gamma)}\right)$,
  where $S_5 = \sum_{x > \gamma}(x_i - \gamma)(y_i - b_0 - b_1(x_i - \gamma))$.

- $\sigma^2 \mid -\sigma^2, Y$ is an inverse gamma distribution $(1/\sigma^2 \mid -\sigma^2, Y \sim gamma\left(\frac{n}{2} + 1, \frac{L_1^\delta + L_2^\delta}{2}\right))$.

- $\gamma \mid \theta_{-\gamma}$ is proportional to $\pi_\gamma = e^{-\frac{L_1^\delta + L_2^\delta}{2\sigma^2}}$, not a standard distribution. We also use an acceptance-rejection method by first drawing

$\gamma^\star$ from a uniform distribution on the range of the predictor (x), and evaluating $M^\star = L_1^\delta + L_2^\delta$ with $\gamma = \gamma^\star$. The maximum of π_γ is reached at $\gamma^{min} = \frac{n_1 b_0 b_1 + n_2 b_0 (b_1 + \delta) - b_1 S_{g1} - (b_1 + \delta) S_{g2}}{n_1 b_1^2 + n_2 (b_1 + \gamma)^2}$, where $S_{g1} = \sum_{x_i \le \gamma^\star} y_i - b_1 \sum_{x_i \le \gamma^\star} x_i - n_1 b_0$ and $S_{g2} = \sum_{x_i > \gamma^\star} y_i - (b_1 + \delta) \sum_{x_i > \gamma^\star} x_i - n_2 b_0$. Then, $\gamma^\star$ is accepted with probability

$$p_a = e^{-\frac{(L_1^\star + L_2^\star) - (L_1^{min} + L_2^{min})}{2\sigma^2}}.$$

In the GitHub companion of the book, we included two comparisons. One uses simulated data where all model parameters are known to compare the Gibbs sampler estimated parameters to the known values. The other compares the two versions of Gibbs sampler using the Everglades data. Qian and Richardson [1997] allowed the residual variance to vary before and after the change point. Also, they used conjugate priors for some of the parameters when deriving the conditional posteriors. As a result, our Gibbs sampler produced slightly different results than reported in their paper. We compare the two key parameters: the exponential of α_0 representing the mean log TP concentration when TP loading is below the change point (or background log TP concentration) and the exponential of γ (the estimated long-term TP retention capacity) (Table 2.1).

The estimated TP retention capacity distribution from Qian and Richardson [1997] is consistently larger than the same estimated using our two alternative formulations. The difference is largely due to a coding error in the C++ program used for generating random variates of γ using the acceptance-rejection method. In the original C++ code, the acceptance probability $p_a = e^{\frac{L_2(\gamma^{min}) - L_2(\gamma^\star)}{2\sigma^2}}$ was coded as $p_a = e^{L_2(\gamma^{min}) - L_2(\gamma^\star)}$. Such coding error is very difficult to discover. We reviewed the original code several times before coding the model in R. The error was discovered only when the comparison made it obvious that we needed to check the acceptance-rejection subroutine/function.

TABLE 2.1: Comparing the estimated background total phosphorus concentration and the change point distributions (selected percentiles) from equations (2.8) and (2.10) to the estimates from Qian and Richardson [1997] (QR).

Model	Parameters	5%	20%	30%	40%	50%	60%	70%	80%	95%
QR	γ	0.614	0.909	1.016	1.078	1.150	1.217	1.288	1.358	1.467
eq. (2.8)	γ	0.264	0.718	0.838	0.901	0.939	0.972	1.002	1.033	1.087
eq. (2.10)	γ	0.272	0.717	0.835	0.897	0.933	0.966	0.998	1.029	1.084
QR	α_1	0.018	0.019	0.020	0.020	0.021	0.022	0.022	0.023	0.025
eq. (2.8)	α_0	0.018	0.019	0.020	0.020	0.021	0.021	0.022	0.023	0.025
eq. (2.10)	α_0	0.018	0.019	0.020	0.020	0.021	0.021	0.022	0.022	0.024

3. Non-parametric monotonic regression

The third example is a non-parametric binary regression problem reported in Qian et al. [2000b]. It is an extension of the first example, in that, the observed data in both examples are modeled as binomial random variables, but the probability of success in this example is a monotonic function of a predictor variable x (i.e., $p = f(x)$). The objective of the paper was to examine the nature of the monotonic function f without imposing additional constraints beyond the assumption of a monotonically increasing function. At each observed predictor variable value (or a grid point) x_j, we observe y_j successes in n_j trials. In this example, we describe the Gibbs sampler using the polychlorinated biphenyls (PCB) in the fish example, where we are interested in how likely that a given sized fish caught in Lake Michigan, a Laurentian Great Lake, would have a PCB concentration exceeding a consumption advisory criterion. Salmonid species are popular sports fish in the area. These predator fish often have high PCB contents due to historical industrial contamination. In this example we use data from lake trout (*Salvelinus namaycush*). Madenjian et al. [1998] documented that lake trout in Lake Michigan shift their diet at a size of about 60 centimeters from small alewife (*Alosa pseudoharengus*) and rainbow smelt (*Osmerus mordax*) to large alewife. Because large alewife typically have much higher PCB concentrations, the rate of PCB accumulation in large lake trout (larger than 60 cm) increases more rapidly as a function of size, compared to small lake trout. In this example, we transform the PCB concentration to a binary variable of whether the concentration is above the consumption advisory level of 1 mg/kg. The details of the Gibbs sampler algorithm were originally described in [Lavine, 1994]. Readers unfamiliar with the multivariate Dirichlet distribution may wish to skip this example.

In this problem, we divide the fish length into bins of small increment. The problem can be summarized as follows:

$$
\begin{aligned}
y_j &\sim bin(p_j, n_j) \\
p_j &= f(x_j)
\end{aligned}
\tag{2.11}
$$

where n_j is the total number of fish in the jth length bin, y_j is the is the number of fish in the jth length bin with PCB concentrations above the criterion, x_j is the mean fish length in the jth length bin, and p_j is the probability of a fish in the jth length bin with concentration exceeding the consumption advisory limit. The response variable is modeled by a binomial distribution and the probability of "success" (PCB concentration above the criterion) is modeled as an undefined function of length (x). A non-parametric regression model is not defined by an algebraic formula with unknown parameters, rather it is defined by distinct values of $f(x_j)$ or f_j, the values of the regression function at x_j. In this case, we limit the function $f(x)$ to be monotonic. As larger fish tend to be older, they are therefore more likely to have a higher PCB concentration than a smaller fish. That is, we assume that the function increases as length increases.

Because f is monotonic and $0 \leq f_j \leq 1$, the transformation between f_j and $s_j = f_j - f_{j-1}$ is one-to-one for $j = 1, \cdots, m$ and $f_0 = 0$ and $f_{m+1} = 1$. The joint distribution of $f_1, \cdots, f_m$ can be described through the distribution of $s_1, \cdots, s_m$. Since $s_j \in (0,1)$ and $\sum_{j=1}^{m+1} s_j = 1$, a plausible prior distribution of $s_1, \cdots, s_{m+1}$ is the Dirichlet distribution. A Dirichlet distribution is the multivariate version of the beta distribution with a density

$$\pi(s_1, \cdots, s_{m+1}) = \frac{\prod_{j=1}^{m+1} \Gamma(a_j)}{\Gamma\left(\sum_{j=1}^{m+1} a_j\right)} \prod_{j=1}^{m+1} s_j^{a_j - 1}. \qquad (2.12)$$

Using the notation of Ferguson [1973], a_j is partitioned into a product of α and d_j to represent two pieces of information:

- D_0, the prior expected shape of f (the best "guess" we have on how the relationship should look) and $d_j = D_{0,j} - D_{0,j-1}$, the increment of D_0 from $j-1$ to j;

- α, our confidence in D_0 (e.g., α can be seen as a measure of faith in the prior guess D_0 measured in units of numbers of observations as suggested by Ferguson [1973]).

When a prior is derived from cross-sectional data, α is often selected based on the sample size and our judgment on how relevant the cross-sectional data set is to the site-specific problem. We use $DP(D_0; \alpha)$ to denote the Dirichlet prior of f, i.e., a Dirichlet distribution of $\{s_1, \cdots, s_{m+1}\}$ with parameters $d_1\alpha, \cdots, d_{n+1}\alpha$.

This non-parametric problem has m parameters $(f_1, \cdots, f_m)$. To derive the Gibbs sampler, we need to derive the full set of conditional probabilities $\pi(f_j | f_{-j})$. Here, we use the subscript $-j$ to denote "all except j." One feature of the Dirichlet distribution is that the conditional distribution of s_j given s_{j-1} and s_{j+1} is a re-scaled beta distribution:

$$\frac{s_j}{s_{j+1} - s_{j-1}} \bigg| s_{j-1}, s_{j+1} \sim beta(d_j\alpha, d_{j+1}\alpha) \qquad (2.13)$$

which is equivalent to

$$\frac{f_j - f_{j-1}}{f_{j+1} - f_{j-1}} \bigg| f_{j-1}, f_{j+1} \sim beta(d_j\alpha, d_{j+1}\alpha). \qquad (2.14)$$

The joint posterior distribution of f_j is proportional to the prior times the likelihood:

$$\pi(f_1, \cdots, f_m | Y) \propto \pi(f_1, \cdots, f_m) L(Y, f_1, \cdots, f_m).$$

To use the Gibbs sampler, we need posterior conditional density

$$\pi(f_j | f_{-j}, Y_j) \propto \pi(f_j | f_{-j}) L(Y, f_1, \cdots, f_m). \tag{2.15}$$

Because f is monotonic, $\pi(f_j | f_{-j}) = \pi(f_j | f_{j-1}, f_{j+1})$, a re-scaled beta distribution (equation (2.14)).

The likelihood function is proportional to

$$L(Y_j | f_1, \cdots, f_m) = \prod_{j=1}^{m} f_j^{y_j} (1 - f_j)^{n_j - y_j}.$$

The maximum of the likelihood is reached when $f_j^\star = y_j / n_j$, the observed frequency of success. One way to draw a random sample from the conditional posterior (equation (2.15)) is to use the acceptance-rejection method (Section 2.3.2). The posterior density is less than $\pi(f_j | f_{-j}) \prod_{j=1}^{m} (f^\star)^{y_j} (1 - f^\star)^{n_j - y_j}$. That is, we choose the target density to be $\pi(f_j | f_{-j})$ (the prior as the instrument distribution), and $M = \prod_{j=1}^{m} (f_j^\star)^{y_j} (1 - f_j^\star)^{n_j - y_j}$. Consequently, a random variate from the conditional posterior can be drawn by first drawing f_j from its conditional prior (a re-scaled beta distribution) and accept the result with probability $\left(\prod_{j=1}^{m} f_j^{y_j} (1 - f_j)^{n_j - y_j} \right) / M$.

R code for this example is in the GitHub companion of the book. The original code was written in C and much of the original data were no longer available to us.

These examples show that (1) conditional distributions are often easier to work with than the joint distribution and (2) even when we face a difficult conditional distribution, we can still draw random samples from it.

2.5   Bayesian Inference Using Markov Chain Monte Carlo

With the Gibbs sampler, sampling from multivariate distributions becomes relatively simple. Many early applications of the Gibbs sampler in Bayesian inference were focused on deriving the complete set of conditional densities from the posterior, as illustrated by the change point model (page 47) and the binary monotonic regression (page 52) examples. With the "Metropolisation" of the Gibbs sampler [Müller, 1991], the derivation of conditional densities is no longer necessary. By Metropolisation, we mean the use of the Metropolis-Hastings method for drawing random samples from conditional posterior densities. We wrap up this chapter by revisiting the snake fungal disease example.

2.5.1 Metropolis-Hastings within a Gibbs Sampler

In the snake fungal disease example, we are interested in estimating the prevalence of the disease (θ) based on a sample of (n) snakes. Among the n snakes, we observed x positive test results. The test is imperfect with a probability of false positive (f_p) and a probability of false negative (f_n). The observed data can be modeled by the binomial distribution:

$$x \sim bin(n, p_+)$$

where $p_+ = \theta(1 - f_n) + (1 - \theta)f_p$ is the probability of observing a positive result. For simplicity, we use three independent beta distribution priors for $\theta, f_p,$ and f_n. The joint posterior distribution density is proportional to

$$\begin{aligned} \pi(\theta, f_p, f_n | x, n) \quad &\propto \quad \pi(\theta)\pi(f_p)\pi(f_n)p_+^x(1 - p_+)^{n-x} \\ &\propto \quad \theta^{\alpha-1}(1-\theta)^{\beta-1} \times f_p^{a_p-1}(1 - f_p)^{b_p-1} \times \\ &\quad f_n^{a_n-1}(1 - f_n)^{b_n-1} \times \\ &\quad (\theta(1-f_n) + (1-\theta)f_p)^x(1 - \theta(1-f_n) - (1-\theta)f_p)^{n-x}. \end{aligned}$$

$$(2.16)$$

The right-hand side of equation (2.16) is proportional to the posterior density up to a normalizing constant. It is also proportional to any of the three conditional densities. That is, $\pi(\theta|f_p, f_n, x, n)$ is proportional to the joint density if we take f_p and f_n as known constants (R code on page 30). As a result, we can use the Metropolis-Hastings algorithm to draw random samples of θ from its conditional posterior density. We can, again, use the uniform distribution as the proposal (or instrumental) distribution as we did in the simple binomial example (page 46). Likewise, we can use the Metropolis-Hastings method to draw random samples of f_p and f_n from their respective conditional densities.

```
### R Code ###
## prior parameters
alpha <- 1; beta <- 1; ap <- 5; bp <- 20; an <- 2;
bn <- 25; n <- 20; x <- 5

post <- function(theta, fp, fn, x, n)
return ((theta^(alpha-1))*((1-theta)^(beta-1)) *
        (fp^(ap-1))*((1-fp)^(bp-1)) *
        (fn^(an-1))*((1-fn)^(bn-1)) *
        ((theta*(1-fn)+(1-theta)*fp)^x) *
        ((1-theta*(1-fn)-(1-theta)*fp)^(n-x)))

set.seed(101)
```

```
n_sims<-4000
theta <- fp <- fn <- numeric()
theta[1] <- rbeta(1, alpha, beta) # initial value
fp[1] <- rbeta(1, ap, bp)
fn[1] <- rbeta(an, bn)
for (j in 2:n_sims){
  ## theta
  th <- runif(1)
  r <- post(th, fp[j-1], fn[j-1], x, n) /
      post(theta[j-1], fp[j-1], fn[j-1], x, n)
  if (runif(1) < r) theta[j] <- th
  else theta[j] <- theta[j-1]
  ## fp
  f_p <- runif(1)
  r <- post(theta[j], f_p, fn[j-1], x, n) /
      post(theta[j], fp[j-1], fn[j-1], x, n)
  if (runif(1) < r) fp[j] <- f_p
  else fp[j] <- fp[j-1]
  ## fn
  f_n <- runif(1)
  r <- post(theta[j], fp[j], f_n, x, n) /
      post(theta[j], fp[j], fn[j-1], x, n)
  if (runif(1) < r) fn[j] <- f_n
  else fn[j] <- fn[j-1]
}

theta <- theta[round(1+n_sims/2):n_sims]
fp <- fp[round(1+n_sims/2):n_sims]
fn <- fn[round(1+n_sims/2):n_sims]

par(mfrow=c(1,3))
hist(theta, prob=T)
curve(dbeta(x, alpha, beta), add=T)
curve(dbeta(x, alpha+5, beta+n-5), add=T, lty=2)
hist(fp, prob=T)
curve(dbeta(x, ap, bp), add=T)
hist(fn, prob=T)
curve(dbeta(x, an, bn), add=T)
### End ###
```

In the above code, we used relatively informative priors for f_p ($beta(5, 20)$) and f_n ($beta(2, 25)$). As we will learn in Chapter 5, informative priors for f_p and f_n are necessary because the model is "non-identifiable." The likelihood function has information on the probability of observing a positive result only. The resulting posterior marginal distributions of f_p and f_n are nearly identical from their respective prior distributions (Figure 2.7).

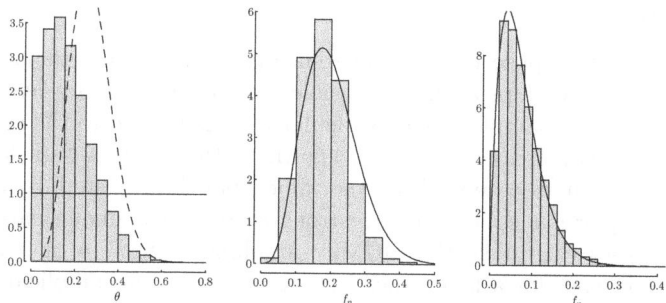

FIGURE 2.7: The Metropolis-Hastings in Gibbs sampler algorithm applied to the snake fungal disease problem to estimate the prevalence θ, false positive probability (f_p) and the false negative probability (f_n) simultaneously. The histograms are the posterior samples, the solid lines are the prior densities, and the dashed line for θ is the posterior of θ when $f_p = f_n = 0$.

2.6 MCMC Software

With the Gibbs sampler and the Metropolis-Hastings algorithm, a generic and efficient computer program is possible. The first popular software package for Markov chain Monte Carlo simulation is a program known as BUGS (Bayesian inference using Gibbs sampler), developed by the Medical Research Council Biostatistics Unit in Cambridge, UK, first released in 1989. The release of BUGS versions v0.5 and v0.6 was accompanied by a well-written user's manual [Spiegelhalter et al., 1996] and a large volume of examples. The standalone Windows operating system version of BUGS, WinBUGS, was expanded in 1998 to implement a general Metropolis-Hastings algorithm. The WinBUGS program was written in Component Pascal and implemented in a Rapid Application Development environment known as BlackBox Component Builder [Lunn et al., 2009]. In 2004, the code behind BUGS and WinBUGS was made available in open-source format. All development of the BUGS software was moved to OpenBUGS, with the development of accessing BUGS from other computing environments (especially R; R2OpenBUGS) as a main objective. At the same time, Martyn Plummer developed a program known as Just Another Gibbs Sampler (JAGS). His aim was to provide a program that is compatible with WinBUGS but without a graphical user interface (GUI). That is, JAGS was designed to be called from other programs. In R, we can call JAGS through the package rjags among others. JAGS is written in C++ and is platform independent.

2.6.1   Stan

These general-purpose Bayesian inference programs make inference of increasingly complicated problems accessible. In the process, we learned the weaknesses of Gibbs sampler. One particular issue is related to the correlated nature of a Markov chain, sometimes known as the random-walk behavior. That is, the current step depends on the value from the last step. In addition, the Gibbs sampler is also sensitive to strong correlations among parameters. These two issues can make the MCMC sampling "stuck" in one region of the parameter space for a long time. As a result, for some complicated models, a Gibbs sampler may require an unacceptably long time to converge. Neal [2011] introduced a hybrid Monte Carlo (HMC) method developed for simulating the state of molecular movement, the same problem studied in Metropolis et al. [1953]. The hybrid method unites the simulation approach of Metropolis et al. [1953] with a deterministic modeling approach using the Hamiltonian dynamics [Alder and Wainwright, 1959]. As a result, the acronym HMC is also referred to as Hamiltonian Monte Carlo. HMC is a Markov chain Monte Carlo algorithm. But HMC avoids the random walk behavior and is less sensitive to correlated parameters. HMC, however, is more difficult to automate because it requires a user to specify an important parameter which determines the efficiency of the algorithm. In other words, when running HMC, a user must hand turn the dial to optimize the parameter. Hoffman and Gelman [2014] developed an adaptive form of HMC that calculates the parameter based on values from initial iterations. They call the algorithm the No-U-Turn Sampler (NUTS). NUTS is implemented in the open-source program **Stan**, named after Stanislaw Ulam, the inventor of Monte Carlo methods [Carpenter et al., 2017].

In the rest of the book, we will use **Stan** as the main computational tool through the R package **rstan**. Stan documentation and examples are widely available. Here, we give a broad summary for a practical purpose. Stan is designed to support full Bayesian inference based on the Bayes' theorem (see Chapter 3). The Bayes' theorem states that the probability density function of an unknown parameter (θ) after observing data ($\pi(\theta \mid Y)$) is proportional to the product of the prior probability density function of the parameter ($\pi(\theta)$) and the likelihood function ($L(Y \mid \theta)$), or

$$\pi(\theta \mid Y) \propto \pi(\theta)L(Y \mid \theta).$$

The goal of a Bayesian inference is to learn about the unknown parameter θ. Using Stan, we aim to sample θ from its posterior distribution. As we discussed in Section 2.4.1, when using the Metropolis-Hastings algorithm, we only need to specify the distribution function up to a proportional constant. As such, the necessary input we need to provide is the prior density functions and the likelihood function. As a result, the most efficient means of writing a Stan model is to (1) explicitly write out the assumed model (the probability distribution of the response variable), (2) the unknown model parameters to be estimated, and (3) prior distributions of model parameters. These steps complete the model formulation step (Figure 1.5). From the specified model, we can group necessary information into three groups – data necessary to specify the likelihood function, parameters to be estimated, and probability distributions (the response variable distribution and prior distributions of the model parameters). These parts correspond to Stan's three minimum code blocks.

A functional Stan code includes at least three parts: a **data** block specifying the necessary input data of a problem, a **parameters** block declaring model parameters, and a **model** block. The **model** block describes the components of the posterior density function, that is, priors and the likelihood function. In the snake fungal disease example (Section 1.1.1 on page 6), the response variable is the number of infected x in a sample of n snakes. Assuming that we know $f_p = 0.07$ and $f_n = 0.05$, the unknown parameter is then θ. The necessary data are then x and n.

The probabilistic assumption of the response variable is the binomial distribution:

$$x \sim bin(p_+, n)$$

where $p_+ = \theta(1 - f_n) + (1 - \theta)f_p$. The binomial distribution determines the likelihood function. Translating this model into Stan code, order the code into **data**, **parameters**, and **model** blocks:

```
### Stan Code ###
data{
  int<lower=1> n;
  int<lower=0> x;
  real<lower=0,upper=1> fp;
  real<lower=0,upper=1> fn;
}
parameters{
  real<lower=0,upper=1> theta;
}
model{
  theta ~ beta(1,1);
  x ~ binomial(n, theta*(1-fn)+(1-theta)*fp);
}
### End ###
```

The **data** block defines the necessary input data and their type (real and integer). The **parameters** block declares **theta** as a real type parameter bounded between 0 and 1. The **model** block specifies the prior distribution of the parameter and the response variable distribution. These two distributions are translated into the log-posterior function (the right-hand side of equation (1.4) without the normalizing constant of the denominator) to develop the HMC algorithm. We can also specify the log-likelihood function (up to a proportional constant) directly using the target increment:

```
### Stan Code ###
model{
   theta ~ beta(1,1);
   target += x*log(theta*(1-fn)+(1-theta)*fp)+
             (n-x)*log(1-theta*(1-fn)-(1-theta)*fp);
}
### End ###
```

To simplify the code, we can add a `transformed parameters` block between the `parameters` and `model` blocks to specify the probability of a positive observation:

```
### Stan Code ###
transformed parameters{
   real <lower=0,upper=1> p_pos;
   p_pos = theta*(1-fn)+(1-theta)*fp;
model{
   theta ~ beta(1,1);
   target += x*log(p_pos)+(n-x)*log(1-p_pos);
}
### End ###
```

Because the binomial distribution function is part of the Stan language, we can directly use the log-probability function:

```
### Stan Code ###
transformed parameters{
   real <lower=0,upper=1> p_pos;
   p_pos = theta*(1-fn)+(1-theta)*fp;
model{
   theta ~ beta(1,1);
   target += binomial_lpmf(x | n, p_pos);
}
### End ###
```

Because the prior $beta(1,1)$ has a constant density value (uniform between 0 and 1), the line `theta ~beta(1,1)` can be omitted. In general, if the prior distribution is not specified in the Stan code, the prior is a "weakly informative" prior (see Section 3.3). For clarity, we usually do not omit the priors, rather explicitly define them in our code.

In practice, we write Stan code following the same thought process used in specifying a statistical model: we first make the probability distribution assumption about the response variable. The assumed model then defines unknown model parameters and the likelihood function. Once the parameters and the likelihood function are defined, the rest will fall into place naturally. We consult the Stan User's Guide (`mc-stan.org/users/documentation/`) on a regular basis. We also find the multiple volumes (as of late 2021, there were 8 volumes) of case studies very helpful (`mc-stan.org/users/documentation/case-studies`). We comment on Stan program details as we explore various models.

2.7 Summary

The Monte Carlo simulation method was first introduced in 1949 [Metropolis and Ulam, 1949] with a number of applications in mind. In addition to estimating the probability of a successful solitaire hand (an intractable combinatorial analysis) using the Monte Carlo simulation, Metropolis and Ulam envisioned a wide range of applications in natural science to solve "integro-differential" equations. In these applications, we should view the Monte Carlo simulation as a two-step process: a step to draw random variates from the intended probability distribution and a step of making inference. In using Monte Carlo simulation, we approximate the infinite population represented by a probability distribution using a finite number of random samples. As a result, we reduce the process of integration and differentiation of a continuous function to summations and subtractions of a large, but finite, number of values. In this chapter, we discussed a number of basic techniques for generating random variates from known probability distributions. These algorithms are part of R, Stan, and many modern statistical software packages. The inverse-CDF and acceptance-rejection methods were presented largely for historical purposes. In nearly all applications, we can rely on Stan to draw MCMC random samples from the target posterior distributions. Statistical inference based on these MCMC samples (e.g., estimating probabilities) is problem-specific, as illustrated by the species apportionment example (Section 2.3.5). How to use MCMC samples to draw statistical inference, in addition to presenting the summary statistics (e.g., mean, standard deviation, selected percentiles) and histograms of the marginal posterior distributions, should be guided by specific inference needs. In many cases, we use various integro-differential equations to describe the quantities of interest and design the simulation accordingly.

Chapter 3

An Overview of Bayesian Inference

In this chapter, we discuss our understanding of using statistics in applied science and provide a detailed summary of the book. We, like our readers, are not statisticians. We learned statistics because statistics is required in our graduate programs and we need to use statistics in our work. A common experience for most non-statisticians with regard to learning statistics is that we often feel good while in statistics classes, but do not remember much once a class is over. Consequently, when we use statistics, we often make mistakes, and these mistakes are often difficult to recognize by ourselves and difficult to accept when they are pointed out to us. For example, the now obvious problem related to the hypothesis testing used in the "nonparametric deviance reduction" method for detecting and quantifying environmental threshold [Qian et al., 2003a] was not obvious to us until we carefully analyzed many similar problems from several different angles (see, for example, Qian [2015], Qian and Cuffney [2012]). Even after we recognized the sources of the problem, documenting them was harder. Only after many years of repeated revision, we finally were able to pinpoint the sources of errors and explain why they were mistakes [Cuffney and Qian, 2013, Qian and Cuffney, 2018]. This experience is not new. When analyzing ecological papers, Peters [1991] recognized that the most common mistake in the "Methods" section is in the statistical methods. But he recommended that "statistics are better learned from direct applications of the statistics in the context of one's own research." He further declared that taking statistics classes is ineffective.

In our view, the difficulties in using statistics and the ineffectiveness of statistics classes are largely due to the disconnect between how statistics are taught and how statistics are used. Using Fisher's framework of statistical inference [Fisher, 1922], the first task of an analysis is to address the **problem of specification** (answering the question "of what population is this (data) a random sample"). Once the model is selected, we know the specifics of the next task of estimating unknown parameters (**the problem of estimation**). The last task is the **problem of distribution**; in the context of classical statistics, this problem is about the sampling distribution of the estimated parameters. It is a problem because in Fisher's time, "very little progress has been made in the study of the distribution of statistics derived from samples" [Fisher, 1922]. Without the distribution of a statistic derived from random samples, we are unable to properly evaluate the estimation uncertainty. Nowadays, we have numerous studies on such distributions. Given the availability of cheap computing power, we can use simulation to approximate such distributions should their theoretical forms be unavailable. To propose a reasonable model, we need advanced knowledge in statistical distribution to know the options, as well as detailed subject matter knowledge to make the model practically meaningful. Statistics professors may not be well versed in many science disciplines represented by their students, and students in introductory statistics classes from applied fields are new to their chosen fields of study. Neither the instructor nor the students may have necessary knowledge and experience to address the problem of specification, the first task of a successful application of statistics. As a result, statistics instruction may be focused on the problem of estimation for a number of specific distributions (or models). In a typical graduate-level statistics or data analysis class, we teach data analysis problems where the normal distribution is the appropriate model for the response variable. The hypothetical nature of statistical inference, therefore, may be unlikely to register in the minds of students.

In Bayesian analysis, we also have these three problems. For the problem of specification, we must specify not only the model for the response variable of interest, but also the prior distributions for all unknown parameters. The problems of estimation and distribution are combined; instead of using the maximum likelihood estimator, parameter estimation is achieved by deriving the posterior distributions of unknown parameters. Naturally, the distribution of the estimated parameters are their posterior distributions. The issue of model assessment and evaluation is addressed with predictive distributions of either future observations or predictive distributions of some known characteristics of the data.

As in Fisher's framework, we evaluate a model by comparing model predictions to data. If the data agree with the model predictions, we consider that the model is supported by the data. The resulting posterior distributions of model parameters become the prior distributions for future applications. Otherwise, we need to reconsider the model, either the model formulation, or the prior distributions, or both. The iterative nature of statistical inference is a common feature of scientific inquiry. In our experience, the lack of standard functions such as the R function for linear model (`lm`) and generalized linear model (`glm`) in Bayesian statistical software is a distinct advantage. It allows us to explicitly write the model into code. As a result, we are always conscious about the problem of specification. The problem of estimation was the main obstacle of applying Bayesian statistics before the advent of Markov chain Monte Carlo simulation methods. Because the posterior distributions are represented by random samples, graphical display of these distributions may be the most logical means of presentation. As a result, we may examine the distribution before calculating point estimates. This practice is advantageous because the spread of the posterior distribution may be more informative about the model than the point estimate alone.

3.1 The General Approach

Technically, only one formula is needed in Bayesian statistics. This formula is the Bayes' theorem. We used Bayes' theorem in Chapter 1 for discrete probability problems. For continuous variable problems, the Bayes' theorem is

$$\pi(\theta|y) = \frac{\pi(\theta)L(y|\theta)}{\int \pi(\theta)L(y|\theta)d\theta} \tag{3.1}$$

where y represents observed data (both for response and predictor variables), θ represents the unknown model parameter vector, and $L(y|\theta)$ is the likelihood function. Just as in a classical statistical modeling problem, the likelihood function is based on the probability distribution assumption about the response variable. Consequently, the problem of specification needs to be addressed first. The model determines the parameters to be estimated. The most challenging aspect of Bayesian applications used to be the derivation of the analytical solution of the posterior distribution, due largely to the integral of the denominator. This difficulty has been largely resolved because of the recent development in Markov chain Monte Carlo simulation (Section 2.4). Using MCMC we can draw random variates of θ directly from the posterior distribution without knowing the denominator. As a result, we often express the posterior as proportional to the product of the prior and the likelihood:

$$\pi(\theta|y) \propto \pi(\theta)L(y|\theta).$$

In the rest of this book, we introduce the use of Bayesian inference in environmental and ecological data analysis with an emphasis on model specification, both response variable model and the prior models. As a necessary prerequisite, we document the process of a traditional Bayesian inference (without using MCMC) in this chapter. The example is then used to illustrate MCMC.

We use MCMC (implemented in Stan through R package rstan) as the main computation tool for estimating the posterior. Regardless of computational methods, our focus is on the justification of the model we use. All examples we use in this book are from published literature. We document the original model development process and provide additional thoughts on how we might improve the analysis.

3.2   Example: Assessing Water Quality Standard Compliance in the Neuse River Estuary

Qian and Reckhow [2007] reported a study of water quality standard compliance assessment for the Neuse River Estuary in North Carolina, along the mid-Atlantic coast of the USA. In a typical standard compliance analysis, we want to determine whether the mean concentration of a regulated constituent is below (or above) the legal criterion. As we can only observe a limited number of concentration measurements, the mean concentration is estimated by the sample average. To infer the unobserved mean concentration, the conventional approach is to use null hypothesis testing, with the null hypothesis being that the water is in compliance [Smith et al., 2001]. Qian and Reckhow [2007] opted for a Bayesian approach, where water quality concentration measurements (y) are assumed to follow a log-normal distribution ($\log(y) \sim N(\mu, \sigma^2)$); the quantity of interest is μ. Using the posterior distribution of μ, we can estimate the probability that the mean is within the legal limit and make a probabilistic decision on the compliance status of the water.

3.2.1   Background

As we discussed in Section 1.4.4, environmental standard compliance assessment is often a process dominated by statistical null hypothesis testing based on limited monitoring data. The uncertainty associated with such tests is often the source of confusion in practice. The errors associated with measurement uncertainty, lags in pollutant concentration changes and/or in biotic response to management actions, and lags in implementation of total maximum daily load (TMDL) plans often lead to conflicting results between water quality model predictions and statistical analysis of monitoring data. As a result, some in the water quality modeling community recommend the use of models to assess progress made in implementing TMDL plans.

An example of this conflict between model and data is the TMDL program implemented to reduce nitrogen loading to the Neuse River Estuary in North Carolina. The Neuse River Estuary was placed on the state of North Carolina's Water Quality Assessment and Impaired Waters List (305(b) and 303(d) Report) in 2000 for chlorophyll *a* standard violation. However, the available chlorophyll *a* data from the estuary do not support the conclusion that the Neuse River Estuary is in danger of water quality standard violation. Furthermore, an earlier study of the estuary and the river basin [Qian et al., 2000a] indicated that nutrient inputs to the estuary have been either steady or decreasing from early 1970 to 2000. The decision to prepare a TMDL for the Neuse River basin apparently was made based on a combination of fish-kill incidents in the estuary in the mid-1990s and modeling studies.

This conflict between the TMDL decision and the compliance of water quality reflects the different interpretations of what is the "true" water quality status. All water quality models have prediction uncertainties, some of which can be quite large. So, which assessment is more reliable: the model forecast or the monitoring data? On the one hand, routine monitoring data are often regarded as "happenstance data" [Berthouex and Brown, 1994] not designed for inference about the water quality status of an entire basin. In other words, they may not have the proper spatiotemporal coverage to reflect the true concentration conditions. In addition, water quality response to management actions tends to have a time lag. As a result, using monitoring data alone will not give us confidence that the estimated water quality status is close to the truth. On the other hand, models are simplifications of the real world and a model's predictions are limited by the model's own structural limitations, as well as by the data used to calibrate the model. For the Neuse River Estuary, we observed large-scale fish-kill incidents in the mid-1990s and the rapid increase in concentrated animal farming in the river basin. These observations along with model predictions indicated a need for reducing nutrient input to the estuary to keep water quality in compliance. Both approaches (using data and using a model) can be justified, and both approaches can be justifiably criticized. It is often impossible to determine which source of information is more reliable. Consequently, the question should be whether we can combine these two sources of information to better support the water quality management decision-making process. Qian and Reckhow [2007] argued that both assessments can, and should, be used to evaluate compliance and the adequacy of management actions. Even though the model will always yield uncertain predictions, it has value in forecasting impacts (otherwise we would not be using it to develop the management plan). Likewise, lags, natural variability, and measurement uncertainty do not prevent deriving useful inferences from measurements, even though adjustments to account for these assessment shortcomings may be required. Consequently, results from water quality models were used to derive prior distribution of μ. Combining the prior and annual data, the posterior distribution of annual chlorophyll a concentrations were derived.

3.2.2 Study Area and Data

The Neuse River Basin has been the subject of intense study in the decade spanning the turn of the 21st century due to large-scale fish-kill events in the mid-1990s. The Neuse River estuary is seen as threatened by eutrophication from rapid urban development in the upper Neuse River Basin and expanded agriculture activity (especially concentrated animal feedlot operations such as modern hog farming) in the middle and lower Neuse River Basin. The state of North Carolina has a chlorophyll a concentration criterion of 40 μg/L to protect designated uses of the estuary. Since in the mid-1990s, chlorophyll a had, on occasion, exceeded this criterion, a TMDL was required for the Neuse with an objective of reducing total nitrogen (TN) loading to the estuary so that compliance with the criterion would be achieved. As part of the TMDL work, a spatially referenced regression on watershed attributes (SPARROW) model was developed for the basin [McMahon et al., 2003]; subsequently, a Bayesian SPARROW model was developed for the same study area [Qian et al., 2005] to estimate the nitrogen loads reaching the estuary. The impact of watershed nitrogen loading to the Neuse River Estuary was assessed largely based on modeling studies.

The data we used are the chlorophyll *a* concentrations measured in the mid-section of the Neuse River Estuary reported in Qian and Reckhow [2007]. The data were from three sources: Institute of Marine Sciences of the University of North Carolina, North Carolina Department of Environmental Quality, and Weyerhaeuser, Inc. Using annual summer chlorophyll *a* concentration data, Qian and Reckhow [2007] estimated the mean concentration distributions incrementally from 1992 to 2000.

3.2.3   The Problem of Specification

The objective of water quality standard compliance assessment is to evaluate whether the mean concentration of the regulated constituent is within the legal limit (in this case, the mean chlorophyll *a* concentration $< 40 \ \mu g/L$). We typically assume that a concentration variable can be approximated by the log-normal distribution, while the log transformed concentration has a normal distribution [Ott, 1995]. That is,

$$\log(y_i) \sim N(\mu, \sigma^2) \tag{3.2}$$

where μ and σ^2 are the mean and variance of the normal distribution; these are the two parameters to be estimated.

3.2.4   The Problem of Estimation and Distribution

In a Bayesian analysis, the problems of estimation and distribution are combined into a single step of deriving the posterior distribution, specifically, characterizing the distribution proportional to the product of the prior density function and the likelihood function. The log-normal distribution from the previous step defines the parameter of interest – μ and σ^2, as well as the likelihood function.

3.2.4.1   The Likelihood Function and Prior Distribution

The likelihood function in this problem is:

$$L = \prod_{i=1}^{n} \frac{1}{\sqrt{2\pi}\sigma} e^{-\frac{(\log(y_i)-\mu)^2}{2\sigma^2}}. \tag{3.3}$$

There are at least two general approaches for deriving a prior distribution. One requires us to quantify our knowledge about the parameters of interest using a probability distribution, and the other is to derive the prior based on certain mathematical requirements. We find that neither approach is practical. Most of us are not accustomed to using probability to express our uncertainty, let alone using a probability distribution to express our understanding of a parameter. Often in a problem such as this, we may have some knowledge about the magnitude of the chlorophyll *a* concentration. If we try hard enough, we may be able to use a simple probability distribution to summarize this knowledge. For example, for a researcher who had measured chlorophyll *a* in the Neuse River estuary for many years, she may tell us a likely range of concentration values and the most likely value. Based on her expert knowledge and the log-normality assumption (eq. (3.2)), we may be able to describe the concentration distribution. For example, we may interpret the most likely value as the median (hence the log mean μ) and the range as covering the middle 95% of all data (in logarithmic scale roughly $\mu \pm 2\sigma$, hence the log standard deviation σ). We will call these values our initial "estimates" $\tilde{\mu}$ and $\tilde{\sigma}^2$.

This process, however, illustrates two issues. First, this is a model-guided process. Without the log-normal distribution assumption, we cannot readily translate the most likely value to $\tilde{\mu}$. Second, this process is subjective. By subjective, we mean that the likely range must be represented as an interval with a certain coverage probability. We use a 95% coverage because it is convenient (as we know that roughly 95% of the probability mass is within 2 (1.96) times standard deviation of the mean). If we assume the range as the middle 90% interval, the estimated standard deviation will be different. But more importantly, we still don't have the prior distribution of μ and σ^2. Going from a rough estimate to a prior distribution requires guidance of statistical knowledge. For this simple problem, we can use the sampling distributions of sample average and sample variance from classical statistics as a reference. The sampling distribution of an average is asymptotically normal with the mean equal to the population mean and the variance equal to the population variance divided by the sample size (the central limit theorem). Perhaps we can propose that the prior distribution of μ is normal. The mean of the prior can be the initial estimate $\tilde{\mu}$. The variance of a sample average is approximately the population variance (σ^2) divided by the sample size (σ^2/n_0). At this point, we must decide the value of n_0. A variance is a measure of uncertainty; the larger the variance the less certain we are about the mean. We can also use variance as a measure of information. A large variance indicates the estimated mean is not informative. In this case, the variance of the mean is dependent on n_0. So, we may suggest that our expert make another decision. She should decide how certain she is with regard to the rough estimate of the mean concentration, and express her uncertainty in terms of n_0: evaluating the information in her estimate as if it was a mean calculated based on n_0 data points. If the mean is based on 5 data points, it is then less informative (more variable) than the mean based on 20 data points.

We must admit that the discussion in the previous paragraph sounds unnatural. We don't think like that and we probably don't know the amount of information in a given number of data points. In fact, we don't have a quantitative definition of information that is applicable for this study. The idea that a prior distribution represents the subjective knowledge of a scientist is appealing, but difficult to implement. Estimating the mean of a normal distribution is the simplest estimation problem in statistics. The difficulty we have in finding a prior distribution is a harbinger of things to come: the process of eliciting a prior distribution is unnatural and uncertain.

Once we have selected n_0 and $\tilde{\mu}$, we have a prior distribution for the mean: $\mu \sim N(\tilde{\mu}, \sigma^2/n_0)$. But σ^2 is also a parameter that is in need of a prior. In most cases, variance is a harder parameter to grasp than the mean is. As a result, finding a probability distribution for the unknown variance is even harder. Because we can learn from observing data, we can, therefore, use the sampling distribution of the estimated variance $\tilde{\sigma}^2$ as a guide. The sampling distribution of a sample variance is a scaled χ^2 distribution:

$$\frac{(n-1)\tilde{\sigma}^2}{\sigma^2} \sim \chi^2(n-1).$$

The population variance σ^2 is unknown and the observed $\tilde{\sigma}^2$ is a fixed value for a given data set. Conceptually, we consider, in classical statistics, $\tilde{\sigma}^2$ a realization of a random variable and σ^2 as non-random. In Bayesian statistics, σ^2 is unknown to us and our uncertainty about the variable is summarized using a probability distribution function. The Bayesian interpretation of the classical sampling distribution would lead to prior distribution of σ^2 to be a scaled-inverse χ^2 distribution:

$$\frac{\sigma^2}{(n-1)\tilde{\sigma}^2} \sim \text{inv-}\chi^2(n-1) \rightarrow \sigma^2 \sim \text{scale-inv-}\chi^2(n-1, \tilde{\sigma}^2).$$

This distribution (scale-inv-$\chi^2(n-1, \tilde{\sigma}^2)$) is the same as a scaled inverse gamma distribution:

$$\sigma^2 \sim \text{inv-}gamma\left(\frac{n-1}{2}, \frac{(n-1)\hat{\sigma}^2}{2}\right).$$

We will see in a moment that parameterizing the prior using the inverse-gamma distribution can greatly simplify the process of deriving the posterior. Because the scaled inverse-χ^2 distribution is the same as the inverse-gamma, we can again use the sampling distribution to guide us in selecting the prior parameters. The degrees of freedom parameter for the inverse χ^2 is the sample size minus 1, and the scale parameter is the observed sample variance. In other words, the scale parameter can be determined based on the likely variance value, an initial guess which we may have learned from previous studies or from literature. The degrees of freedom parameter $\nu = n - 1$ is a measure of our confidence in the initial guess. The larger the sample size (or ν), the higher the confidence. An inverse-gamma distribution is commonly parameterized as inv-gamma(α, β).

Through this long and winding process, we now have the following:

1. The response variable distribution is log-normal:

$$\log(y) \sim N(\mu, \sigma^2)$$

which leads to the likelihood function:

$$L = \frac{1}{(2\pi)^{n/2}\sigma^n} e^{-\frac{\sum_{i=1}^{n}(y_i - \mu)^2}{2\sigma^2}}.$$

2. The prior distribution of μ, conditional on σ^2, is

$$\mu \sim N(\mu_0, \sigma^2/n_0)$$

with a density function

$$\pi(\mu|\sigma^2) = \frac{\sqrt{n_0}}{\sqrt{2\pi}\sigma} e^{-\frac{(\mu - \mu_0)^2}{2\sigma^2/n_0}}. \tag{3.4}$$

3. The prior distribution of σ^2 is

$$\sigma^2 \sim \text{inv-gamma}(\alpha, \beta)$$

with a density function

$$\pi(\sigma^2) = \frac{\beta^\alpha}{\Gamma(\alpha)} (1/\sigma^2)^{\alpha+1} \exp\left(-\beta/\sigma^2\right). \tag{3.5}$$

3.2.4.2 Deriving the Posterior Distribution

Using Bayes' theorem, the posterior distribution of μ and σ^2 is

$$\pi(\mu, \sigma^2|y) \propto \pi(\mu|\sigma^2) \times \pi(\sigma^2) \times L.$$

The process of deriving the posterior distribution is algebraically tedious, similar to the process of deriving the conditional distributions in the change point example in Section 2.4.2.1 on page 47. We will work out this particular case to illustrate the process. To simplify the process, we use $\bar{y} = \sum_{n=1}^{n} y_i/n$ and $s^2 = \sum_{n=1}^{n}(y_i - \bar{y})^2/n$ to represent the sample average and sample variance, respectively. These are the sufficient statistics of a normal distribution. Next, we want to remove the summation sign from the likelihood function:

$$\begin{aligned} \sum_{i=1}^{n}(y_i - \mu)^2 &= \sum_{i=1}^{n}((y_i - \bar{y}) - (\mu - \bar{y}))^2 \\ &= ns^2 + n(\bar{y} - \mu)^2. \end{aligned}$$

Now we can simplify the likelihood function:

$$L \propto \left(\tfrac{1}{\sigma^2}\right)^{n/2} e^{-\frac{ns^2+n(\bar{y}-\mu)^2}{2\sigma^2}}$$
$$= \left(\tfrac{1}{\sigma^2}\right)^{n/2} e^{-\frac{\frac{1}{2}ns^2}{\sigma^2}} e^{-\frac{(\bar{y}-\mu)^2}{2\sigma^2/n}}.$$

Rearranging the product of the priors and the likelihood by grouping similar terms:

$$\pi(\mu,\sigma|y) \propto \left(\tfrac{1}{\sigma^2}\right)^{1/2}\left(\tfrac{1}{\sigma^2}\right)^{\alpha+1}\left(\tfrac{1}{\sigma^2}\right)^{n/2} e^{-\frac{\beta+ns^2/2}{\sigma^2}} e^{-\frac{n(\bar{y}-\mu)^2}{2\sigma^2}} e^{-\frac{n_0(\mu-\mu_0)^2}{2\sigma^2}}$$
$$\propto \left(\tfrac{1}{\sigma^2}\right)^{\alpha+(n+1)/2+1} e^{-\frac{\beta+\frac{1}{2}ns^2+\frac{1}{2}\frac{nn_0}{n+n_0}(\bar{y}-\mu_0)^2}{\sigma^2}} e^{-\frac{\mu-\frac{n\bar{y}+n_0\mu_0}{n+n_0}}{2\sigma/(n+n_0)}}.$$

The joint posterior distribution of μ and σ^2 is proportional to the product of three exponents. Conditional on μ (i.e., when μ is a known constant), the conditional posterior of σ^2 is an inverse-gamma distribution with parameters $\alpha_n = \alpha + n/2$ and $\beta_n = \beta + \frac{1}{2}ns^2 + \frac{1}{2}\frac{nn_0}{n+n_0}(\bar{y}-\mu_0)^2$. Similarly, the conditional posterior distribution of μ is a normal distribution with mean of $\mu_n = \frac{n\bar{y}+n_0\mu_0}{n+n_0}$, which is a weighted average of $\bar{y}$ and μ_0, and variance of $\sigma^2/(n+n_0)$. In other words, the posterior joint distribution of μ,σ^2 is a normal-inverse-gamma distribution with parameters $\mu_n, n_n = n+n_0, \alpha_n$, and β_n.

Because we used the classical sampling distributions as a reference at the beginning, we can again use the sampling distribution to better understand the prior and the posterior. In setting the prior of σ^2, the scaled inverse-χ^2 distribution is directly borrowed from the sampling distribution of $\hat{\sigma}^2$. As a result, the two parameters $\nu = n-1$ and $\tau^2 = \tilde{\sigma}^2$ represent the degrees of freedom and the observed variance. When used as a prior, we can interpret τ^2 as an initial guess of the variance and ν as the measure of confidence in the guess (measured in number of data points). When re-parameterizing the prior using the inverse gamma distribution, we set $\alpha = \nu$ and $\beta = \nu\tau^2$. In other words, we can view α as the measure of confidence and the ratio $\beta/(\alpha-1)$ (the mean of the inverse gamma distribution) as the initial guess of the variance. The conditional prior of the mean is easier to interpret. The prior is centered around mean μ_0 and the variance is the population variance divided by n_0, which can be interpreted again as the measure of our confidence in the initial guess (μ_0). The posterior distribution of the mean is also a conditional normal, and is the weighted average of $\bar{y}$ and μ_0.

3.2.4.3   Predictive Distribution

With the posterior distribution of μ and σ^2, we can now make an inference about the distribution of y. The distribution of y is a conditional normal:

$$y|\mu,\sigma^2 \sim N(\mu,\sigma^2).$$

The predictive distribution is

$$\pi(y) = \int_\mu \int_\sigma^2 \pi(\mu,\sigma^2)\pi(y|\mu,\sigma^2)d\mu d\sigma^2.$$

This leads to a non-standard t-distribution with mean $m_t = \mu_n$, variance $\sigma_t^2 = \frac{\beta_n(n_n+1)}{\alpha_n n_n}$, and degrees of freedom $\nu = 2\alpha_n$. This is a generalized t-distribution, a location-scale family of distribution. The mean (location) and standard deviation (scale) parameters relate a non-standard t-distribution random variable (y) to a standard t-distribution variable t:

$$y = \mu_t + \sigma_t t.$$

Inference on y can be made using the standard t-distribution variable t. For example, the q quantile of y is $y_q = \mu_t + \sigma_t t_q$, where t_q is the q quantile of t (in R, $\mathtt{qt(q, df=nu)}$). Furthermore, let $f(t)$ be the density function of the standard t-distribution; the density function of y is $f\left(\frac{y-\mu_t}{\sigma_t}\right)/\sigma_t$.

3.2.5 Application in the Neuse River Estuary

When applied to the Neuse River Estuary example, several empirical models were used to develop the prior (i.e., providing estimates of α, β, μ_0, and n_0). Qian and Reckhow [2007] used two different water quality models to predict the concentrations of total nitrogen (TN) and chlorophyll a (Chla) to (1) develop and apply a prior and (2) sequentially update the distribution of Chla. For TN, one model underpredicts the concentrations and the other slightly overpredicts. Both models over predict Chla concentrations. Assuming that a concentration variable can be approximated by the log-normal distribution, the model-predicted log TN and log Chla are used to derive the prior parameters. These models provide the estimated mean log TN and log Chla concentrations and the estimated log variances. The estimated means of log TN and log Chla were used as estimates of μ_0^{TN} and μ_0^{Chla}, and the estimated prior parameter μ_0 for TN and Chla, respectively. The estimated variances are used as estimates of the ratio of $\beta/(\alpha - 1)$. (In Qian and Reckhow [2007], the normal distribution was parameterized using the mean and precision, the inverse of variance. As a result, the prior of the mean and precision is the normal-gamma distribution.) The parameters n_0 and α were estimated based on the sample sizes used to fit the two models.

```
#### R Code ####
## function for normal-inverse-gamma conjugate priors
NIGpost <- function(x, alpha, beta, n0, mu0){
    x_bar <- mean(x)
    n <- length(x)
    s2 <- sd(x)^2
    return(list(nn=n+n0, mu=(n*x_bar+n0*mu0)/(n+n0),
            alpha = alpha+n/2,
            beta = beta+0.5*(n*s2 + (n*n0)*(x_bar-mu0)^2/(n+n0))))
}
```

```
## Processing data
tmp <- (neuse$Year>=1992 & neuse$Year <= 2000 &
        neuse$SECTION=="UPPER") |
        neuse$SECTION=="MIDDLE"
neuse2 <- neuse[tmp,]

par(mar=c(3,3,1,1), mgp=c(1.25, 0.125,0),las=1, tck=0.01)
hist(log(neuse2$TOTN), prob=T, nclass=20,
    axes=F, xlab="Total Nitrogen (mg/L)",
    ylim=c(0,1.5), main="")
axis(1, at = log(c(10, 100, 250, 500, 1000, 2500, 5000)),
                labels=c(10, 100,250, 500, 1000, 2500, 5000))
pst <- list(alpha =32,
            beta = 28,
            nn = 45,
            mu = 7.6)
### End ###
```

At this point, we have all the necessary data and R functions for sequentially updating the distribution of Chla and TN and graphically present the updated predictive distributions.

```
pr_mut <- pst$mu
pr_sigmat <- (pst$beta/pst$alpha)*(1+1/pst$nn)
pr_df <- pst$alpha*2
## prior
curve(dt((x-pr_mut)/pr_sigmat, df=pr_df)/pr_sigmat, add=T, lwd=3)

## sequential updating
for (i in 1992:2000){
    tmp <- neuse2$Year==i & !is.na(neuse2$TOTN)
    pst <- NIGpost(log(neuse2$TOTN[tmp]),
                    pst$alpha, pst$beta, pst$nn, pst$mu)
    mu_t <- pst$mu
    sigma_t <- (pst$beta/pst$alpha)*(1+1/pst$nn)
    df_t <- pst$alpha*2
    curve(dt((x-mu_t)/sigma_t, df=df_t)/sigma_t,
          lty=i-1990, add=T)
}
### End ###
```

The updated TN and Chla distributions are in Figures 3.1 and 3.2.

When reviewing Qian and Reckhow [2007], we realized that the sequential updating process may not be the most appropriate interpretation of the U.S. Clean Water Act. The law requires a periodic assessment of waters in the U.S. because the water quality status changes over time. We are to evaluate the

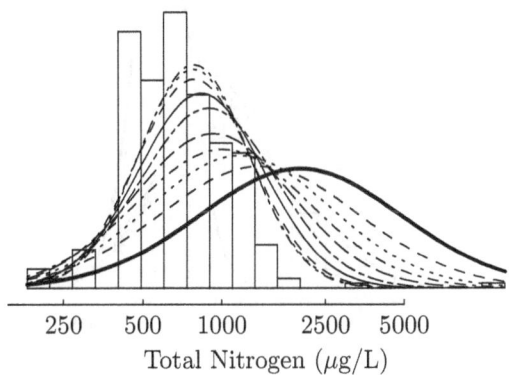

FIGURE 3.1: Total nitrogen (TN) concentration data are presented in the histogram and sequentially estimated TN concentration distributions are shown in dashed lines. The thick black line is the TN distribution based on the prior.

status of water quality over a time period. The estimated parameters from the sequential updating process quantify the predictive distributions of TN and Chla over the entire time period up to the time of updating. Thus the previous model assumed that the variability of TN and Chla remained largely stable over time. This process is not for detecting changes over time. If periodic assessments are intended to identify changes in water quality, an estimate of the long-term concentration distribution would not serve the purpose well. Because most water quality assessments are done on an annual basis, we should estimate annual mean distributions of TN and Chla in this case.

We again use data from 1992 to 2000. That is, we have to estimate nine annual distributions. Naturally, we can estimate these nine annual distributions separately, each time using only data from the specific year. Let y_{ij} be the ith observation from the jth year. Estimating annual distribution separately can be represented by

$$y_{ij} \sim N(\mu_j, \sigma_j^2). \tag{3.6}$$

When parameters μ_j and σ_j^2 are estimated separately using only data from the jth year, we assume that data from each year are unrelated. Since the data were measured from samples taken from the same water body, one should expect some connections among years because of the shared environment (e.g., weather and climate conditions, land use patterns in the watershed).

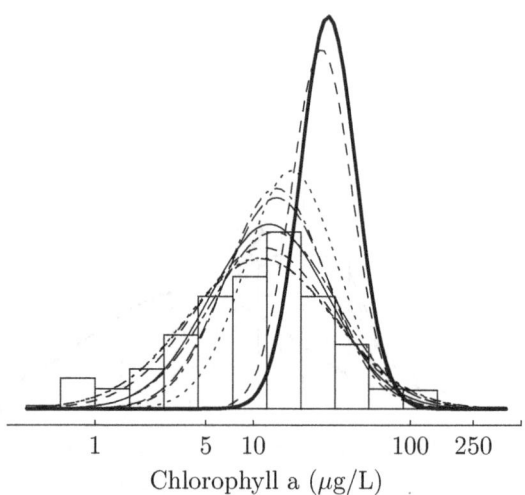

Chlorophyll a (μg/L)

FIGURE 3.2: Chlorophyll a (Chla) concentration data are presented in the histogram and sequentially estimated Chla concentration distributions are shown in dashed lines. The thick black line is the Chla distribution based on the prior.

However, without detailed knowledge of the area, especially knowledge of what happened in the past, we may not be able to identify how the water quality status would change over time. As a result, selecting priors for μ_j and σ_j^2 for each year would be difficult. We will come back to this example later in Chapter 4.

3.3   Specifying Prior Distributions

A distinct feature of the Bayesian inference is its capability of incorporating existing knowledge in the form of a prior distribution. However, specifying a prior distribution is a highly technical problem. The difficulty is similar to the difficulty in the model specification problem. Specifically, deriving a prior distribution requires knowledge in both statistics (what probability distributions are relevant) and subject matter (how to quantify oft-qualitative knowledge). In a study of fish response to lake acidification in the Adirondack lakes in New York State, Reckhow [1987, 1988] used a logistic model to predict the probability of a lake supporting brook trout (*Salvelinus fontinalis*) using the lake's average pH level. The prior distributions of the regression model parameters were constructed based on a fisheries expert's answers to questions like the following:

> Given 100 lakes in the Adirondacks that have brook trout popula-
> tions in the past, and if all 100 lakes have pH = 5.6 and calcium
> concentration = 130 μeq/L, what number do you now expect to
> continue to support the brook trout population?

This question was repeated twenty times with a variety of pH-calcium pairs to produce 20 predicted responses. The estimated model coefficients from fitting the 20 responses to the 20 pairs of predictor values were used to develop prior distributions of the same parameters. Not only labor-intensive and time consuming, eliciting prior distribution by interviewing experts is often impossible in many cases where simple and unambiguous questions are not possible.

In the Neuse River example, the goal was to evaluate water quality compliance of the Neuse River Estuary where earlier process-based models predicted nitrogen enrichment [Qian and Reckhow, 2007]. As such, we naturally use model predicted total nitrogen (TN) and chlorophyll a (Chla) concentrations as the basis for formulating prior distributions. Even in arguably the simplest Bayesian application of quantifying a normal (log-normal) distribution, Qian and Reckhow [2007] found that specifying a prior requires more careful thinking than expected. They opted to use predictions from models that were largely empirical – regression models based on simple processes. These models predicted the means and standard deviations of TN and Chla. In addition, they also chose to use the conjugate family of priors and interpreted the meaning of prior distribution parameters based on the relationship between the prior and posterior distribution parameters. The interpretation is then used as a guide for selecting these prior parameters.

The concept of conjugate prior was introduced as an algebraic convenience. When a conjugate prior distribution is used, we can derive the closed-form expression of the posterior distribution. The posterior and prior distributions belong to the same family of distributions. As a result, we avoid the potentially difficult numerical integration.

The simplest conjugate prior is the beta distribution for the binomial distribution parameter p (Figure 1.1). In a binomial distribution problem, the response variable is the number of successes y from n trials. The likelihood function is proportional to

$$p^y(1-p)^{n-y}.$$

Using a beta prior with parameter α, β, that is, $\pi(p) = \frac{\Gamma(\alpha+\beta)}{\Gamma(\alpha)\Gamma(\beta)}p^{\alpha-1}(1-p)^{\beta-1}$, the posterior distribution is proportional to

$$p^{\alpha-1}(1-p)^{\beta-1} \times p^y(1-p)^{n-y} = p^{y+\alpha-1}(1-p)^{(n-y)+\beta-1}.$$

Because the expression is a probability distribution function, we can easily verify that the posterior distribution of p is a beta distribution with parameters

$\alpha_n = y + \alpha$ and $\beta_n = (n - y) + \beta$. The first shape parameter of the posterior distribution is the number of successes plus the first shape parameter of the prior and the second shape parameter of the posterior distribution is the number of failures plus the second shape parameter of the prior distribution. As such, we can interpret the prior distribution as based on α successes and β failures. One way to propose a prior is to first provide an initial guess of the probability of success, which represents the expected value (i.e., $p_0 = \alpha/(\alpha + \beta)$). Then, express our confidence in the initial guess in terms of prior "sample size" ($n_0 = \alpha + \beta$). That is, we guessed the magnitude of the probability p_0 as the ratio of the number of successes (α) over the total prior sample size (n_0). With p_0 and n_0, we can estimate α and β.

In Chapter 5, we use the Poisson distribution to model count variables. The Poisson distribution has one parameter, which represents the expected value (and variance) of the count variable. The density function is $\pi(y \mid \lambda) = \frac{e^{-\lambda}\lambda^y}{y!}$. Upon observing $y_1, \cdots, y_n$, the likelihood function is

$$L = \frac{e^{-n\lambda}\lambda^{\sum_{i=1}^n y_i}}{\prod_{i=1}^n y_i!}.$$

The conjugate prior of λ is the gamma distribution (with a shape parameter α and rate parameter β). Its density function is $\pi(\lambda \mid \alpha, \beta) = \frac{\beta^\alpha}{\Gamma(\alpha)}\lambda^{\alpha-1}e^{-\beta\lambda}$. The posterior distribution function is proportional to

$$\begin{aligned}\pi(\lambda \mid y_1, \cdots, y_n) &\propto \lambda^{\alpha-1}e^{-\beta\lambda} \times e^{-n\lambda}\lambda^{\sum_{i=1}^n y_i} \\ &= e^{-(n+\beta)\lambda}\lambda^{\sum_{i=1}^n y_i + \alpha - 1}.\end{aligned}$$

The posterior distribution is also a gamma distribution with the shape parameter $\alpha_n = \sum_{i=1}^n y_i + \alpha$ and the rate parameter $\beta_n = n + \beta$. As such, we can interpret the prior parameters α as the total count and β as an imaginary (prior) data set sample size. Alternatively, we can first elicit an initial guess of the expected number $m_0 (= \alpha/\beta)$, then use β a measure of the confidence we have in the guess (m_0), expressed as the sample size used to derive the initial guess.

For the Neuse River problem, the response variables (log concentrations of TP and Chla) are normal random variables. For a normal distribution problem, the conjugate prior for the mean and variance is the normal-inverse-gamma distribution: $\pi(\mu, \sigma^2) = N(\mu_0, \sigma^2/\nu) \cdot IG(\alpha, \beta)$, where $\mu_0, \nu, \alpha, \beta$ are the prior distribution parameters. The posterior distribution of μ and σ^2 is also a normal-inverse-gamma distribution, with parameters

$$\mu_n = \frac{n\bar{x}+\nu\mu_0}{n+\nu}, \quad n_n = n + \nu,$$
$$\alpha_n = \alpha + n, \quad \beta_n = \beta + \frac{ns^2}{2} + \frac{\nu n(\mu_0 - \bar{x})^2}{2(\nu+n)}$$

where n is the sample size of the data, $\bar{x}$ is the sample average, and s^2 is the sample variance. From the posterior distribution parameters, we can make the following interpretations:

- The parameter μ_0 is an initial guess of the mean because the posterior parameter μ_n is the weighted average of μ_0 and the sample average.

- The parameter ν can be interpreted as the prior "sample size," or the quantification of the certainty we have on the initial guess of the mean (μ_0) because the posterior parameter n_n is the sum of ν and the data sample size.

- The parameter α seems to represent the prior sample size with respect to our prior information on the variance (because $\alpha_n = \alpha + n$).

- The parameter β is related to the magnitude of the prior variance, measured as the sum of squares. As the mean and mode of the inverse gamma distribution are $\beta/(\alpha - 1)$ and $\beta/(\alpha + 1)$, respectively, we can derive the prior parameters by first eliciting the most likely value (which would be close to β/α, then deciding the confidence we have in the initial value in terms of the prior sample size.

In Qian and Reckhow [2007], models used to predict TN and Chla are regression based. As a result, model predictive uncertainty can be estimated using Monte Carlo simulation Qian [2016, Chapter 9]. Using Monte Carlo simulation, we obtain random samples of the predicted mean and random samples of the predicted variance. Using these random samples, Qian and Reckhow [2007] estimated the prior distribution parameters using the method of moments.

Using conjugate priors allows us to conveniently organize prior information when available and accumulate information from data in the same form. As we discussed above, many conjugate prior distributions can be interpreted in ways that can connect their values to our experiences. In our discussion, we assumed that we can often estimate the magnitude of the parameter of interest based on our experience, including previous studies on similar topics. The level of confidence in such magnitude estimates is harder to conceptualize. In our discussion, we emphasize the use of "prior sample size" as a measure of our certainty or confidence in the prior magnitude estimate.

Frequently, we have no real information on the parameter of interest. Some also argue that we should allow the data to speak for itself. As a result, the class of "non-informative" priors is often appealing. In many cases, a non-informative prior is a uniform distribution and the density function is expressed as proportional to 1. As such, the posterior distribution is the normalized likelihood function. Such non-informative or flat priors can be problematic, especially when functions of distribution model parameters are of interest [Seaman III et al., 2012] and very informative. For example, the commonly used Jeffrey's prior [Jeffreys, 1946] for the normal distribution parameters μ and σ is $\pi(\mu, \sigma) \propto 1/\sigma^2$, which implies a uniform distribution between $-\infty$ and $+\infty$ for both μ and $\log(\sigma)$. When using MCMC software such as BUGS, priors must be proper (i.e., the density function must integrate to 1 over its range). As approximations, we often use $N(0, 10000)$ and $Gamma(0.01, 0.01)$

as priors for μ and σ. Statistical problems of such "diffuse" priors are well-documented [Gelman, 2006]. Specifically for the defused gamma prior for log standard deviation, the prior favors large values of σ. As a result, the prior can be highly informative.

Gelman et al. [2008] proposed a number of "weakly informative" priors for regression models. The goal was to purposely provide less information than we have (just like non-informative priors) yet achieve numerical stabilization. Many such weakly informative priors are implemented in Stan as default priors. The "weakly informative" priors of Gelman et al. [2008] were constructed assuming that response variables are scaled to have mean 0 and standard deviation 0.5. When the response variable of a regression model is not scaled, the weakly informative prior on model coefficients can be highly informative. In other words, weakly informative is relative. See the lilac first bloom example in Section 7.2 for an example.

3.4   Summary

In applying statistics, whether classical or Bayesian statistics, we follow the general procedure similar to Fisher's three statistical problems. We first identify the variable of interest (the response variable) and make a probabilistic distribution assumption about it. The proposed model consists of unknown parameters that need to be properly described in the form of prior distributions. The problem of parameter estimation is the process of deriving the posterior distributions of the model parameters, which is proportional to the product of the prior density and the likelihood function. The likelihood function is derived based on the probability distribution of the response variable (and the independence assumption). A "proper" prior is a probability distribution that represents what we know about the parameter and facilitates the characterization of the posterior distribution. In the Neuse River Estuary example, we chose to use the conjugate family of priors – where both the prior and the posterior are in the same family of probability distribution. The conjugate family of priors are available to a limited number of parameters. When using them, we should understand how to choose the prior parameters to reflect our understanding of the parameter. We used the Neuse River Estuary example to illustrate this process.

In a typical Bayesian analysis, the process of deriving the posterior distribution is often characterized by tedious algebraic maneuvers to factor out specific patterns of familiar distribution functions. The algebraic manipulation is to avoid the potentially difficult integrals. Not all model parameters can have posterior distributions among the list of known distribution functions. As a result, Bayesian inference was limited to relatively simple models, particularly the exponential family of distributions where the conjugate family of distributions can be found.

Although we are no longer limited by the computational difficulties because of simulation-based methods such as MCMC, the steps we illustrated in this chapter are still the proper steps of developing a useful model.

Chapter 4

Environmental Monitoring and Assessment – Normal Response Models

In the last chapter, we used the Neuse River Estuary water quality assessment as an example to illustrate the basic process of the Bayesian inference. Technically, the Bayesian inference process differs from the classical or frequentist's approach only in the use of a prior distribution. When a flat prior (i.e., $\pi(\theta) \propto 1$) is used, the difference between the two approaches lies in the interpretation of the likelihood function. The frequentist's approach uses the likelihood function to obtain a point estimate, while the Bayesian approach normalizes the likelihood function to derive the posterior distribution. The frequentist's point estimate is the mode of the likelihood profile, while the Bayesian point estimate is often the mean or the median of the posterior distribution. If the likelihood function profile is symmetric, the two approaches will lead to the same point estimate.

Moving forward with the Neuse River Estuary water quality assessment example, we illustrated the concept of updating: the transition of the prior distribution to the posterior distribution upon the observation of data. In our example, we started with a prior derived from water quality model outputs. The model-predicted total nitrogen (TN) concentrations did not agree with the observed values. Nevertheless, the Bayesian approach allows us to gradually update the predicted TN concentration distributions. Once we have several years of observations, our predicted (posterior distribution of) TN concentrations are very close to the observed TN concentration distribution as presented by a histogram (Figures 3.1 and 3.2). This process of updating is the key characteristic of the Bayesian approach. It is a process of learning from experience (observing data): we first summarize the experience (assuming a probability distribution which led to the likelihood function) and then generalize the experience for predicting future experience via the Bayes' theorem. As remarked by Jeffreys [1961], the process of generalization is the most important part because "events that are merely described and have no apparent relation to others may as well be forgotten, and in fact usually are." The updating procedure as a general methodology is a distinct scientific method that is universal in all scientific endeavors. It represents a common feature of science, just as Karl Pearson elegantly expressed that "the unity of all science consists alone in its method, not in its material" [Pearson, 1900].

In the Neuse River Estuary water quality assessment example, we used the conjugate family of priors (the normal-inverse-gamma distribution). This approach was used to avoid computational difficulties in Bayesian analysis before the advent of MCMC. When using the conjugate family of priors, we have the analytic form of the posterior distribution. The conjugate family of priors is flexible enough for many practical applications. In our experience, the conjugate family of priors is a convenient choice even when the applications are more complicated than the simple cases under which a conjugate prior is derived. However, as we discussed in Chapter 2, the use of MCMC changes the mode of inference of a probability distribution from using the analytic formula of the probability density function to using random samples from the target probability distribution. This change is not natural as the use of random sample requires a different view of the probability density. We will make this transition here.

4.1   A Simulation-Based Inference

The Neuse River Estuary example is a Bayesian approach to a hypothesis testing problem, where the estuary TN concentrations predicted chlorophyll *a* concentrations are compared to the water quality standards. It is a hypothesis testing problem because of a study by Smith et al. [2001], who pointed out the statistical issues of an early rule for deciding whether a water body is impaired. The rule in question is known as the 10% rule, which declares a water body to be impaired if more than 10% of the water samples from the water body have concentrations above the water quality criterion in question. The Neyman-Pearson lemma guarantees that a properly designed null hypothesis test would outperform the 10% rule. As a result, Smith et al. [2001] suggested that the 10% rule should be replaced by a binomial test with the null hypothesis that the water is in compliance (or the probability of observing a concentration value above the criterion is less than or equal to 0.1). To use the binomial test, water quality data (measured pollutant concentrations) are first transformed to binary, either 0 (below the criterion) or 1 (above the criterion). This transformation results in a test of whether the 0.9 quantile of the pollutant concentration distribution is above the water quality standard. As we argued in the Neuse River Estuary example, the U.S. Clean Water Act defines the criterion with respect to the mean concentration. As such, directly estimating the concentration distribution is closer to the spirit of the Clean Water Act. An estimation-oriented method, such as the Bayesian approach, can provide both a point estimate of the mean concentration, as well as the posterior distribution of the mean parameter to summarize the uncertainty. The posterior distribution can be used to determine whether the mean is likely higher or lower than the relevant water quality standard. The 10% rule is intended to ensure a high level of confidence in compliance. We can achieve the same by using the posterior distribution of the mean to estimate the probability that the mean is less than the observed water quality standard. For example, we may consider that the water body is in compliance only when the probability is above 0.9.

The use of the normal-inverse-gamma prior allows the updating process to be confined to tractable analytic forms; however, as discussed in Chapter 2, an MCMC algorithm draws random samples from the target posterior distribution and we use these random samples to infer the characteristics of the posterior distribution. When observing data from the first year in the Neuse River Estuary example, the updating process is expressed in the following steps:

- At the observational level, the likelihood function is based on the response variable distribution (equations (3.2) and (3.3)).

- At the model parameter level, we define the prior distribution of μ and σ^2 in equations (3.4) and (3.5).

- The posterior distributions of the parameters are proportional to the product of the likelihood function and prior density function(s). When using the conjugate family of priors, we can derive the analytic form of the posterior density function (which is a density from the same family of distributions). Using a sampling approach, we directly work with the product of the prior density function and the likelihood function and define an algorithm to draw random samples from the posterior.

As we discussed in Chapter 2, an MCMC algorithm can be derived based on a function that is proportional to the target density function. As the posterior density function is proportional to the product of the prior density and the likelihood function, the above two equations are sufficient to derive an MCMC algorithm.

The use of MCMC enables us to implement more realistic and increasingly complicated models, because we are not limited to using conjugate families of priors or restricted to models with analytic solutions. Additionally, with the relatively easy-to-use computer language of Stan, Bayesian applications are as simple as writing down the likelihood model equations and the priors. For example, equations (3.2)–(3.5) can be easily translated into Stan (see the next section). As a comparison, we implement the Neuse River Estuary example using Stan to illustrate our preferred workflow.

4.1.1   Using Stan through R Package `rstan`

Using Stan we divide our R script into three parts. The first part is the Bayesian model written in the Stan language (the Stan model). The second part consists of R code to create necessary input data and initial values for the Stan model, which are passed to the Stan engine through the R function `stan` from package `rstan`. The resulting MCMC output is processed through the third code block, where the MCMC samples are almost always converted into random variable objects using the package `rv`.

Setting up `rstan`

Stan can be set up to run multiple MCMC chains in parallel to take advantage of multicore computer processors found in almost all modern personal computers. The following code detects the number of available cores and sets the number of chains to the minimum of the number of cores and 8, if more than 8 cores are available.

```
### R Code ###
packages(rv)
packages(rstan)

rstan_options(auto_write = TRUE)
options(mc.cores = min(c(parallel::detectCores(), 8)))

nchains <- min(c(parallel::detectCores(), 8))
niters <- 50000
nkeep <- 2500
nthin <- ceiling((niters/2)*nchains/nkeep)
### End ###
```

The Stan model

The basic model of the Neuse River Estuary example is a normal distribution model with unknown mean (μ) and variance (σ^2):

$$
\begin{aligned}
y_i &\sim N(\mu, \sigma^2) \\
\mu &\sim N(\mu_0, \sigma^2/n_0) \\
\sigma^2 &\sim IG(\alpha, \beta)
\end{aligned}
$$

The first line of the model describes the response variable distribution as a normal distribution with mean (μ) and variance (σ^2), which is the basis for the likelihood function. The next two lines are the prior distributions of the two parameters. The model requires input data, including the observed log concentrations y_i and prior parameters μ_0, n_0, α, and β. The target parameters are μ and σ^2. A functional Stan model consists of a minimum of three blocks: `data`, `parameter`, and `model`. These three blocks can be stored in a character string object:

```
### R Code ###
stan_mod <- "
  data{
    int N; // observation count
```

```
    real y[N]; //response variable data
    real mu0; // prior parameters
    real n0;
    real alpha;
    real beta;
  }
  parameters{
    real<lower=0> sigma_sq;
    real mu;
  }
  model{
    sigma_sq ~ inv_gamma(alpha, beta);
    mu ~ normal(mu0, sqrt(sigma_sq/n0));
    y ~ normal(mu, sqrt(sigma_sq));
  }
"
```
End

The first two lines in the model block define the prior distributions and the third line defines the likelihood function. Stan uses the log-probability function to construct the posterior. There are several alternatives to write the likelihood. We can use a `for` loop:

Partial Stan Code

```
  ...
  model{
  ...
  for (i in 1:N)
    y[i] ~ normal(mu, sqrt(sigma_sq));
  }
```
End

Using a `for` loop in this case has no computational advantage. In some cases, for example when the distribution parameter is indexed by i, a `for` loop is necessary. We can also use the **target +=** statement to specify the log-likelihood:

Partial Stan Code

```
  ...
  model{
  ...
  for (i in 1:N)
    target += normal_lpdf(y[i] | mu, sqrt(sigma_sq));
  }
```
End

or

```
### Partial Stan Code ###
  ...
  model{
  ...
    target += normal_lpdf(y | mu, sqrt(sigma_sq));
### End ###
```

When the likelihood function is not a standard function included in Stan, we can write out the log-likelihood function (up to a proportional constant, in this case, $-\log(\sigma) - (y_i - \mu)^2/(2\sigma^2)$) directly:

```
### Partial Stan Code ###
  ...
  model{
  ...
  for (i in 1:N)
    target += -log(sigma_sq)/2-(y[i] - mu)^2/(2*sigma_sq);
  }
### End ###
```

Once the model is written, we compile it using the function stan_model:

```
fit <- stan_model(model_code = stan_mod)
```

The compilation process checks the syntax of the Stan model and translates the Stan modeling language to C++ code. The C++ code for the model plus other auxiliary code is compiled into a dynamic shared object (DSO) and then loaded.

Organizing input data and running the model

Values of the input data in the **data** block, as well as initial values of model parameters (in the **parameter** block), need to be organized and fed to the Stan program. Input data and initial values are passed into Stan as components of a list. We normally use a function to process input data and initial values:

```
### R Code ###
stan_in <- function(data=neuse, yVAR="SURFCHLA",
                    Sub=NULL, chains=nchains,
                    mu0=0,n0=1,alpha=0.1,beta=0.1){
    if (is.null(Sub))
        y <- log(data[,yVAR])
    else y <- log(data[Sub, yVAR])
```

```
    y <- y[!is.na(y)]
    stan_data <- list(N=length(y), y=y, mu0=mu0, n0=n0,
                      alpha=alpha, beta=beta)
    stan_inits <- list()
    for (i in 1:chains)
        stan_inits[[i]] <- list(sigma_sq=runif(1),
                                mu=rnorm(1))
    return (list(data=stan_data, inits=stan_inits,
                pars=c("mu", "sigma_sq"),
                n.chains=chains))
}

input.to.stan <- stan_in(Sub=neuse$Year==1992)
fit2keep <- sampling(fit, data = input.to.stan$data,
                     init = input.to.stan$inits,
                     pars = input.to.stan$para,
                     iter = niters, thin=nthin,
                     chains = input.to.stan$n.chains)
### End ###
```

The compiled model `fit` is called by the function `sampling`, along with
the necessary input data, initial values, and a list of parameters to draw
samples. In situations where the model is used more than once, separating the compiling and sampling processes will avoid the need for
`rstan` to re-compile the same code multiple times. The function `stan`
(part of the `rstan` package) includes the functionality of both compiling
(`stan_model`) and MCMC sampling (`sampling`). We prefer the separate
steps of compiling and sampling because we often use the same model
repeatedly.

Processing Stan output

Stan output in the object `fit2keep` contains MCMC samples of all
parameters. The default method for `print` is to print the summary of
saved parameters:

```
### R Output ###
print(fit2keep)
```

MCMC samples are extracted using the function `extract`:

```
### R Code ###
fitcoef <- rvsims(as.matrix(as.data.frame(
           extract(fit2keep, permute=T,
                   pars=c("mu", "sigma_sq")))))
### End ###
```

We use various functions from the `rv` package to summarize, visualize, and process Stan output. For example, the sequential updating process can be coded as a series of repeated Stan runs, where between runs MCMC samples are processed to produce prior parameters for the next updating, perhaps using the method of moments. For example, the first two moments of the normal-inverse-gamma distribution are (when $\alpha > 2$):

$$E(\mu) = \mu_0 \qquad Var(\mu) = \frac{\beta}{(\alpha-1)n_0}$$
$$E(\sigma^2) = \frac{\beta}{\alpha-1} \quad Var(\sigma^2) = \frac{\beta^2}{(\alpha-1)^2(\alpha-2)}.$$

Solving for the four unknown parameters we have:

$$\hat{\mu}_0 = E(\mu) \qquad \hat{n}_0 = \frac{E(\mu)}{Var(\mu)}$$
$$\hat{\alpha} = 2 + \frac{E^2(\sigma^2)}{Var(\sigma^2)} \quad \hat{\beta} = (\hat{\alpha} - 1)E(\sigma^2).$$

```
### R Code ###
priors_normal <- function(fit_coef=summary(fitcoef)){
    mu <- fit_coef$name=="mu"
    sig2 <- fit_coef$name=="sigma_sq"
    ex <- fit_coef$mean[mu]
    vx <- fit_coef$sd[mu]^2
    esig2 <- fit_coef$mean[sig2]
    vsig2 <- fit_coef$sd[sig2]^2
    return(list(mu0 = ex, n0 = ex/vx,
                alpha=(alpha <- 2+esig2^2/vsig2),
                beta=(alpha-1)*esig2))
}


prior1993 <- priors_normal()
input.to.stan <- stan_in(Sub=neuse$Year==1993,
                    mu0=prior1993$mu0,
                    n0=prior1993$n0,
                    alpha=prior1993$alpha,
                    beta=prior1993$beta)
fit <- stan_model(model_code = stan_mod)
fit2keep <- sampling(fit,
                data = input.to.stan$data,
                init = input.to.stan$inits,
                pars = input.to.stan$para,
            iter = niters, thin=nthin,
                chains=input.to.stan$n.chains)
### End ###
```

A distinct advantage of Stan is its strong diagnostic capability, reflected in its warning messages. These warning messages often indicate potential problems in model formulation. We illustrate this advantage using the snake fungal disease as an example. The likelihood function is

$$L = (\theta(1 - f_n) + (1 - \theta)f_p)^x (1 - \theta(1 - f_n) - (1 - \theta)f_p)^{n-x}$$

and the log-likelihood function is

$$LL = x\log(\theta(1 - f_n) + (1 - \theta)f_p) + (n - x)\log(1 - (\theta(1 - f_n) + (1 - \theta)f_p)).$$

The priors are $f_p \sim beta(a_p, b_p)$, $f_n \sim beta(a_n, b_n)$, and $\theta \sim beta(\alpha, \beta)$. The model block of the Stan model is then:

```
### Partial Stan Code ###
...
model{
  real ppos;
  ppos = theta*(1-fn)+(1-theta)*fp;
  theta ~ beta(alpha,beta);
  fp ~ beta(ap, bp);
  fn ~ beta(an, bn);
  target += x*log(ppos) + (n-x)*log1p(-ppos);
}
### End ###
```

We encourage readers to run this example on their own computers and experience the warning messages.

As we mentioned in Section 2.5.1, this model is non-identifiable. Using Stan running MCMC with multiple chains, we are able to diagnose potential issues with the model. In this case, the Stan model encountered numerous divergent transitions indicating that the model results may not be reliable. A divergent transition is usually an indication of "degenerate" geometry of the posterior distribution. The term degenerate means that the posterior distribution of certain parameters was poorly defined, which can mean a widely spread distribution or complicated correlations among variables. Such complexity makes efficient HMC sampling difficult, which, in turn, hampers our ability to numerically compute the posterior distribution effectively. Stan's warning of divergent transitions is often an indication of problematic model formulation. Later in Chapter 5, we will revisit this model and discuss the model in more detail, especially the strong correlation between θ and f_p.

4.2 Examples of Analysis of Variance

Analysis of variance (ANOVA) is the most commonly used statistical model. However, ANOVA is also among a few statistical models that are still using the computational method developed before the computer was available. The general approach of ANOVA is to divide the total variance of the response variable into within- and among-group variances. By comparing the within-group variance and the among-group variance, we can make inferences about the differences among group means. Using a statistical modeling approach, within-group variance can be expressed as the distribution of the response variable for each group:

$$y_{ij} \sim N(\mu_j, \sigma_1^2) \tag{4.1}$$

where y_{ij} represent the ith observation in the jth group, μ_j is the group mean, and σ_1^2 is the within-group variance. The among-group variance can be expressed as the distribution of μ_j:

$$\mu_j \sim N(\theta, \sigma_2^2) \tag{4.2}$$

where θ is the overall mean and σ_2^2 is the among-group variance.

Alternatively, we can view ANOVA as a problem of estimating multiple means simultaneously. Equation (4.1) can be seen as the straightforward distributional assumption of the $j = 1, \cdots, J$ response variables. We are interested in estimating the unknown means μ_j. If we do not have additional information on how the means differ from each other, we can simply impose a common prior distribution for all means as expressed in equation (4.2).

No matter how we interpret the formulation, the difference between a Bayesian model and an ANOVA model lies in the estimation methods. In ANOVA, the focus is the between- and within-group variances, and the estimation method is limited to what computational tools Fisher had at his disposal when he developed the method in the 1920s. Using a Bayesian approach, we need to provide prior distributions of the unknown parameters $(\theta, \sigma_1^2, \sigma_2^2)$ and derive the posteriors, including group means μ_j's. The emphasis is on the estimation of these parameters, rather than testing the null hypothesis that all group means are equal to each other. As this is one of the most basic multivariate problems, we will derive the Bayesian solutions incrementally.

The objective is the estimation of $\mu_j, \theta, \sigma_1^2$, and σ_2^2. We need only assign prior distributions for θ, σ_1^2, and σ_2^2. As these are normal distribution parameters, we can use the typical conjugate family of priors:

$$
\begin{aligned}
\sigma_1^2 &\sim IG(\alpha, \beta) \\
\mu_j &\sim N(\theta, \sigma_2^2) \\
\theta | \sigma_2^2 &\sim N(\mu_0, \sigma_2^2/n_0) \\
\sigma_2^2 &\sim IG(a, b).
\end{aligned}
$$

In Bayesian hierarchical modeling literature, the common prior distribution of μ_j is often known as the "hyper-distribution" and the parameters of the distribution (θ, σ_2^2) are known as the "hyper-parameters." The likelihood function is based on the normal distribution assumption of equation (4.1):

- y_{ij} conditional on μ_j and σ_1^2:

$$\prod_{j=1}^{J}\prod_{i=1}^{I_j}\frac{1}{\sqrt{2\pi}\sigma_1}e^{-\frac{(y_{ij}-\mu_j)^2}{2\sigma_1^2}}.$$

- The prior density of μ_j (conditional on θ) is defined by equation (4.2):

$$\prod_{j=1}^{J}\frac{1}{\sqrt{2\pi}\sigma_2}e^{-\frac{(\mu_j-\theta)^2}{2\sigma_2^2}}.$$

The prior density of σ_1^2 is the inverse gamma distribution density, and the prior density of θ and σ_2^2 is normal-inverse-gamma density.

- The product of the likelihood and the prior densities is proportional to the joint posterior distribution of $\mu_j, \theta, \sigma_1^2$, and σ_2^2. The analytic result can be derived by algebraically rearranging the product. Details of the process are presented in Box and Tiao [1973]. Here, we present the steps of using Stan to numerically solve for the posteriors.

4.2.1   The Seaweed Grazer Example

This example is a typical study designed for ANOVA. The data and study design were detailed in Ramsey and Schafer [2012]. Qian [2016] used the data to discuss the multilevel modeling, which is mathematically equivalent to the Bayesian approach outlined by equations (4.1) and (4.2) when using non-informative (flat) priors for θ, σ_1^2, and σ_2^2 (i.e., $\pi(\theta, \sigma_1^2, \sigma_2^2) \propto 1/\sigma_1^2 \cdot 1/\sigma_2^2$) [Clayton, 1996].

The study was designed to estimate the effects of three seaweed grazers on seaweed regeneration. These grazers are small fish (f), large fish (F), and limpets (L). The experiments were carried out in eight inter-tidal zones along the Pacific coast in Oregon, USA. These eight sites were selected to represent various levels of wave energy. The experiment design includes 12 plots of rock surfaces per site cleared of seaweeds and physical and/or chemical treatments were applied to limit access to these plots. For example, a paint stripe around the plot would prevent limpets from accessing the plot; a fine mesh net will allow only small fish to access the plot. However, when large fish are allowed to access a plot, small fish can access as well. Consequently, the experiment designed six levels of treatment: C – no grazers were allowed access (control), f – only small fish were given access, fF – both small and large fish were allowed, L – only limpets were allowed, Lf – small fish and limpets were allowed, and LfF all grazers are allowed. The treated plots were revisited to measure the fraction of the plot surface covered with regenerated seaweed.

We start by considering the treatment as the only factor (a one-way ANOVA problem). The logit-transformed recovery fraction is assumed to have a normal distribution as in equation (4.1). Equation (4.2) defines the priors for μ_j. Combined with the conjugate priors for σ_1^2 and θ, σ_2^2, the model is expressed in Stan's model section:

```
### Stan Code ###
stan_aov <- "
data{
  int N;
  int J;
  real y[N];
  int treatment[N];
  real<lower=0> alpha;
  real<lower=0> beta;
  real<lower=0> a;
  real<lower=0> b;
  real<lower=0> n0;
  real<lower=0> mu0;
}
parameters{
  real<lower=0> sigma1sq;
  real<lower=0> sigma2sq;
  real theta;
  real mu_j[J];
}
model{
  sigma1sq ~ inv_gamma(alpha, beta);
  sigma2sq ~ inv_gamma(a, b);
  theta ~ normal(mu0, sqrt(sigma2sq/n0));
  for (j in 1:J){
    mu_j[j] ~ normal(theta, sqrt(sigma2sq));
  }
  for (i in 1:N){
    y[i] ~ normal(mu_j[treatment[i]], sqrt(sigma1sq));
  }
}
"

fit <- stan_model(model_code = stan_aov)
### End ###
```

Now we organize the input data, generate necessary initial values, and define the variables we want to monitor using the following function:

```
### R Code ###
input_Stan <- function(data=seaweed, chains=nchains,
                       a, b, alpha, beta, mu0, n0){
  y <- car::logit(data$COVER)
```

```
trt <- as.numeric(ordered(data$TREAT))
J <- max(trt)
N <- length(y)
stan_data <- list(N=N, J=J, y=y, treatment=trt,
                  a=a, b=b, alpha=alpha,
                  beta=beta, mu0=mu0, n0=n0)
stan_inits <- list()
for (i in 1:chains)
  stan_inits[[i]] <- list(sigma1sq=runif(1),
                          sigma2sq=runif(1),
                          mu_j=rnorm(J),
                          theta=rnorm(1))
para=c("mu_j","sigma1sq","sigma2sq", "theta")
return(list(data=stan_data, inits=stan_inits,
            paras=para, n.chains=chains))
}
### End ###
```

With the data processed, we can run the Stan model. For comparison with ANOVA, we use relatively "non-informative" priors:

```
### R Code ###
input.to.stan <- input_Stan(a=0.1, b=0.1,
                            alpha=0.01, beta=0.01,
                            mu0=0, n0=1)
fit2keep <- sampling(fit, data = input.to.stan$data,
              input.to.stan$inits,
              pars = input.to.stan$para,
              iter=niters, thin=nthin,
              chains=input.to.stan$n.chains)
### End ###
```

The object `fit2keep` is of class **stanfit** and contains the output from fitting the Stan model (MCMC samples). The posterior draws of the parameters listed in the **pars** argument can be extracted using the function `extract(fit2keep)`.

By default, the function extracts draws from all monitored parameters after the warm-up with samples from all chains merged. The results are stored in a list with names of components corresponding to the names of parameters. To use the package rv, the resulting list should be converted into a matrix:

```
### R Code ###
mcmcdraws <- rvsims(as.matrix(as.data.frame(
    extract(fit2keep))))
### End ###
```

The object `mcmcdraws` is a random variable vector of length 10 (six treatment means, residual standard deviation, the two hyper-parameters, and the "log-likelihood" `lp__`). The log-likelihood is recorded for model diagnostics. It is the product of posterior densities of all observations, up to a constant. The constant is related to sample size and the probability model.

Compared to the conventional ANOVA model, the estimated treatment means are shrunk toward the overall mean (Figure 4.1). That is, the Bayesian estimated $\hat{\mu}_j$'s are closer to the overall mean than the ANOVA estimated $\bar{x}_j$. The shrinkage effect is a desired feature of the Bayesian ANOVA. Mathematically, the Bayesian ANOVA is a generalization of the conventional ANOVA. The ANOVA null hypothesis model corresponds to the Bayesian model when assuming $\sigma_2^2 = 0$; when estimating treatment effects, the ANOVA model corresponds to the Bayesian model when $\sigma_2^2 = \infty$ [Gelman, 2005]. That is, when σ_2^2 is infinity, we estimate μ_j's separately where the sample average (MLE) is the best estimator. In reality, σ_2^2 is somewhere between 0 and ∞. Equations (4.1) and (4.2) provide the basis for estimating σ_2^2 from the observed data.

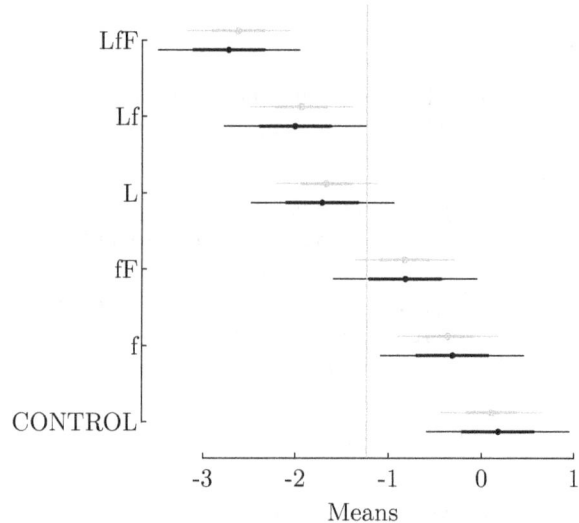

FIGURE 4.1: Estimated treatment means are compared between the conventional ANOVA (black lines and dots) and the Bayesian model (grey lines and dots). The thick lines are the interquartile range, the thin lines are 95% credible intervals and the dots are the estimated means.

Within classical statistics, we can view ANOVA as a special case of the mixed effect model. For example, in the seaweed example, we view the six treatment effects as fixed because these are the only treatments designed. If these treatments were randomly selected among many possible treatments, we would call them random effects. The random-effects model using the maximum likelihood estimator is equivalent to the Bayesian ANOVA (hierarchical model) using flat priors [Clayton, 1996].

In our Stan code, the Bayesian ANOVA model is parameterized by $\mu_j, \theta, \sigma_1^2$, and σ_2^2. The treatment effects (the difference between a treatment mean and the overall mean) can be derived in a separate code group (`generated quantities`). For example, the effect of large fish cannot be directly estimated because the experiment cannot exclude access from small fish when large fish had access to a plot. The large fish effect is then estimated as the average of two differences: $\mu_F = \frac{1}{2}(\mu_{fF} - \mu_f + \mu_{LfF} - \mu_{Lf})$. Likewise, the effect of small fish is represented in two differences and can be estimated by the average of $\mu_f - \mu_C$ and $\mu_{Lf} - \mu_L$, and the effect of limpets should be the average of $\mu_L - \mu_C$, $\mu_{Lf} - \mu_f$, and $\mu_{LfF} - \mu_{fF}$. As the treatment is ordered alphabetically (i.e., C, f, fF, L, Lf, LfF), the effects of individual grazers can be coded as follows:

```
### Partial Stan Code ###
generated quantities{
  real muf;
  real muF;
  real muL;
  muf = 0.5*(mu_j[2]-mu_j[1] + mu_j[5]-mu_j[4]);
  muF = 0.5*(mu_j[3]-mu_j[2] + mu_j[6]-mu_j[5]);
  muL = (mi_j[4]-mu_j[1] + mu_j[5]-mu_j[2] + mu_j[6]-mu_j[3])/3;
}
### End ###
```

In ANOVA, we make inferences about treatment effects based on the comparison of the among-group and within-group variances (more specifically, the mean sum of squares). In a Bayesian ANOVA, we no longer aim at testing the null hypothesis of no treatment effects. Rather, we are more interested in estimating these treatment effects. Comparing the among- and within-group variances is, nevertheless, useful in providing an estimation of the signal to noise ratio. The within-group variance is σ_1^2 and the among-group variance can be approximated using sample variances of groups means. That is, we can express the ANOVA model as

$$y_{ij} = \mu_j + \varepsilon_{ij}$$

and the total variance of y is

$$Var(y_{ij}) = Var(\mu_j) + Var(\varepsilon_{ij}).$$

During each MCMC sampling iteration (k), we approximate $Var(\mu_j)$ by using the sample variance of $\{\mu_1^{(k)}, \mu_2^{(k)}, \cdots, \mu_J^{(k)}\}$. The variance component calculation can be carried out in the `derived quantity` code block in the Stan model or after the Stan model run using various functions from the package `rv`. The variance components can be conveniently displayed using the R function `mlplot` from package `rv` (Figure 4.2).

```
### R Code ###
drawnames <- names(mcmcdraws)
mujs <- mcmcdraws[substring(drawnames, 1, 2)=="mu"]
muj_var <- rvsims(apply(mujs, 1, var))
sigma1var <- rvsims(unlist(mcmcdraws[drawnames=="sigma1sq"]))
var_comp <- sqrt(c(muj_var, sigma1var))
names(var_comp) <- c("Treatment", "Residuals")

mlplot(var_comp, xlab="standard deviation")
### End ###
```

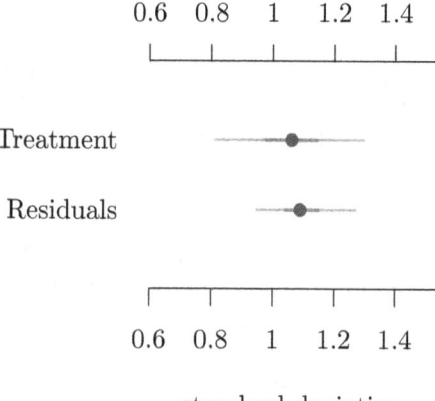

FIGURE 4.2: Variance component plot compares variance explained (in standard deviation) by treatment and residuals.

The study was conducted in eight locations, representing different exposures to wave energy. As such, including the block effect will increase the ANOVA test's power. With the second factor, the two-way ANOVA model is better expressed in terms of treatment and block effects:

$$y_{ijk} = \mu + \delta_j^t + \delta_k^b + \varepsilon_{ijk}$$

Assuming that the treatment effects δ_j^t and block effects δ_k^b are additive, we impose common priors for the two effects:

$$\delta_j^t \sim N(0, \sigma_2^2)$$
$$\delta_j^b \sim N(0, \sigma_3^2).$$

Using default non-informative priors from Stan, the model is coded as follows.

```
### Stan Code ###
stan_aov2 <- "
data{
  int N;
  int J;
  int K;
  real y[N];
  int treatment[N];
  int blck[N];
}
parameters{
  real<lower=0> sigma1sq;
  real<lower=0> sigma2sq;
  real<lower=0> sigma3sq;
  real theta;
  real delta_j[J];
  real delta_k[K];
}
model{
  delta_j ~ normal(0, sqrt(sigma2sq));
  delta_k ~ normal(0, sqrt(sigma3sq));
  for (i in 1:N){
    y[i] ~ normal(theta+delta_j[treatment[i]]+delta_k[blck[i]],
              sqrt(sigma1sq));
  }
}
generated quantities{
  real mu;
  real trt[J];
  real blk[K];
  mu = theta+mean(delta_j[])+mean(delta_k[]);
  for (j in 1:J){
    trt[j] = delta_j[j]-mean(delta_j[]);
  }
  for (k in 1:K){
    blk[k] = delta_k[k]-mean(delta_k[]);
  }
}
"
### End ###
```

The Bayesian estimated treatment and block effects are both shrunk towards 0 (Figure 4.3). The variance components show a similar distribution as the two-way ANOVA table (Figure 4.4). As discussed in Qian [2016], the difference between Bayesian estimated means and ANOVA estimated means is small because the data were collected with ANOVA as the intended analysis method and the among-treatment and among-block differences are very obvious. The same cannot be said for the next example.

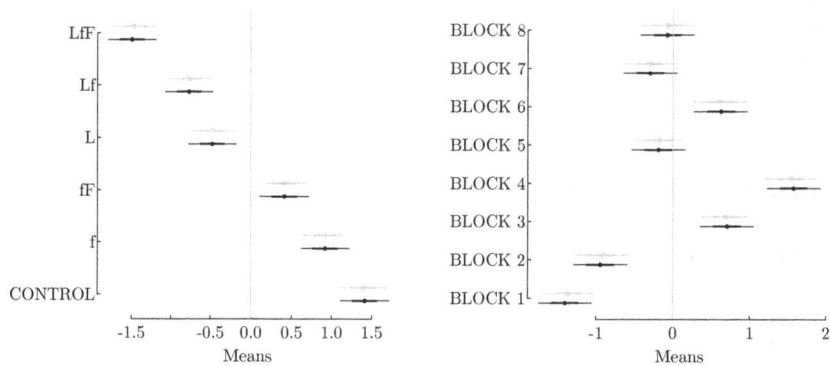

FIGURE 4.3: Estimated treatment (left panel) and block (right panel) effects using the conventional ANOVA (black lines) and Bayesian model (gray lines) are compared to show the shrinkage effect.

4.2.2   The Gulf of Mexico Hypoxia Example

Although the classical ANOVA is focused on testing the null hypothesis of no difference, the ANOVA test itself is almost always a starting point of an analysis. This is because when the ANOVA null hypothesis is rejected, we are naturally interested in the nature of the treatment effects, which is a multiple comparisons problem. In the classical ANOVA framework, multiple comparisons are conducted by adjusting the significance level of each comparison to achieve a family-wise type I error probability of 0.05. When the null hypothesis is not rejected, we cannot readily conclude that there is no treatment effect because failure to reject the null does not definitely show that the alternative is false. In many cases, we have reason to believe that the null hypothesis of no difference is unlikely to be true (which is why we were able to write a convincing proposal to win the research funding for the study). Consequently, the objective of the experiment or data collection is largely to quantify the differences among multiple treatment levels. This is why we find that using the Bayesian hierarchical modeling (BHM) approach (e.g., equations (4.1) and (4.2)) is the most logical approach. BHM is an estimation method. The shrinkage effect of BHM automatically reduces the magnitude

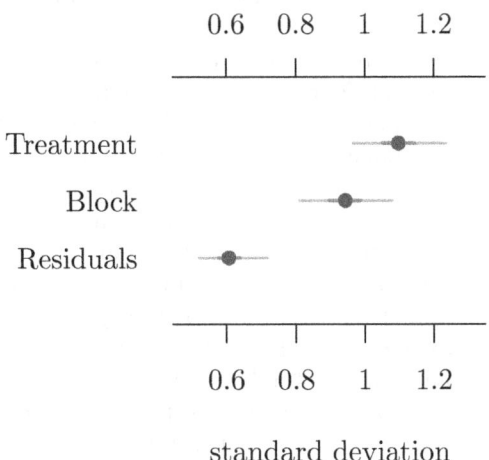

FIGURE 4.4: Variance component plot for the two-way ANOVA model.

of any given difference. Compared with inflating the confidence interval to address the multiple comparison problem, a shrinkage estimator such as BHM adjusts the estimated differences based on the relative balance between within- and among-group variances.

The analysis of the data from studying the effects of the Gulf of Mexico hypoxia on the benthic macroinvertebrate community is such an example. Using data from Baustian et al. [2009], Qian et al. [2009] reformulated the ANOVA analysis to focus on the estimation of the effects of seasonal hypoxia in the benthic community in the Gulf of Mexico.

4.2.2.1 Study Background

Hypoxia occurs when the dissolved oxygen level near the bottom drops below 2 milligrams per liter (mg/L). A continuous band of hypoxia parallel to the coast of the U.S. state of Louisiana was discovered in the 1980s. The hypoxic band occurs on an annual basis west of the Mississippi River along the Louisiana coast and onto the northeastern coast of Texas. The hypoxic condition is commonly attributed to two causes: stratification of the water column (which prevents bottom-to-top circulation) and nutrient input from the Mississippi and Atchafalaya rivers (which promotes high primary productivity that ultimately leads to high organic loading onto the seabed and subsequent high benthic respiration rates). Under hypoxic conditions, benthic infaunal communities decline in density and species richness. Many species of benthic infauna are primary prey items for some regionally important fisheries (e.g., Atlantic croaker - *Micropogonias undulatus*) [Baustian et al., 2009].

The study was designed to understand the effects of hypoxia on the benthic infauna community. Data were derived from sediment core samples taken in 15 locations over an approximately 5,000 km^2 area off the central coast of Louisiana near Terrebonne Bay from August 2–12, 2003. Five of these sampling sites were located within the hypoxic zone about 10 km from the nearest coast, four were located immediately to the north of the hypoxic zone (toward the Louisiana coastline, inshore sites), and six were located to the south of the hypoxic zone (away from the Louisiana coastline, offshore sites). Each sediment core sample was divided into three parts for analysis of benthic macroinvertebrate species composition, which was then used to derive species abundance (total number of individuals per square meter) and species richness (total number of species), the two response variables of interest. The average dissolved oxygen concentration in the hypoxic zone was < 1 mg/L, substantially lower than the dissolved oxygen concentration outside the zone (3–5 mg/L) [Baustian et al., 2009].

4.2.2.2 Prior Analysis

To study the effects of hypoxia on the benthic macroinvertebrate community measured by the total abundance and the species richness, ANOVA was used initially to estimate the differences in means of the two response variables among the three zones. Because of the large differences among sites within each zone, ANOVA did not show a statistically significant difference among the three zones (i.e., p-values of the ANOVA tests were larger than 0.05) [Baustian et al., 2009]. The use of ANOVA in this case is, however, questionable. ANOVA is intended for analyzing experimental data for causal inferences based on randomized experiments which generate independent measurements of the response variable from treatments and controls. When ANOVA is applied to observational field data, where samples or sampling stations are considered replicated experimental units and categorized into discrete groups presumed to differ with respect to some independent, or "treatment," variables, the results of ANOVA can be ambiguous when the independence assumption of the response data is not met. In addition, the sampling design was nested and unbalanced and the background variability was high. As a result, the test is of low statistical power.

Using the same data, Qian et al. [2009] focused on estimating the effects of hypoxia, rather than testing if there was an effect. They used three alternative models to explore whether other factors, such as water depth, can also affect the two response variables. The first model considers the sampling design, especially the nested nature of the replicated core samples. That is, the three measurements taken from each sediment core should be modeled differently:

$$y_{ijk} \sim N(\mu_{jk}, \sigma_{y_k}^2) \tag{4.3}$$

where y represents the response variable (log abundance or log species richness), the index ijk represents the ith observation from the jth sediment core from zone k, μ_{jk} is the core mean, and $\sigma^2_{y_k}$ are zone-specific residual variance. Because of the relatively large variance from sediment core to sediment core within each of the three zones, we further model the sediment core means as exchangeable only within their respective zones:

$$\mu_{jk} \sim N(\theta_k, \sigma^2_z) \qquad (4.4)$$

where θ_k represents the mean of zone k and σ^2_z is among sediment core variance. We are interested in the mean of each zone, θ_k. More specifically, we are interested in the differences between the hypoxic zone mean and the means of the other two zones. Let $k = 2$ be the hypoxic zone, $k = 1$ be the inshore zone, and $k = 3$ be the offshore zone, and we want to estimate $\delta_1 = \theta_2 - \theta_1$ and $\delta_2 = \theta_2 - \theta_3$. To complete the model, we now impose a common prior with mean (μ_{hyp}) and variance (σ^2_{hyp}) for θ_i:

$$\theta_k \sim N(\mu_{hyp}, \sigma^2_{hyp}) \qquad (4.5)$$

This formulation seems to be straightforward. However, the study design used only three zones. That is, we are estimating the hyper-parameters based on three zone-means. We expect to have numerical difficulties even though the model is theoretically sound. In Qian et al. [2009], the model was implemented in WinBUGS and they replaced equation (4.5) with a non-informative flat prior: $\theta_k \sim N(0, 1000)$ in the WinBUGS code because of the numerical issues. This change led to a different model, implying that the three zones are entirely different (with a very large among-zone variance). Without a hyprt-distribution, the three zone means (θ_k) were estimated separately (no shrinkage effect).

4.2.2.3 Implementation in Stan and Alternative Models

We implemented the model represented by equations (4.3) through (4.5) in Stan using Stan's default "weakly informative" priors for the standard deviations and hyper-mean. The Stan code of the model is relatively straightforward (see online companion). Although the model convergence diagnostic statistic $\hat{R}$ suggests the model converges after 500,000 iterations, the multiple chains mixed poorly and had divergent transitions after warm-up (250,000 iterations). Divergent transitions indicate that the posterior distribution has a complex "geometry" that made it difficult for the HMC algorithm to explore it. Consequently, results from simulations with a large number of divergent transitions may not be reliable. The warning often is an indicator of model formulation or data issues. In this case, we believe that the numeric issue is caused by the small number of zones. Estimating a variance based on three "data points" is always difficult because the data do not provide sufficient information. To avoid such a problem, we need either more data (in this case, more zones) or to reformulate the model to allow the use of more informative prior models. We do not have information on among-zone variance of species richness or abundance. However, we can transform the response variable to make it easier to consider more informative prior distributions. For example, we can center the response variable $(y - \bar{y})$ so that the hyper-mean is likely centered around 0. We could also standardize the response variable $((y - \bar{y})/sd(y))$ so that the standard deviations in the model can be reasonably modeled using, for example, half-normal $N(0, 1)$ or $N(0, 0.5)$. For this problem, standardizing the response variable did not resolve the numeric problem. The problem lies in the model's inability to estimate the hyper-parameters. The scatter plot of the posterior samples of σ_{hyp} against μ_{hyp} shows a funnel-shaped cloud (Figure 4.5, left panel). This is an example of Neal's funnel [Neal, 2003], a common problem with some hierarchical models with non-informative priors of μ_{hyp} and σ_{hyp}, while the data do not provide much information on the hyper-parameters. When σ_{hyp} is small (small among-group differences), μ_{hyp} is limited to a small range (the neck of the funnel); when σ_{hyp} is large (large among-group differences), the variation of μ_{hyp} becomes large. Stan has difficulties in sampling the "neck" area of the funnel. When using the half normal ($N(0, 1)$) as the prior for σ_{hyp}, the model runs much faster, but we still have the same problem (Figure 4.5, right panel). Furthermore, we believe that hypoxia can be detrimental to benthic organisms, which implies that the among-zone variance should be large. As a result, using a prior that limits σ_{hyp} to be small is contradictary to what we believe. Alternatively, we can set a prior with low values of σ_{hyp} to avoid the neck area. For example, we can use an inverse gamma distribution with a mode away from 0. However, a prior that inflates σ_{hyp} contradicts the spirit of the study – if the result is overly dependent on the prior, we cannot determine how much the differences among the three zones are due to our prior on σ_{hyp}.

The problem is likely due to the small number of zones and, perhaps, large among-core variances within each zone. As a result, the estimated zone means (θ_k) do not constrain the hyper-distribution tightly. One frequently used method to improve Stan's sampling efficiency is to reparameterize the Stan model and avoid sampling μ_{hyp} and σ_{hyp} altogether. Specifically, we introduce a new parameter ($\eta_k \sim N(0, 1)$) and parameterize θ_k as:

$$\theta_k = \mu_{hyp} + \sigma_{hyp}\eta_k$$

This reparameterization does not change the model, but avoided directly sampling θ_k. In Stan, we set θ_k as transformed parameters:

Partial Stan Code

```
...
parameters{
...
  real eta[I];
transformed parameters{
  real theta[I];
```

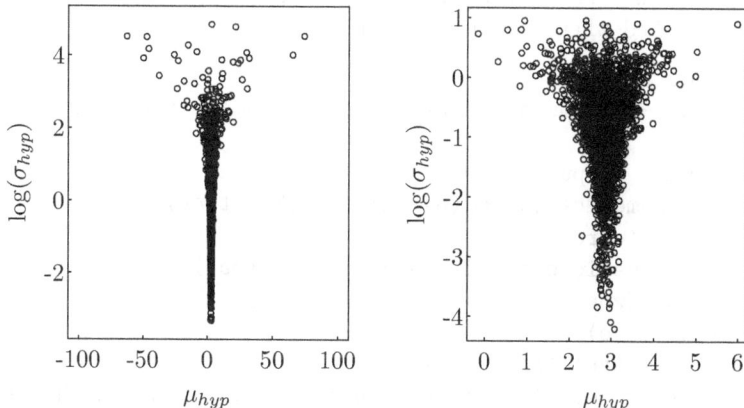

FIGURE 4.5: Scatter plots of posterior samples of σ_{hyp} against μ_{hyp} from the richness model show funnel-shaped data cloud suggesting the model has difficulties in estimating the two hyper-parameters. The left panel was from the model using the default non-informative prior for σ_{hyp} and the right panel was from the model with the prior of σ_{hyp} set to be half-normal $N(0, 1)$.

```
for (i in 1:I)
   theta[i] = mu_hyp+sigma_hyp*eta[i];
}
### End ###
```

This approach reduced the correlations among θ_k's and greatly improved the sampling speed. It, however, does not change the funnel-shaped posterior geometry of $\log(\sigma_{hyp})$ and μ_{hyp}. The funnel-shaped posterior distribution geometry made the inference on the hyper-parameters difficult. In this problem, we believe that the data did not have enough information to properly quantify the hyper-parameters (because of the small number of groups).

We propose two alternative models for this problem by avoiding the hyper-parameters. First, we simplify the problem to a one-way ANOVA problem with sediment cores as the only factor variable. Inference about differences among the three zones are estimated by regrouping the estimated core means. Specifically, we eliminate equation (4.5) and change equation (4.4) to:

$$\mu_{jk} \sim N(\mu_{hyp}, \sigma_{hyp}^2) \tag{4.6}$$

As a result, the hyper-distribution is estimated based on 15 group-level (sediment cores) means.

Using MCMC, we draw posterior random samples from the joint distribution of μ_{jk}. With the MCMC samples, we can numerically estimate the marginal distribution of zonal means and their differences. The numerical process of estimating these marginal means and differences among means is greatly simplified when using the R package **rv**.

```
#### R Code ####
rich_stan2 <- rvsims(as.matrix(as.data.frame(extract(fit2keep))))

## processing output
core <- as.numeric(ordered(benthic.data$Station))
n.core <- max(core)
zone <- as.numeric(ordered(benthic.data$Area))
n.zone <- max(zone)
oo <- order(core)
ind <- cumsum(table(core[oo]))
Core.zone <- zone[oo][ind] ## each core belongs to which zone
core.mus <- rich_stan2[1:15]
zone1.Rmu <- mean(core.mus[Core.zone==1])
zone2.Rmu <- mean(core.mus[Core.zone==2])
zone3.Rmu <- mean(core.mus[Core.zone==3])

deltaR1 = zone2.Rmu-zone1.Rmu
deltaR2 = zone2.Rmu-zone3.Rmu
deltaR3 = zone1.Rmu-zone3.Rmu
### End ###
```

Second, following the discussion of modeling nested multilevel structure in Bates [2010, Chapter 2], we revise the model to explicitly model the zonal effect through a nested two-way ANOVA. The key to this approach is to label the cores as nested in zones. That is, each sediment core is labeled uniquely and linked to the zone it belongs to. For example, we used a column **core** and a column **zone** to label each observation and both are included as factor variables in the model:

```
y    core   zone
1.1  A1     inshore
2.1  A1     inshore
3.1  B2     inshore
1.2  C4     hypothic
2.1  C4     hypothic
5.4  D5     hypothic
... ...    ...
### End ###
```

Using the following R code idiom, we can reference cores and zones:

```
#### R Code ####
core <- as.numeric(ordered(core))
zone <- as.numeric(ordered(zone))
### End ###
```

The resulting objects core and zone are numeric integer vectors ranging from 1 to the numbers of unique cores and zones, respectively. The kth value of core or zone (e.g., 2) represents the core or zone number (e.g., 2) from which the kth observation was made. They are directly used in the model:

$$
\begin{aligned}
y_i &\sim N(\mu_i, \sigma_y^2) \\
\mu_i &= \mu_0 + \alpha_{k[i]} + \beta_{j[i]} \\
\alpha_k &\sim N(0, \sigma_z^2) \\
\beta_j &\sim N(0, \sigma_c^2)
\end{aligned}
\tag{4.7}
$$

where i is the index of observation, k is the index of zone, and j is the index of core. The notation $k[i]$ denotes that the ith observation is located in the kth zone (directly represented by zone in the code) and $j[i]$ represents that the ith observation is from the jth core (core). This formulation estimates the overall mean μ_0 and the effects of core (β) and zone (α). As a result, we can set their prior mean to be 0. Furthermore, if we standardize the response variable, we can use a half-normal distribution ($N(0, 0.5)$) as the prior for σ_z and σ_c.

When the goal is to compare zone averages, we find the second alternative is still problematic because (1) we still have numeric issues estimating a variance variable from three "data points" (although the concentrated prior helped) and (2) the core effects (β's) do not sum to 0 for cores within the same zone. In other words, the MCMC model will be much slower and the output needs to be processed in the same way as in the first alternative.

As in Qian et al. [2009], we present the results graphically. Marginal distributions of relevant parameters can be expressed by using a simplified boxplot, where the median is represented by a dot, the 50% credible interval is a thick line connecting the 25th and the 50th percentiles, and the 95% credible interval is a line connecting the 2.5th and the 97.5th percentiles. In the following figures, we refer to the model represented in equations (4.3)–(4.5) as the original model, the first alternative model (equations (4.4) and (4.6)) as alternative model 1, and the second alternative model (equation (4.7)) as alternative model 2. Figures 4.6 and 4.7 compare the estimated posterior distributions of the means of log richness and log abundance for all sediment cores (μ_{ij}). The three models resulted in similar marginal means and 95% credible intervals.

Figures 4.8 and 4.9 compare estimated marginal posterior distributions of zone means (θ_i) of log richness and log abundance. The estimated zone means from the three models overlap, especially when using the original model. Overlapping confidence intervals are often used as an indication of no statistically significant differences. The pairwise differences (δ's) show, however, a different picture (Figures 4.10 and 4.11). The prominent difference among the three models is the estimation uncertainty represented by the widths of the 95% credible intervals. The overall patterns are consistent among the three models, and both richness and abundance in the hypoxic zone are lower than the same in the other two zones. The reduced uncertainty in the two alternative models is largely due to the simplified model structure that made the MCMC

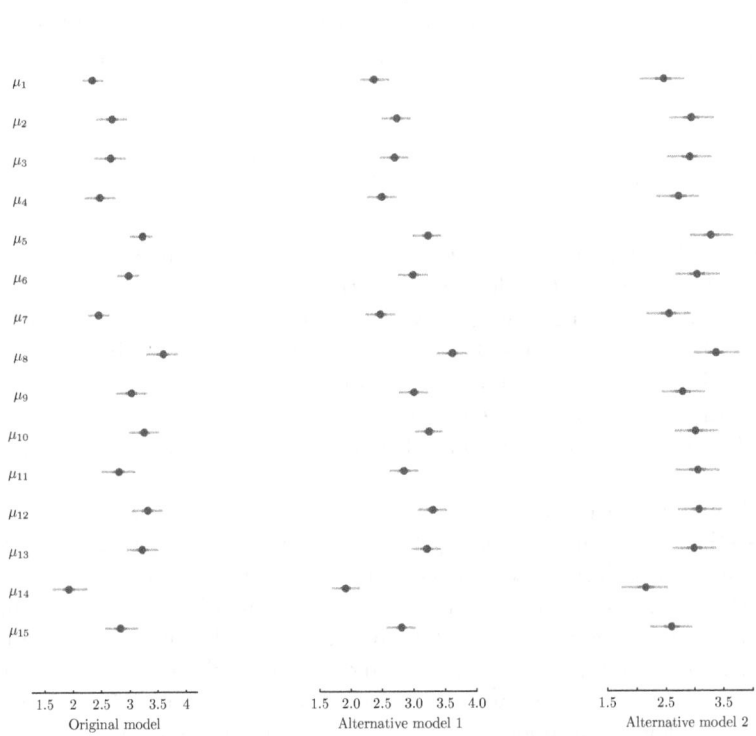

FIGURE 4.6: Estimated richness core means are compared among three model formulations.

sampling more efficient. The reduced estimation uncertainty made it possible to state that all three pairs of differences are statistically significant (with $p < 0.05$), although we prefer not to use the term "statistically significant" (see Section 8.4).

4.3   Regression Models

Regression models with normal response variables are the same as the ANOVA problems, except the normal means are linear or nonlinear functions of continuous predictor variables. From the perspective of fitting a Bayesian model, a regression model is a natural extension of the ANOVA model.

log Abundance

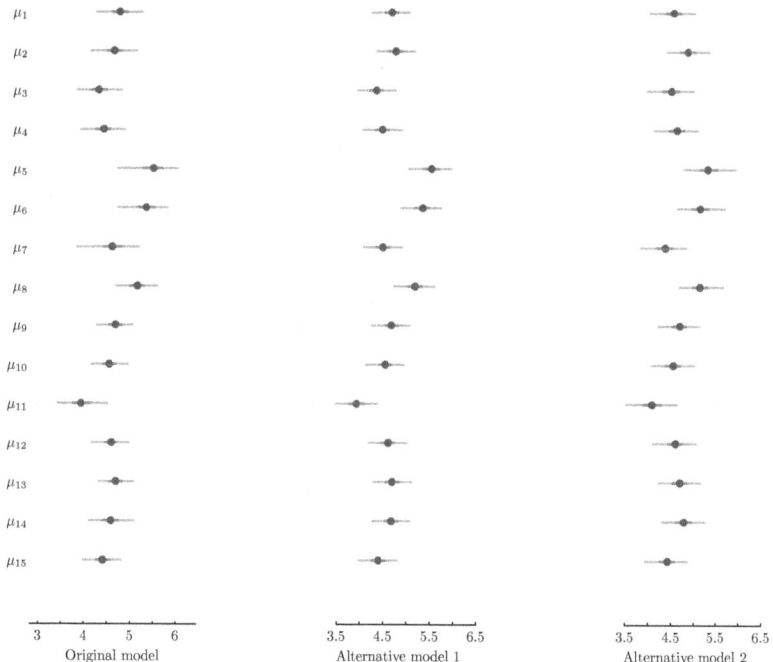

FIGURE 4.7: Estimated total abundance core means are compared among three model formulations.

In many cases, we find that the classical least squares method for fitting linear and nonlinear regression models is satisfactory. The advantage of the Bayesian framework lies in its flexibility to increase a model's complexity to suit the need of a problem. In this section, we illustrate this point with examples.

4.3.1 Linear Regression Example

For all practical purposes, we see no need for implementing Bayesian linear regression as the classical linear model is a well-studied topic and the least-squares estimator is often very efficient. Unless we have specific prior information on the model coefficients [Reckhow, 1987, 1988, e.g.,], the classical regression analysis will lead to similar results and the conventional simulation approach based on classical sampling distributions is satisfactory. Furthermore, simulations based on classical sampling distribution theories can be

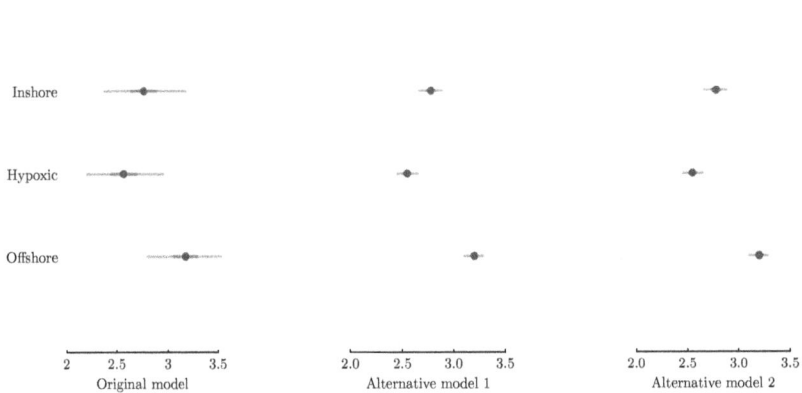

FIGURE 4.8: Estimated richness zone means are compared among three model formulations.

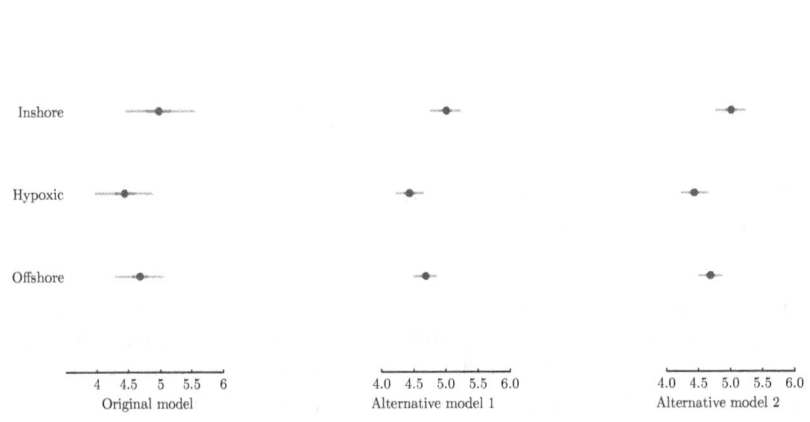

FIGURE 4.9: Estimated total abundance zone means are compared among three model formulations.

used to generate Bayesian posterior samples of regression model coefficients [Qian, 2016, Chapter 9].

As an example, we use the PCB in Lake Michigan fish data of Stow and Qian [1998] to illustrate the use of R function lm() and a simulation algorithm as a short cut for Bayesian linear regression.

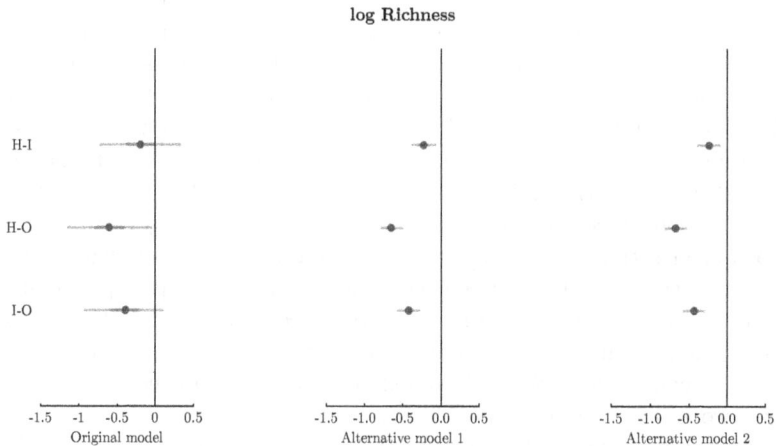

FIGURE 4.10: Estimated pairwise differences in zone mean richness.

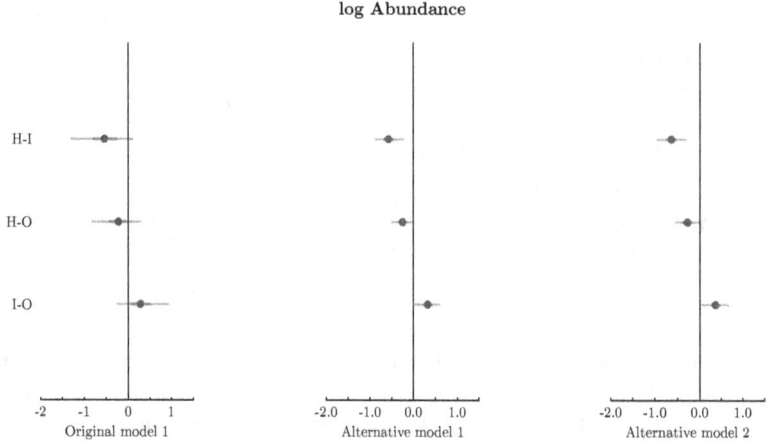

FIGURE 4.11: Estimated pairwise differences in zone mean total abundance.

Stow and Qian [1998] aimed at providing a size-based fish consumption advisory to help anglers decide whether to eat their catch from Lake Michigan. Salmonid species are popular sports fish in the area. These predatory fish often have high PCB contents due to historical industrial contamination. PCBs are very stable mixtures of chemicals that are resistant to extreme temperature and pressure. They were widely used in electrical equipment like capacitors and transformers, as well as in hydraulic fluids, heat transfer fluids, lubricants, and plasticizers. PCBs are probable carcinogens and are known to have adverse health effects, especially for pregnant women and young children. Although the production and use of PCB was outlawed in 1974 in the Great Lakes region, PCBs accumulated in soil and lake sediments continue to find their way to enter into the aquatic food chain. PCB concentrations in large salmonids are often quite high as a result of bio-magnification. Fish consumption advisories issued by local and state agencies are often based on PCB concentrations. For example, the state of Wisconsin's advisory in the 1990s contained the following five consumption categories based on fish PCB concentration: (a) at concentrations below 0.05 mg/kg, fish can be eaten without restriction; (b) between 0.05 and 0.2 mg/kg consumption should be restricted to no more than one meal per week; (c) from 0.2 to 1.0 mg/kg consumption is limited to no more than one meal per month; (d) concentrations between 1 and 1.9 mg/kg result in a limit of no more than one meal every two months; and (e) people are advised not to eat any fish with PCB concentrations greater than 1.9 mg/kg [WDH and WDNR, 1997]. Because anglers cannot readily know the PCB concentration of their catch, the advisory translates these concentration-based consumption categories into fish size ranges for the important recreational species. However, PCB concentrations among individual fish are highly variable, even among similar-sized fish of the same species. A regression model linking fish size (length) and its PCB concentration can be used as the basis of a risk assessment. That is, using the regression model to derive a predictive distribution of PCB concentration for a given sized fish. The predictive distribution is then used to estimate the probability of PCB concentration exceeding various levels of concentration threshold to allow consumers to decide whether to eat their catch.

The basic regression model uses fish size to predict the log PCB concentration. In the Bayesian notation, the regression model is:

$$\log(PCB_i) \sim N(\beta_0 + \beta_1 Size_i, \sigma^2)$$

where β_0 and β_1 are the regression intercept and slope, respectively, and σ^2 is the residual variance. In general, the regression model can be more parsimoniously expressed in vector-matrix notation. That is, the regression model is

$$\boldsymbol{y} \sim N(\boldsymbol{X\beta}, \sigma^2 \boldsymbol{I_n})$$

where $\boldsymbol{y}$ is a vector of length n (the sample size), $\boldsymbol{\beta}$ is the model coefficient vector with length k, $\boldsymbol{X}$ is the $(n \times k)$ design matrix, and $\boldsymbol{I_n}$ is the $n \times n$ identity matrix.

The conjugate family of priors for $\boldsymbol{\beta}, \sigma^2$ is the multivariate normal-inverse-gamma distribution. The prior for σ^2 is

$$\sigma^2 \sim IG(a_0, b_0)$$

and the conditional prior for $\boldsymbol{\beta}$ is multivariate normal:

$$\pi(\boldsymbol{\beta}) \propto (\sigma^2)^{-k/2} e^{-\frac{1}{2\sigma^2}(\boldsymbol{\beta}-\boldsymbol{\mu_0})^T \boldsymbol{\Gamma_0}(\boldsymbol{\beta}-\boldsymbol{\mu_0})}.$$

Or, $\boldsymbol{\beta} \sim N(\boldsymbol{\mu}_0, \sigma^2 \boldsymbol{\Gamma}_0^{-1})$.

The joint posterior distribution of $\boldsymbol{\theta} = \{\boldsymbol{\beta}, \sigma^2\}$ is the product of the prior and likelihood:

$$\pi(\boldsymbol{\beta}, \sigma^2 | \boldsymbol{y}, \boldsymbol{X}) \propto \pi(\boldsymbol{y} | \boldsymbol{X}, \boldsymbol{\beta}, \sigma^2) \pi(\boldsymbol{\beta} | \sigma^2) \pi(\sigma^2). \tag{4.8}$$

After rearranging the right-hand side of equation (4.8), we can express the posterior of $\boldsymbol{\beta}$ and σ^2 to show that the posterior distribution is also a normal-inverse-gamma distribution:

$$
\begin{aligned}
\pi(\boldsymbol{\beta}, \sigma^2 | \boldsymbol{y}, \boldsymbol{X}) &\propto \pi(\boldsymbol{\beta} | \sigma^2, \boldsymbol{y}, \boldsymbol{X}) \pi(\sigma^2 | \boldsymbol{y}, \boldsymbol{X}) \\
\boldsymbol{\beta} | \sigma^2, \boldsymbol{y}, \boldsymbol{X} &\sim N(\boldsymbol{\mu}_n, \sigma^2 \boldsymbol{\Gamma}_n^{-1}) \\
\sigma^2 | \boldsymbol{y}, \boldsymbol{X} &\sim IG(a_n, b_n)
\end{aligned}
\tag{4.9}
$$

where

$$
\begin{aligned}
\boldsymbol{\Gamma}_n &= (X^T X + \boldsymbol{\Gamma}_0), \quad \boldsymbol{\mu}_n = (\boldsymbol{\Gamma}_n)^{-1}(X^T X \hat{\boldsymbol{\beta}} + \boldsymbol{\Gamma}_0 \boldsymbol{\mu}_0), \\
a_n &= a_0 + n/2, \qquad b_n = b_0 + (\boldsymbol{y}^T \boldsymbol{y} + \boldsymbol{\mu}_0^T \boldsymbol{\Gamma}_0 \boldsymbol{\mu}_0 - \boldsymbol{\mu}_n^T \boldsymbol{\Gamma}_n \boldsymbol{\mu}_n)/2
\end{aligned}
$$

and $\hat{\boldsymbol{\beta}} = (X^T X)^{-1} X^T \boldsymbol{y}$ (the least squares estimate).

Often, we use a non-informative prior for $\boldsymbol{\beta}$ and σ^2:

$$\pi(\boldsymbol{\beta}, \sigma^2) \propto \sigma^{-2}$$

which is close to setting $\boldsymbol{\mu}_0 = 0$, $\boldsymbol{\Gamma}_0 = I_k$, and $a_0 \to 0, b_0 \to 0$ in equation (4.9). The posterior marginal distributions of $\boldsymbol{\beta}$ and σ^2 are identical to the respective classical statistics sampling distributions. That is, the marginal posterior distribution of $\boldsymbol{\beta}$ is a multivariate Student-t (MVT) distribution

$$\boldsymbol{\beta} | \boldsymbol{y}, \boldsymbol{X} \sim MVT(\hat{\boldsymbol{\beta}}, s^2 (\boldsymbol{X}^T \boldsymbol{X})^{-1}, n - k) \tag{4.10}$$

where $s^2 = \frac{(\boldsymbol{y} - \hat{\boldsymbol{y}})^T (\boldsymbol{y} - \hat{\boldsymbol{y}})}{n-k}$ (the residual variance). From the joint Student-t distribution, we can derive the marginal posterior distribution for individual coefficients:

$$\beta_j | \boldsymbol{y}, \boldsymbol{X} \sim t(\hat{\beta}_j, s^2 c_{jj}, n - k)$$

where c_{jj} is the jth diagonal element of the un-scaled variance-covariance matrix $((\boldsymbol{X}^T \boldsymbol{X})^{-1})$. In other words, $\frac{\beta_j - \hat{\beta}_j}{s \sqrt{c_{jj}}} \sim t(df = n - k)$. In nearly all statistical software, estimated regression model coefficients are linked to their respective estimation standard errors (which are $s\sqrt{c_{jj}}$), t-statistics (which are the t-statistic for testing the null hypothesis of $\beta_j = 0$ or $t_j = \frac{\hat{\beta}_j - 0}{s \sqrt{c_{jj}}}$), and p-values (the two-sided tail area of t_j, or in R `2*(1-pt(abs(tj), n-k))`).

The posterior marginal distribution of σ^2 is a scaled inverse chi-squared distribution

$$\sigma^2 | \boldsymbol{y}, \boldsymbol{X} \sim Scaled\text{-}\chi^{-2}(\nu, \tau^2). \tag{4.11}$$

That is, $\sigma^2/(\nu s^2)$ is a $\chi^{-2}(\nu)$ random variable, where $\nu = n-k$ is the degree of freedom and $\tau^2 = s^2$ is the scale parameter. The scaled inverse chi-squared distribution and the inverse gamma distribution describe the same distribution. Specifically, the density of $\chi^{-2}(\nu, \tau^2)$ is the same as the density of $IG(\alpha = \nu/2, \beta = \nu\tau^2/2)$. Because the inverse gamma distribution is more intuitive for some, the conjugate prior for a normal distribution variance is often specified as $IG(a_0/2, b_0/2)$ and the posterior of σ^2 as inverse gamma $(a_n/2, b_n/2)$, such that $a_n = a_0 + n$ and $b_n = b_0 + (\boldsymbol{y}^T\boldsymbol{y} + \boldsymbol{\mu}_0^T\boldsymbol{\Gamma}_0\boldsymbol{\mu}_0 - \boldsymbol{\mu}_n^T\boldsymbol{\Gamma}_n\boldsymbol{\mu}_n)/2$.

The R functions `sim` (from package `arm`) and `posterior` (from package `rv`) draw random samples of σ^2 and $\boldsymbol{\beta}$ from their posterior distributions (equations (4.10) and (4.11)) from a linear model object fitted with linear model function `lm()`.

Let's now use data from the PCB in one species of fish, lake trout, as an example to explore using R functions `lm()` and `posterior` for Bayesian regression. The data for lake trout were discussed in detail by Qian [2016], including the use of simulation to explore the posterior distributions of $\boldsymbol{\beta}$ and σ^2. Because many quantities used in Bayesian regression posteriors are calculated and stored in the linear model (`lm()`) output, we start the Bayesian regression model by first fitting a simple linear regression model:

```
#### R Code ####
lake.lm1 <- lm(log(pcb) ~ length, data=laketrout)
### End ###
```

The linear model object `lake.lm1` includes the fitted model coefficients ($\hat{\boldsymbol{\beta}} = (\boldsymbol{X}^T\boldsymbol{X})^{-1}\boldsymbol{X}^T\boldsymbol{y}$) and the summary function returns a list, including the unscaled covariance matrix ($(\boldsymbol{X}^T\boldsymbol{X})^{-1}$, `cov.unscaled`) and $s = \sqrt{\frac{(\boldsymbol{y}-\hat{\boldsymbol{y}})^T(\boldsymbol{y}-\hat{\boldsymbol{y}})}{n-k}}$ (`sigma`).

Random samples from the posterior distributions of σ^2 and $\boldsymbol{\beta}$ can be generated by generating χ^2 random variates, followed by multivariate normal random variates:

```
#### R Code ####
nsims <- 5000
summ <- summary(lake_lm1)
beta_hat <- coef(lake_lm1)
V_beta <- summ$cov.unscaled
n <- sum(summ$df[1:2])
k <- summ$df[1]
sigma <- summ$sigma


## random numbers of sigma
rsigma <- sigma * sqrt((n - k)/rchisq(nsims, n-k))
hist(rsigma)


## random numbers for beta
```

```
beta <- array(NA, c(nsims, k))
dimnames(beta) <- list(NULL, rownames(beta_hat))
for (i in 1:nsims){
    beta[i, ] <- MASS::mvrnorm(1, beta_hat, V_beta *
                                rsigma[i]^2)
}
### End ###
```

This process of drawing random numbers from the posterior distributions is implemented in the function `posterior` from package `rv`.

```
#### R Code ####
require(rv)
setnsims(5000)
lakeM1_rv <- posterior(lake.lm1)
### End ###
```

The function returns a list of two "random variable" (rv) objects:

```
#### R Output ####
> lakeM1_rv
$beta
          name  mean     sd    1%   2.5%    25%    50%    75%  97.5%    99%
(Intercept) -1.95 0.170 -2.36 -2.28  -2.07  -1.95  -1.84  -1.62  -1.55
   size_cm   0.05 0.003  0.04  0.04   0.04   0.05   0.05   0.05   0.05

$sigma
      mean    sd    1%  2.5%   25%   50%   75%  97.5%   99%
[1]   0.8  0.022  0.75  0.75  0.78  0.79  0.81   0.84  0.85
### End ###
```

The `rv` object `sigma` consists of 5000 random samples from the posterior distribution of σ. But these samples are represented by a scalar object. Likewise, the `rv` object `beta` represents a matrix of random samples of the two regression coefficients. The object is presented as a vector of two random variables and can be used in R as a vector.

To evaluate the risk of PCB exposure, we are interested in the PCB concentration distribution for a given sized fish – the posterior predictive distribution of log PCB concentration of a fish with a given size $\tilde{x}$: $\pi(\tilde{y}|\tilde{x}, Y) = \int_{\Theta} \pi(\beta_0, \beta_1, \sigma^2|Y)d\Theta$. To be consistent with the matrix notation, we use $\tilde{x}$ to represent the design matrix of new covariates (e.g., size of multiple fish). The distribution of the predicted log-PCB $\tilde{y}$ is called the posterior predictive distribution. It is a multivariate Student-t distribution:

$$\tilde{y}|\tilde{x} \sim t(\tilde{x}\hat{\beta}, s^2(I + \tilde{x}(X^T X)^{-1}\tilde{x}^T), n - k).$$

The predictive distribution can be evaluated using the random numbers generated from the posterior distributions of β and σ.

```
#### R Code & Output ####
tildeX <- c(50, 60, 70, 80, 90)
lakeM1_rv <- posterior(lake.lm1)
lakeM1_pred <- rvnorm(1,
    lakeM1_rv$beta[1]+lakeM1_rv$beta[2]*tildeX,
    lakeM1_rv$sigma)

lakeM1_pred

     mean   sd   1%   2.5%   25%  50%  75% 97.5% 99% sims
[1] 0.34 0.81 -1.57 -1.22 -0.21 0.34 0.88   1.9 2.2 5000
[2] 0.81 0.79 -1.00 -0.74  0.27 0.80 1.34   2.4 2.7 5000
[3] 1.25 0.80 -0.66 -0.33  0.71 1.25 1.80   2.8 3.1 5000
[4] 1.71 0.80 -0.16  0.12  1.18 1.72 2.25   3.3 3.5 5000
[5] 2.16 0.79  0.37  0.64  1.62 2.16 2.69   3.7 4.0 5000
### End ###
```

The probability of PCB concentration exceeding a threshold, for example 1 mg/kg, is obtained by using the function `Pr`:

```
### R code ###
Pr(exp(lakeM1_pred) > 1)
### End ###
```

As we stated earlier, the Bayesian regression estimator using non-informative priors is similar to the least-squares estimator. The 95% equal-tail credible intervals of the Bayesian predictive distribution of PCB concentrations are represented by the 2.5% and 97.5% quantiles. The 95% predictive confidence intervals from the classical regression model is calculated based on the sampling distribution, which is implemented in the generic R function `predict()`:

```
#### R code & output ####
tildeX <- data.frame(size_cm=c(50, 60, 70, 80, 90))
lm1_pred <- predict(lake.lm1, newdata=tildeX), se.fit=T,
                    interval="prediction")

> lm1_pred$fit
$fit
        fit         lwr       upr
1 0.2879076 -1.2353261 1.811141
2 0.7774833 -0.7444259 2.299392
3 1.2670590 -0.2552655 2.789384
4 1.7566348  0.2321564 3.281113
5 2.2462105  0.7178472 3.774574
### End ###
```

4.3.2 Nonlinear Regression Models

A general analytic result (e.g., using conjugate priors) for a Bayesian nonlinear regression problem is impossible because the likelihoods that admit conjugate distributions correspond to data distributions that are members of the exponential family. Having a non-linear function of the parameters in the log-likelihood makes it impossible for deriving conjugate priors for model coefficients. As a result, Bayesian nonlinear regression is largely a post-MCMC phenomenon. In principle, implementing a nonlinear regression model using MCMC should be the same as implementing a linear model except the mean function is a nonlinear one. Using the nonlinear regression calibration problem discussed in Qian [2016] as an example, we illustrate the use of MCMC for a nonlinear regression problem. Furthermore, we use this example to discuss the missing data problem related to nearly all modern analytic chemistry analyses.

4.3.2.1 Calibration-Curve Methods

In statistics, the problem of calibration refers to the problem of estimating the unknown predictor variable values based on observed response variable data in a regression problem. Calibration is used in nearly all instrumental methods for measuring the concentration of an analyte. In a typical calibration method, concentrations of the analyte are measured indirectly through an intermediate process, where a number of standard solutions with known concentrations are used in a controlled reaction with another chemical. The reaction results in color or other changes that can be automatically quantified by a sensor. The resulting readings of the sensor are used as the response variable data and the known concentrations of the standard solutions are used as the predictor variable data to fit an empirical (regression) model. The model can be linear or nonlinear, depending on the nature of the chemical reaction. In all cases, the measured instrumental response is a monotonic function of the analyte concentration. The fitted model is often called the standard curve or the calibration curve. Samples with unknown concentrations are put through the same reaction process and the sensor readings are recorded. These readings are used to estimate the unknown concentrations, most commonly, using the inverse function of the regression model. Only a limited number of samples can fit into a typical instrument. As a result, the number of standard solutions is limited to a small number to allow more analyte samples to be fit into the instrument. In a typical specialized lab, a large number of similar analysis are run on a regular basis. Each time when the same analysis is repeated, a new calibration curve is fit, because the sensors used in these instruments can be influenced by many environmental factors such as temperature and humidity. Consequently, statistical features of a calibration curve are an important consideration.

In statistical terms, a calibration curve is an empirical relationship between the instrumental responses and the analyte concentration. A calibration problem consists of two steps. First, a regression model $y_i = f(x_i, \boldsymbol{\theta}) + \epsilon_i$ is fit, where x_i is the known concentration of a standard solution, y_i is the measured instrumental response, $f(\cdot)$ is a linear or nonlinear function with parameter vector $\boldsymbol{\theta}$, and ϵ is the model error term often assumed to be a normal random variable with mean 0 and a constant variance. Fitting the standard curve with data from the standard solutions results in the estimated model parameters $\hat{\boldsymbol{\theta}}$. Second, instrumental responses (y_0) of the solution with unknown analyte concentration (x_0) are used to derive an estimate of the unknown concentration $(\hat{x}_0)$, typically using the inverse function of the resulting standard curve: $\hat{x}_0 = f^{-1}(y_0, \hat{\boldsymbol{\theta}})$. Statistical calibration studies are aimed at finding an estimator for x_0, including its sampling distribution. A typical standard curve is either a linear ($y_i = \beta_0 + \beta_1 x_i + \epsilon_i$ and $\boldsymbol{\theta} = \{\beta_0, \beta_1\}$) or a sigmoid curve (e.g., the four-parameter logistic function, $y_i = \theta_4 + (\theta_1 - \theta_4)/\left[1 + (x_i/\theta_3)^{\theta_2}\right] + \epsilon_i$ and $\boldsymbol{\theta} = \{\theta_1, \theta_2, \theta_3, \theta_4\}$).

In most calibration problems, the sample size used to fit the calibration curve is usually small (e.g., $i = 1, \cdots, 6$). A regression model fit with a small sample size may often show favorable goodness-of-fit statistics (e.g., R^2, often used as a quality control criterion) but is inherently unreliable when the fitted model is used as a tool for measuring unknown concentrations. Furthermore, the sampling distribution of the estimated unknown concentration from a linear calibration curve has an infinite expected variance (regardless of the sample size used to fit the calibration curve). In other words, increasing the sample size in fitting the calibration curve is unlikely to reduce the estimation uncertainty [Osborne, 1991]. Although no general theoretical results are available for nonlinear calibration problems, we do not expect better outcomes than the linear calibration ones.

The calibration-curve method commonly used to measure concentrations of cyanobacterial toxin (various congeners of microcystin, or MC) is an enzyme-linked immunosorbent assay (ELISA), in which microcystin molecules in standard solutions react with the enzyme-linked antibody attached to the inner wall of the testing wells resulting in changes in the color of the solution. The change in color is recorded by a sensor. The instrument-recorded values (known as the optical density) are linked to the MC concentration through a nonlinear regression model.

Typically, measurement is done using a commercial test kit, which comes in the form of a testing plate with 96 wells (small test tubes) coated with the necessary chemicals on the inner walls of these wells. The kit comes with standard solutions with known MC concentrations. Typically, two replicates of six standard solutions are used in each plate to produce data needed for fitting the calibration curve. Properly processed water samples with unknown MC concentrations are put in the remaining 84 wells. In other words, a commercial kit can be used to analyze up to 42 water samples.

4.3.2.2 The Toledo Water Crisis of 2014

On August 1, 2014, one drinking water sample from the drinking water treatment plant of the City of Toledo, Ohio, USA, was found to have a microcystin (MC) concentration nearly 2.5 μg/L, exceeding the drinking water quality standard of 1 μg/L. The lab reanalyzed the water samples two times to confirm the abnormally high concentration on the same day. The city issued a "Do-Not-Drink" advisory on the following day, affecting nearly 500,000 residents for three days.

On August 2, 2014, the City of Toledo tested drinking water samples collected throughout the city. Additional water samples were also analyzed by labs operated by Lake Superior State University, Ohio Environmental Protection Agency, and U.S. EPA. All tests showed that MC concentrations were below the threshold MC concentration of 1 μg/L.

Microcystins are a class of over 50 toxins (congeners) produced by certain freshwater cyanobacteria (commonly known as blue-green algae). They can cause serious liver damage. A U.S. EPA report cites a study showing that 80 percent of samples in Canada and U.S. were positive for microcystins and 4.3 percent were above the World Health Organization (WHO) guideline of 1 μg/L [U.S. EPA, 2015].

4.3.2.3 ELISA Test Data

Raw data from a total of six ELISA tests were made available to the public after the Toledo Water Crisis.[1] The first test that reported the high MC concentration was performed in the afternoon of August 1, 2014. Immediately, two more sets of tests were carried out and completed around 9:15 pm on the same day. On August 2, 2014, the Toledo Water Treatment Plant used three additional test kits to analyze drinking water samples collected throughout the city and performed three more sets of tests. We use data from these six tests to illustrate the Bayesian nonlinear modeling and the Bayesian missing data problem.

The software accompanying the test kit provides the option to use the four-parameter logit function as the calibration curve. Because the test kit comes with standard solutions including one with a concentration of 0, the four-parameter logistic function used by the test kit is defined in the concentration scale (equation (4.12)). The zero-concentration solution is meant for calculating the baseline instrumental response.

$$y = \theta_4 + \frac{\theta_1 - \theta_4}{1 + (x/\theta_3)^{-\theta_2}} + \epsilon \tag{4.12}$$

In equation (4.12), θ_1 and θ_4 are the lower (when $x \to \infty$) and upper (when $x = 0$) bounds of the curve, θ_3 is the x value when the expected value of y is $(\theta_1 + \theta_2)/2$, and $\theta_2 > 0$ is the shape parameter. This model can be fit

---

[1]https://tinyurl.com/4363xd9f

using the R function `nls` with the self-starter function in Qian [2016, Chapter 6]. We note that the four-parameter logistic function defined in Qian [2016, equation (6.4)] $\left(y = \alpha_4 + \frac{\alpha_1 - \alpha_4}{1+(x/\alpha_3)^{\alpha_2}} + \varepsilon\right)$ uses α_4 as the lower bound and α_1 as the upper bound of the curve. There is no advantage of using the Bayesian method if fitting the model is the only goal. The advantage of the Bayesian estimation method is in the estimation of unknown concentrations. That is, the unknown concentration of x_0 associated with the observed response of y_0. When using the fitted coefficients (i.e., $\hat{\boldsymbol{\theta}}$), the inverse solution of x_0 does not exist when the observed y_0 is outside of the range defined by the estimated θ_4 and θ_1. Furthermore, the estimator of x_0 based on the inverse function of equation (4.12)

$$\hat{x}_0 = \hat{\theta}_3 \left(\frac{\hat{\theta}_1 - y_0}{y_0 - \hat{\theta}_4}\right)^{-1/\hat{\theta}_2}$$

can be unstable when the measured response y_0 approaches either $\hat{\theta}_1$ or $\hat{\theta}_4$, suggesting a potentially high variance in the estimated x_0.

The current practice is to first fit the calibration curve and then estimate the unknown concentrations. An oft-encountered problem in practice is that the water sample response y_0 can be larger than the estimated upper bound $\hat{\theta}_4$ or less than the estimated lower bound $\hat{\theta}_1$, resulting in a negative base of the exponential term in the inverse function. Concentrations for these water samples are reported as censored (or failed quality control), either less than the lowest non-zero standard solution concentration or larger than the largest standard solution concentration. The measurements (y_0's) are, however, not censored. Using only data from the standard solutions disregards information from the measured responses of water samples. In this case, the collection of y and y_0 should be used to inform the potential range of the curve. In statistics, this problem is addressed by treating x_0 as a missing data point to be estimated together with model coefficients, by specifying the likelihood function as a function of model coefficients and the unknown concentration values.

Let $y_1, \cdots, y_k$ be the k response (optical density) values measured from the k known concentrations $x_1, \cdots, x_k$, and $y_{01}, \cdots, y_{0J}$ be the J measured optical density values of the J samples with unknown concentrations $x_{0j}, \cdots, x_{0J}$. The likelihood function based on equation (4.12) is:

$$L = \prod_{i=1}^{k} \left(\frac{1}{\sqrt{2\pi}\sigma} e^{-\frac{(y_i - f(\boldsymbol{\theta}, x_i))^2}{2\sigma^2}}\right) \times \prod_{j=1}^{J} \frac{1}{\sqrt{2\pi}\sigma} e^{-\frac{(y_{0j} - f(\boldsymbol{\theta}, x_{0j}))^2}{2\sigma^2}} \tag{4.13}$$

where $\boldsymbol{\theta}$ represents the vector of model coefficients and σ^2 is the residual variance.

Using the maximum likelihood method to simultaneously estimate $\boldsymbol{\theta}$ and x_0 is computationally challenging. In a Bayesian missing data problem, we multiply the likelihood function by priors of $\boldsymbol{\theta}$ and $\boldsymbol{x}_0$ to derive the joint posterior distribution of x_0 and $\boldsymbol{\theta}$. As Stan works with log-likelihood (a sum of two summations):

$$LL = -(k+J)\log(\sigma) - \frac{\sum_{i=1}^{k}(y_i - f(\boldsymbol{\theta}, x_i))^2 + \sum_{j=1}^{J}(y_{0j} - f(\boldsymbol{\theta}, x_{0j}))^2}{2\sigma^2}.$$

In Stan, the simplest way to write the likelihood function is to use the `normal_lpdf` function, one for standard solutions and one for water samples with unknown concentrations.

The four-parameter logistic function is quite flexible, which made nonlinear regression with non-informative flat priors quite difficult for MCMC. For example, in equation (4.12), θ_1 is the lower bound of the curve and θ_4 is the upper bound (i.e., $\theta_1 < \theta_4$), the negative exponent (i.e., $\theta_2 > 0$) defines a rapid descending curve as concentration x increases. The same curve can be parameterized by using θ_1 as the upper bound and θ_4 as the lower bound of the curve (i.e., set $\theta_1 > \theta_4$, as in equation (6.4) of Qian [2016]), as long as the exponent is positive (changing $(\frac{x}{\theta_3})^{-\theta_2}$ to $(\frac{x}{\theta_3})^{\theta_2}$ in the denominator of the equation). In programming the Stan model, we need to explicitly define whether θ_1 or θ_4 is the lower bound of the curve. In our Stan model, we explicitly define θ_1 as the lower bound of y (close to 0) and introduce $\delta = \theta_4 - \theta_1$ as the positive distance between the upper and lower bounds. The four-parameter logistic function is defined using $\theta_1, \delta, \theta_2$, and θ_3. All of them are positive. The upper bound θ_4 is modeled as a transformed parameter ($\theta_4 = \theta_1 + \delta$) in Stan. The reparameterized model to beis expressed as $y = \theta_4 - \frac{\delta}{1+(x/\theta_3)^{-\theta_2}} + \epsilon$. The limited number of unique known concentration values made it necessary to use proper informative prior distributions of model coefficients to ensure numerical stability. Based on the description of the test kit, we know that all four coefficients are of limited magnitude, typically well within 2. The response y is between 0 (when the concentration approaches infinity) and approximately 1 or 2 (when the concentration is 0), depending on the type of the instrument (plate readers) for reading the optical density. As such, the prior for θ_1 can be a truncated normal distribution with mean 0 and a small standard deviation (e.g., 0.5). We can also use positive half-normal $N(0,2)$ for θ_2 and θ_3. The prior for δ can be a truncated normal (e.g., $N(1,1)$). The unknown water sample MC concentrations are unlikely to have a large variance, especially most of the water samples are treated drinking water. We used the positive half of $N(0, 2.5)$, a relatively wide distribution compared to the commonly seen MC concentrations.

```
### Default ELISA model
### Stan Model (single test kit)
ELISA1 <- "
data {
int<lower=0> N; // sample size (standard solutions)
int<lower=0> M; // observed ODs from water samples
real y[N]; // response data
```

```
real x[N]; // predictor data
real<lower=0> dlf[M]; // dilution factor
real y0[M]; // water sample response
int MM; // # of unique water samples
int ws[M]; // water samples (with replicates)
}
parameters {
real<lower=0> delta;
real<lower=0> th1;
real<lower=0> th2;
real<lower=0> th3;
real<lower=0> sigma;
real<lower=0> x0[MM];
}
transformed parameters{
real mu[N];
real mu0[M];
real<lower=0> th4;
th4 = th1 + delta;
for (i in 1:N){
  mu[i] = th4 - (delta)/(1+(x[i]/th3)^(-th2));
}
for (i in 1:M){
  mu0[i] = th4 -
          (delta)/(1+((x0[ws[i]]/dlf[i])/th3)^(-th2));
  }
}
model {
x0 ~ normal(0,2.5);
delta~normal(1,1);
th1~normal(0,0.5);
th2~normal(0,2);
th3~normal(0,2);
target += normal_lpdf(y | mu, sigma);
target += normal_lpdf(y0 | mu0, sigma);
}
"
```

End

In the code, we used an integer variable ws[i] to indicate that observation i is associated with water sample ws[i]. In the data, most water
samples had replicates. Some water samples were diluted in anticipation of
high MC concentrations. For each observed optical density value, we use
dlf to record their dilution factor (dlf=1 without dilution). As each water sample has only one unknown concentration, the unknown concentration enters in the code as x0[ws[i]]/dlf[i]. (Later in Section 4.3.2.4, the

four-parameter logistic function is defined in log concentration, the code is changed to x0[ws[i]]-log(dlf[i]).) That is, our program will return only one concentration value for each unique water sample. In the ELISA kit, the default model calculates a concentration value for each optical density observation. For each water sample, the test kit will return two concentration values if no dilutions were included. For each additional dilution of the same water sample, the ELISA kit will return two additional concentration values.

The classical nonlinear regression for this problem is computationally much simpler in R because of the self-starter function developed in Qian [2016]. However, there is no efficient computational method for the maximum likelihood estimator of the unknown concentrations. The current practice in analytic chemistry of using the inverse function to calculate the missing concentration does not account for the large predictive uncertainty of a regression model fit with a small sample size. This high level of uncertainty was shown to be reflected in the highly variable estimates [Qian et al., 2015a]. Furthermore, when a water sample has an optical density (y_0) above (or below) the estimated upper bound $\hat{\theta}_4$ (or lower bound $\hat{\theta}_1$), the inverse function fails. When a concentration is reported as larger than the largest concentration of the standard solutions (in Toledo's test kit, it is 5.550 μg/L), the estimate is often reported as a sample which failed the quality control measure. The same water sample will be diluted and included in the next batch of water samples in a subsequent test. From a statistical modeling perspective, the "failure" lies in the disregard of the information in the measured response y_0 when developing the calibration curve.

Comparing the estimated water sample concentrations using the current nonlinear regression (through inverse function method) and the Bayesian model, we note that the difference between the two sets of concentrations is small (Figure 4.12). Although the Bayesian model fitting process is a few minutes longer, the added computational time is well compensated considering that the Bayesian method would avoid the "censorship" problem, thereby avoiding re-run water samples with "censored" results with dilution.

4.3.2.4 Alternative Parameterization

The four-parameter logistic function can also be defined on the log-concentration scale and the expression is:

$$y = A + \frac{B - A}{1 + e^{\frac{x_{mid} - z}{s_{cal}}}} \tag{4.14}$$

where y is the observed optical density, $z = \log(x)$ is the log MC concentration, model coefficients A and B define the upper and lower bounds of the curve, s_{cal} is the scale parameter (similar to θ_2 in equation (4.12)) defining the shape of the curve, and x_{mid} is the location parameter (similar to θ_3 in equation (4.12)) defining the predictor location where the response is at the middle of the interval bounded by B and A. Nummer et al. [2018] compared the estimation

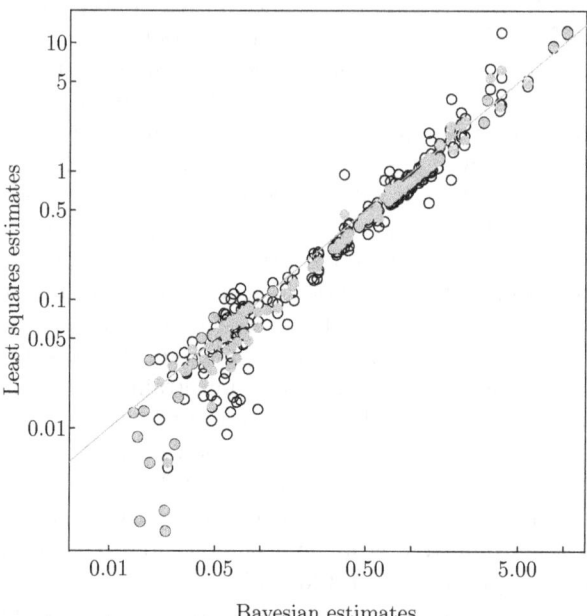

FIGURE 4.12: A scatter plot compares the estimated water sample MC concentrations based on the least-squares and inverse-function method (y-axis) and the Bayesian nonlinear missing value method (x-axis, the posterior mean). The Bayesian method returns one estimate for each unique water sample (filled gray circles), while the least-squares method returns multiple estimates (for replicates and dilutions, open circles).

uncertainties between the two forms of four-parameter logistic functions and concluded that using equation (4.14) had reduced the estimation uncertainty in the least squares estimated MC concentrations. The improved estimation is likely because the sigmoid curve of equation (4.14) in the ELISA problem is of less curvature than is the curve of equation (4.12) [Nummer et al., 2018]. One practical issue was that the function is undefined at concentration of 0. For the data in this example, we attempted three numerical approaches.

- The limit of y (Limit). In the logarithmic scale, the limit of y when the concentration approaches 0 (or $z \to -\infty$) is A. We can define y to be A when the concentration is 0:

$$y = \begin{cases} A + \epsilon & \text{if } x = 0 \\ A + \dfrac{B-A}{1+e^{\frac{x_{mid}-z}{s_{cal}}}} + \epsilon & \text{otherwise} \end{cases}$$

However, this modification creates a discontinuity in the function. (Nummer et al. [2018] recommended that the ELISA kit manufacturer should include a low concentration standard solution to replace the one with a concentration of 0.)

- Regarding 0 as a small value (0.0001). We replace 0 with a small value (e.g., 0.0001). This approach is not ideal as we must decide what value is small enough and yet does not introduce numerical problems.

- Removing 0 concentrations (NAs). We will have a different collection of instrumental response values. The removal may directly influence the estimated upper bound (A) if the removed values include the maximum observed response variable value. Furthermore, the already small sample size for the regression model will be smaller.

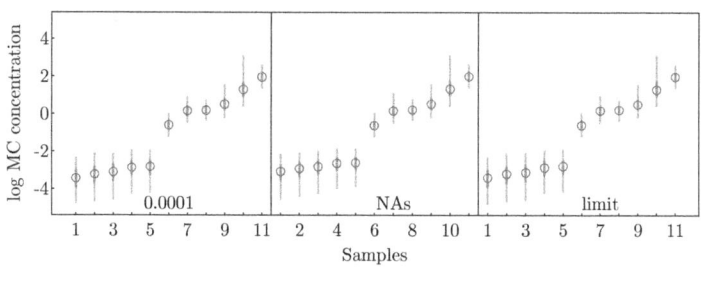

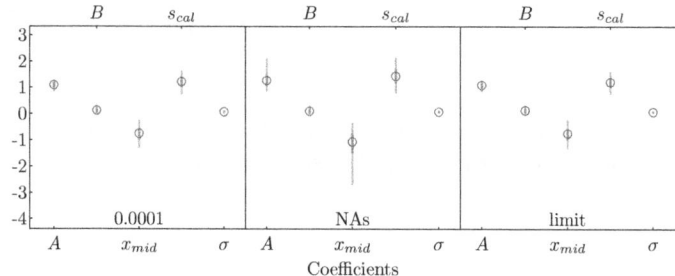

FIGURE 4.13: Marginal posterior distributions of model coefficients (bottom row) and the unknown MC log concentrations from 11 water samples (top row) are compared among three alternative computational approaches of incorporating 0 concentration solutions.

Using data from the second ELISA test conducted in the evening of August 1, 2014 (with 11 unique water samples), we compared the three numerical treatments. The estimated marginal posterior distributions of model coefficients and the predictive distributions of concentrations of the 11 water samples are similar (Figure 4.13). The only noticeable difference is that the estimated model coefficients with 0 concentration removed are of slightly wider marginal posterior distributions, especially of A and x_{mid}. For each test, a quality control sample with an MC concentration of 0.75 μg/L was included. We compared the estimated quality control sample concentrations for each of the six tests using the three alternative methods, as well as the model of equation (4.12) (Figure 4.14). All models resulted in comparable results. The result, however, should not be viewed as showing that the ELISA standard curve should be fit to the concentration scale, because all three treatments of the 0 concentration samples are not ideal, especially removing 0 from the data, which reduced the already small sample size. The experiment presented in Nummer et al. [2018], where existing standard solutions were diluted to create a series of water samples with known MC concentrations (including a solution with a low MC concentration of 0.05 μg/L), was designed for such comparisons.

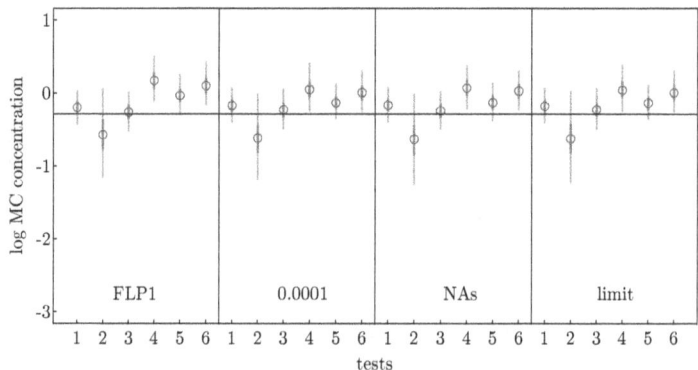

FIGURE 4.14: Marginal posterior distributions of MC concentration of the quality control sample for six ELISA tests are compared.

4.4   Fitting a Hierarchical Model Sequentially

When reviewing Qian and Reckhow [2007], we realized that the sequential updating process we discussed in Chapter 3 (page 73) may not be the appropriate interpretation of the U.S. Clean Water Act (CWA). The law requires a periodical assessment of waters in the United States because water quality status changes over time. As such, we are to evaluate the status of water quality over a time period. The estimated parameters using the updating process we discussed in Chapter 2 quantify the predictive distributions of total nitrogen and chlorophyll-a concentrations based on all available data up to the year when updating was done, rather than detecting changes from year to year (Figure 4.15). If periodical assessments are intended to identify temporal changes in water quality, an estimate of the long-term concentration distribution would not serve the purpose well. Because most water quality assessments are done based on annual summer samples, we should estimate annual distributions of TN and Chla in this case.

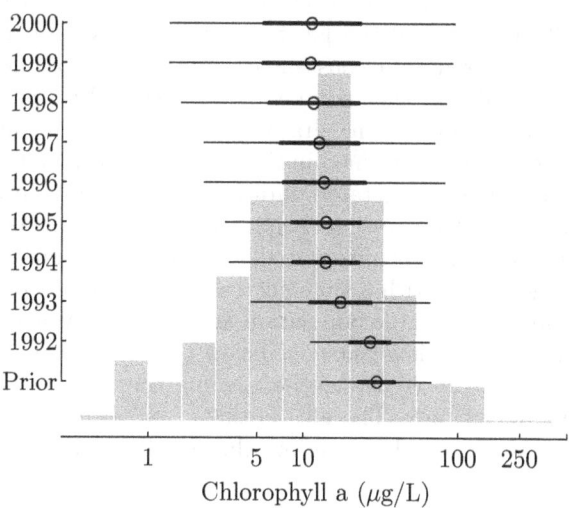

FIGURE 4.15: Sequentially updated estimate of the long-term chlorophyll *a* concentration distributions are compared to all available data from 1992 to 2000 (shaded histogram). The annual updated estimates represent the posterior distribution updated using data up to the time of updating. The posterior distributions are represented by their means (open circles), middle 50% credible intervals (thick lines), and 95% middle credible intervals (thin lines).

More importantly, our estimation should address the legal requirement of a compliance assessment. In this case, the specific law governing the assessment is Section 303(d) of CWA. The U.S. Environmental Protection Agency (EPA) is responsible for the enforcement of the law through developing regulatory rules. Statistics is an important part of the compliance assessment process as we are interested in making inference about the underlying levels of pollution using a limited number of samples. The U.S. EPA defines the process in terms of magnitude, duration, and frequency (MDF), recognizing that the compliance assessment process is a process of making a binary decision under uncertainty.

Discussions about the MDF framework for standard compliance assessment are often unclear, especially with regard to the underlying statistical reasons. The earliest (and the most explicit) discussion of MDF appeared in

Stephan et al. [1985], which explained that the magnitude is the pollutant concentration associated with protecting the designated uses of the water body. For many pollutants, this magnitude is determined based on toxicity studies as the concentration level that will not impair a water body's ability to support aquatic life. The duration or averaging period is defined as the length of time over which one averages environmental measurement of the pollutant when determining whether a water body complies with the standard. The duration was introduced to bridge the difference between the natural conditions, where concentration fluctuates, and the lab test conditions, where the test organisms are usually exposed to a constant concentration. Specifically, Stephan et al. [1985] explained that the arithmetic means should be used to represent the exposure of organisms in a natural water (where concentrations vary) to compare the magnitude determined in the lab. When using an average as the estimate of the mean over the stated duration, we inevitably introduce uncertainty to the assessment process. A sample average is an unbiased estimate of the population mean. That is, if repeatedly sampled to obtain a large number of sample averages, each with a different value, the average of these sample averages will approach the true population mean. For a given sample average, we are uncertain whether it is above or below the true mean. As a result, an allowed frequency of sample averages exceeding the standard is specified to account for this uncertainty. The idea is that if only a small fraction of the sample averages are above the criterion, the true mean is likely to be below the criterion.

Specifying the appropriate frequency component of a criterion can be challenging due largely to the lack of a consistent definition. Stephan et al. [1985] explained that such frequency is to provide a time for an ecosystem to recover from occasional exceedances and suggested that "most aquatic ecosystems can probably recover from most exceedances in about 3 years." (We did not find any reference supporting this statement.) Accordingly, a default frequency of no more than one exceedance in 3 years is recommended [Stephan et al., 1985]. However, Stephan et al. [1985] also explained that the recommended acceptable exceedance frequency of no more than once in 3 years is equivalent to a recurring probability as used in describing flow and precipitation (e.g., a 100-year flood has a recurring frequency of 1 in 100 years or the probability of such flood occurring in a year is 0.01). Using this probabilistic interpretation, we can interpret the frequency component as a specific quantile of the sampling (or posterior) distribution of a sample average. For example, one exceedance in three years represents a frequency of $F = 1/3$ and no more than one exceedance in three years suggests that the $1 - F$ quantile of the sampling distribution is less than or equal to the respective standard. From a Bayesian estimation perspective, we should use the posterior distribution of the annual mean.

Let y_{ij} be the ith observation from the jth year. Estimating annual distribution separately can be represented by

$$y_{ij} \sim N(\theta_j, \sigma^2). \tag{4.15}$$

In assessing water quality compliance for each year, we estimate the probability of θ_j exceeding the designated environmental standard. When parameters θ_j and σ_j^2 are estimated separately using only data from the jth year, we often have small sample sizes which lead to large estimation uncertainty. Furthermore, we assume that data from each year are unrelated. Data were measured from samples taken from the same water body; there should be some connections among years because of the shared environment (e.g., weather and climate conditions, land use patterns in the watershed). However, without detailed knowledge of the area, especially knowledge of what happened in the past, we may not be able to identify how the water quality status would have changed over time. As a result, selecting priors for θ_j and σ_j^2 for each year is a difficult task. As in most cases discussed in this chapter, we are ignorant of how the means and variances change over the years. A natural way to model this level of ignorance is to impose a common prior on θ_j and a common σ^2 for all years. That is, using a Bayesian hierarchical model represented by equations (4.15) and (4.16).

$$\theta_j \sim N(\mu, \tau^2) \tag{4.16}$$

The normal distribution on the right-hand side of Equation (4.16) is the "hyper-distribution," similar to the ANOVA problem in the Seaweed grazer example (see equation (4.2) on page 92). It represents the distribution of annual mean concentrations. When fitting the model using data from multiple years, we can use weakly informative priors on both μ and τ^2. The resulting posterior distributions of μ and τ^2 specify the prior distribution of each year's mean. Because the prior is specified from existing data, this approach is also known as the empirical Bayes approach. When data from the next year are available, we can naturally use the hyper-distribution specified by μ and τ^2 as the prior. In other words, the annual assessment process can be simplified as a Bayesian modeling process using informative priors specified based on data from previous years. The updated distributions of μ and τ^2 are then the priors for the following year's assessment. We now simplify the notation by dropping the index for the year (j). The observed log concentration data follow a normal distribution:

$$y_i \sim N(\theta, \sigma^2).$$

The prior distribution of θ is

$$\theta \sim N(\mu, \tau^2).$$

Using conjugate priors for μ, τ^2 and σ^2, we can specify the full Bayesian model by adding the following:

$$
\begin{aligned}
p(\sigma^2) &\sim IG(a, b) \\
p(\tau^2) &\sim IG(\alpha, \beta) \\
p(\mu|\tau^2) &\sim N(\mu_0, \tau^2/n_0).
\end{aligned}
$$

Box and Tiao [1973] derived the conditional posterior distributions of μ and θ (both are normal). Although the analytic form of the joint marginal posterior of σ^2 and τ^2 is available, it cannot be represented by any known probability distribution. Box and Tiao [1973] suggested that the marginal distributions of σ^2 and τ^2 can be approximated by the scaled inverse-χ^2 distribution. As a result, using the normal-inverse-gamma conjugate family of priors for μ and τ^2 is reasonable. In practice, we can estimate the necessary prior distribution parameters $(\mu_0, n_0, \alpha, \beta, a, b)$, initially, by using model estimates as in Qian and Reckhow [2007] or data from multiple years under a hierarchical model. Using MCMC, we obtain posterior samples of μ, τ^2, and σ^2. These samples allow us to calculate their means and variances. Using the method of moments we can estimate the prior distribution parameters for the next year. Thus, we have a sequential updating process, where the annual mean distribution, as well as the hyper-parameters, are updated over time. For any given year, the environmental standard compliance assessment should be based on the posterior distribution of θ. The updating process can start with a relatively vague joint prior for τ^2 and μ. As a comparison, we fit a hierarchical model using all available data from 1979 to 2000. Using the Stan default non-informative priors for the three parameters (σ^2, μ, τ^2), we estimate the annual means (θ_j). The sequential updating method differs from the hierarchical model in that the within-year variance (σ) is estimated based on annual data. In other words, equation (4.15) should be $y_{ij} \sim N(\theta_j, \sigma_j^2)$. We start the updating process by using a relatively vague prior: $\alpha = 0.5, \beta = 0.5$, and $\mu_0 = 1, n_0 = 2$. The sequentially estimated annual means are very close to the Bayesian hierarchical model estimated annual means (Figure 4.16).

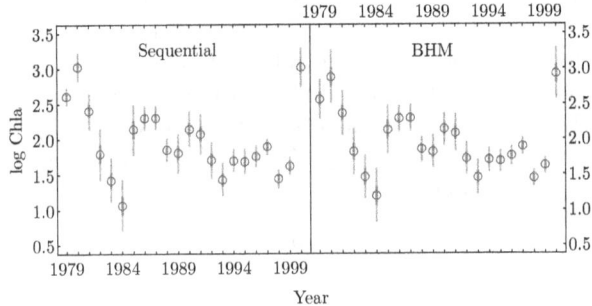

FIGURE 4.16: Sequentially updated estimates of annual chlorophyll a concentration distributions using the sequential updating process (left panel) and the Bayesian hierarchical model (BHM; right panel) are compared.

By sequentially updating the hyper-distribution parameters, we now have a process that is more in line with the legal requirement. The sequentially updated posterior distributions of μ and τ^2 move toward the same posterior distribution estimated using all available data together (based on equations (4.15) and (4.16)). The estimated annual mean distributions from the two methods are very close, which suggests that the hyper-parameter distribution is a natural choice of prior distribution for the assessment process in the future years. The hyper-distribution in this case represents the among-year distribution of annual mean concentrations. We treat years as exchangeable because we cannot determine how annual means differ from each other. A well-defined informative prior benefits the environmental standard compliance assessment in two ways: a proper prior distribution has been shown to improve the accuracy of the estimated posterior distribution of θ_j and the improved estimate can lead to reduced sample size requirement.

Following the same idea of using years as exchangeable units to pool data from multiple years, we can also pool data from multiple similar waters if we can consider them exchangeable with regard to their mean concentrations in a given year. We will return to this idea later in Chapter 6.

4.5 A Mixture of Two Normal Distributions

The statistical models we covered so far in this chapter share a common feature. The association between data of the response variable and observations of the predictor variable(s) is unambiguous. For example, in a two-sample t-test problem, each response variable data point is unambiguously linked to one of the two groups. In a regression problem, the response variable data are paired with predictor variable observations. In some problems, the association itself is in question. For example, in setting the target for an environmental restoration project, we need to know the natural background level of a pollutant in a study area. When we do not know definitely whether or not data collected from the vicinity of study area were influenced by the source of pollution, the first task of data analysis is to estimate the natural background concentration levels without a clear separation between sampling sites that represent the background condition and sites that are influenced by the pollution. Setting a remediation goal by estimating the background level of distribution is a routine analysis in U.S. EPA's "superfund" remediation projects. The uncertainty about the source of the response variable data is common. For example, sex differences in the size of certain animals (e.g., fish, birds) can be difficult to study because their sex is difficult to identify. Statistical analyses of this type of problem have long been part of modern statistics, starting in the late 19th century [Newcomb, 1880, Pearson, 1894]. The seminal book by Titterington, Smith, and Makov [Titterington et al., 1985] summarized the more than 100 years of development in analyzing such data.

In this section, we use an example of estimating background soil contaminant concentrations to discuss the simplest mixture distribution problem: a mixture of two normal distributions. We present the problem, the traditional hypothesis-testing-based approach for the problem, and our estimation approach based on mixture of two normal distributions.

4.5.1   Estimating Background Contaminant Concentrations

Characterizing background concentrations of contaminants is part of the U.S. EPA's risk assessment and risk management process in compliance with the Comprehensive Environmental Response, Compensation, and Liability Act (CERCLA) of 1980 [U.S. EPA, 1989]. Locations affected by CERCLA are commonly known as "superfund" sites. These are sites contaminated with hazardous substances and are required to undergo remedial investigation and remedial action (cleanups) to protect human health and the environment from current and potential threats posed by uncontrolled release of hazardous substances. Because the same hazardous substances associated with a release can occur naturally in the environment or as a result of anthropogenic impacts not associated with site-related activities, EPA recommends that risk assessments consider whether site-specific concentrations fall within the range of local background conditions or whether they may be indicative of site-related contamination [U.S. EPA, 2002]. Background information is important to risk managers because the CERCLA program generally does not clean up to concentrations below natural or anthropogenic background levels.

A large quantity of data is often available at hazardous waste sites for characterizing background concentrations using statistical analysis. The extent of areas affected by the targeted toxic release is often unclear at the start of a cleanup project. As a result, we know that some of the data are potentially from contaminated areas. Separating potentially contaminated data from data indicative of local background is the first task of the risk assessment process. The U.S. EPA and the U.S. Naval Facilities Engineering Command (NAVFAC) suggested a statistical approach for evaluating each available data point and removing potentially contaminated data points one at a time [U.S. EPA, 2002]. This approach is based primarily on statistical tests of discordancy, supplemented by visual examination of the sample distribution.

A typical test for outliers is based on the normality assumption. An observation is deemed to be an outlier if the observation is extremely large (or small) based on the estimated normal mean and standard deviation using all observations except the one at hand. With a large number of data points, this process is time consuming. In addition, repeatedly using hypothesis testing is always a questionable practice.

The question answered by a discordance test is whether a data point is from the contaminated area of the superfund site. A discordancy test is only effective when the number of "outliers" in the sample is small relative to the total sample size. But the exact number of contaminated observations is rarely known. When the number of contaminated samples is large, the problem of outlier detection becomes one of discrimination between two classes of data. From a practical viewpoint, evaluating the background concentration of a contaminant does not require us to identify whether or not each data point was from a contaminated location. As such, using a direct estimation approach should be far more effective than applying the hypothesis testing-based approach on individual observations.

The example used here is from Qian and Lyons [2006], who introduced the use of the mixture model approach for estimating background soil concentrations of two heavy metals (lead and mercury) from a U.S. federal facility in Missouri, USA. In the early 2000s, the facility was regulated for hazardous waste release under the Resource Conservation and Restoration Act (RCRA) and CERCLA. The data set includes soil metal concentrations collected by multiple studies in a total of 30 sampling areas from 1990 to 2003. Data from 24 sampling areas were included in the study for characterizing the background levels of various metals. There are 731 observations of lead (Pb) soil concentrations (with 33 measurements below method detection limits) and 837 observations of mercury (Hg) soil concentrations (with 627 measurements below detection limits). There were at least 4 measurements of both metals from each sampling area. We use the lead soil concentration data in this example, and leave the mercury data for readers as an exercise.

A concentration variable is often modeled by the log-normal distribution. Consequently, we model the log transformed contaminant concentration data from a sampling area as random samples from one of the two normal distributions, one is the background concentration distribution $\pi_b = N(\mu_b, \sigma_b^2)$ and the other is the contaminated concentration distribution $\pi_c = N(\mu_c, \sigma_c^2)$. In our example, soil samples were taken from multiple sampling areas in the vicinity. We assume that the background distribution is the same for the entire study site, while the contaminated concentration distribution is sampling-area-specific.

Because we do not know for sure whether a concentration is from π_b or π_c, the concentration distribution can be expressed as:

$$x = \log(Conc) \sim r\pi_c + (1 - r)\pi_b$$

where r is a Bernoulli random variable $r \sim Bern(p)$ with p being the probability that the sample is from π_c. Conditional on the density functions of the two distributions π_b and π_c, we can assess the relative likelihood of a given data point being from one distribution over the other (the likelihood ratio of the two distributions). For example, if $\pi_b = N(0, 1)$ and $\pi_c = N(4, 4)$ and the observed concentration is 2, the likelihood that the observation is from the background distribution is 0.054 (the density of N(0,1) evaluated at $x = 2$), and the likelihood of the observation being from the contaminated distribution is 0.121. The probability of the observation being from the contaminated distribution can be estimated as $p = 0.121/(0.121 + 0.054) = 0.69$. This probability is a conditional probability of observing $x = 2, \mu_b = 0, \sigma_b^2 = 1, \mu_c = 4$, and $\sigma_c^2 = 4$. The conditional distribution of r is

$$r \sim Bern(p).$$

These steps form a Gibbs sampler. Because r is not directly observed, this is an example of the data augmentation method.

In general, we represent the mixture using p:

$$\pi(x_i) = p \times N(x_i|\mu_c, \sigma_c^2) + (1-p) \times N(x_i|\mu_b, \sigma_b^2). \qquad (4.17)$$

Here we use $\pi(x)$ to represent the density function of the log concentration x and $N(x|\mu_c, \sigma_c^2)$ to represent the normal distribution density function of x with mean μ_c and variance σ_c^2. The goal is to estimate $p, \mu_c, \sigma_c^2, \mu_b$, and σ_b^2. The log likelihood function is

$$LL = \prod_{i=1}^{n} \pi(x_i) = \sum_{i=1}^{n} \log\left(p \times N(x_i|\mu_c, \sigma_c^2) + (1-p) \times N(x_i|\mu_b, \sigma_b^2)\right).$$

In Stan, this likelihood function can be effectively coded using the incremental log density `target += log_likelihood`. The incremental log likelihood is the log of the sum of $p \times N(x_i|\mu_c, \sigma_c^2)$ and $(1-p) \times N(x_i|\mu_b, \sigma_b^2)$. We can use the Stan function `log_sum_exp` to evaluate the log likelihood. The function `log_sum_exp` is an efficient computation algorithm to calculate the log of sum of exponentials:

$$\log\_sum\_exp(a, b) = \log(e^a + e^b).$$

To take advantage of this efficient computation algorithm, we can express $\log(A + B)$ as $\log\left(e^{\log(A)} + e^{\log(B)}\right)$. As such, our log-likelihood increment is then

```
target+=log_sum_exp(log(p)+normal_lpdf(x | mu_c,sigma_c),
                    log(1-p)+normal_lpdf(x | mu_b, sigma_b))
```

Because the mixture distribution problem is common in statistics, Stan includes a function `log_mix` to further simplify the code syntax:

```
target += log_mix(p, normal_lpdf(x | mu_c, sigma_c),
                     normal_lpdf(x | mu_b, sigma_b))
```

Although we do not use the `log_sum_exp` function in this example, we will repeatedly use it later in the book.

Making the code more generic, we use `mu1` and `mu2` to represent the two mean concentrations:

```
#### Stan Code ####
mixture1 <- "
data{
    int N; // sample size
    vector[N] x;
}
parameters{
```

```
    real mu1;
    real mu2;
    real<lower=0> sigma1;
    real<lower=0> sigma2;
    real<lower=0,upper=1> p;
}
model {
    sigma1 ~ normal(0,5);
    sigma2 ~ normal(0,5);
    mu1 ~ normal(0,5);
    mu2 ~ normal(0,5);
    target += log_mix(p, normal_lpdf(x|mu1, sigma1),
                         normal_lpdf(x|mu2, sigma2));
}
"
```

End

This model, however, is unidentifiable because the two normal distributions are interchangeable. For example, if $\mu_c = 2, \mu_b = 1$, and $p = 0.7$ is a set of viable solutions, $\mu_c = 1, \mu_b = 2$, and $p = 0.3$ is equally viable. The two combinations would result in the same likelihood value. For example, using the soil lead data in our example, the Stan model was run using two parallel chains and, in one run, one chain results in $\mu_1 > \mu_2$ and the other $\mu_1 < \mu_2$ (Figure 4.17). The two chains do not mix well, leading to a poor convergence diagnostic statistic ($\hat{R}$). This result suggests a potential way to improve the model stability. The two normal distribution means can be set to be ordered. That is, one mean is set to be larger than the other.

For this example, we can naturally set μ_1 to be the background concentration and express the concentration in contaminated area as $\mu_1 + \delta$ and change the incremental log density in Stan code to:

```
    target += log_mix(p, normal_lpdf(x|mu1, sigma1),
                         normal_lpdf(x|mu1+delta, sigma2));
```

When running with multiple chains, we may still encounter either convergence or divergent transition issues because a very small μ_1 can be compensated by a large δ as shown in one of our runs (Figure 4.18) and properly matched mixture probability value.

Specifically for this example, the sampling areas were selected because they are less likely to be contaminated. As such, we can further constrain the model by assuming that concentration values are more likely representing the background level than representing contaminated levels. That is, we can limit $p > 0.5$. With this additional limit, we now have a stable model (Figure 4.19) and the results are reasonable.

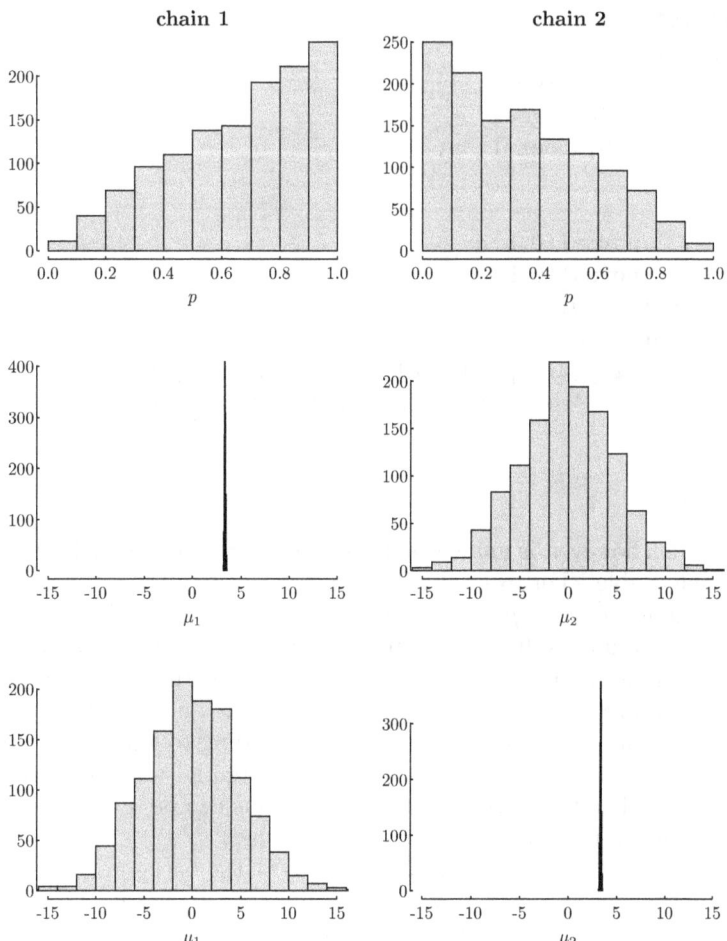

FIGURE 4.17: MCMC samples from two parallel chains of the parameters p, μ_1, and μ_2 show the identification problem of a mixture model.

```
### R output ###
        mean   sd 2.5%   25%   50%   75% 97.5% n_eff  Rhat
mu1     3.33 0.06 3.22  3.29  3.33  3.37  3.45  2532  1
delta   1.60 1.20 0.07  0.64  1.35  2.33  4.39  2480  1
sigma1  1.54 0.04 1.46  1.51  1.54  1.56  1.62  2086  1
sigma2  3.92 3.01 0.14  1.50  3.23  5.74 11.01  2453  1
p       0.78 0.14 0.52  0.66  0.79  0.90  0.99  2575  1
### End ###
```

Qian and Lyons [2006] modeled δ as specific to a sampling area. That is, the contaminated soil contaminant concentrations are assumed to vary by

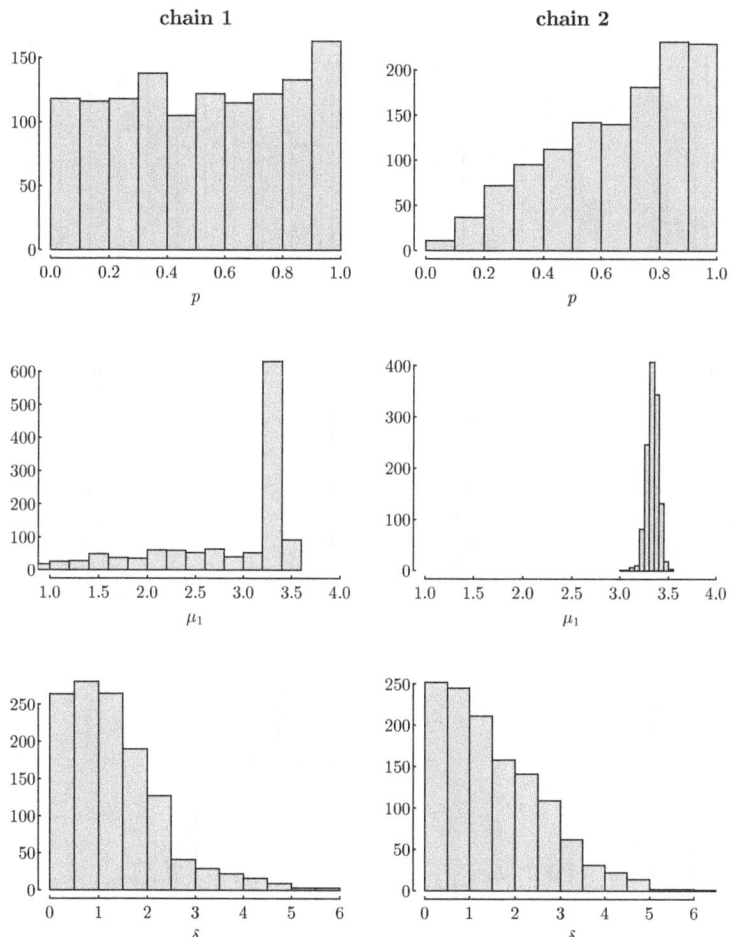

FIGURE 4.18: The identification problem is limited by imposing constraints on the relationship between the two means ($\mu_2 = \mu_1 + \delta$ and $\delta > 0$. But the identification problem is not completely resolved.

sampling areas as these areas had varying distances to the main facility that released the contaminant. The area-specific δ's are further modeled using a hierarchical model:

$$\delta_j \sim N(\mu_\delta, \sigma_\delta^2)$$

A hierarchical structure does not improve the model identification problem. However, it allows us to learn more about the study areas and provide necessary information for setting clean-up priority among the areas of interest. The estimated background concentration distribution from the hierarchical model is lower than the estimate combining all data together (Figure 4.20).

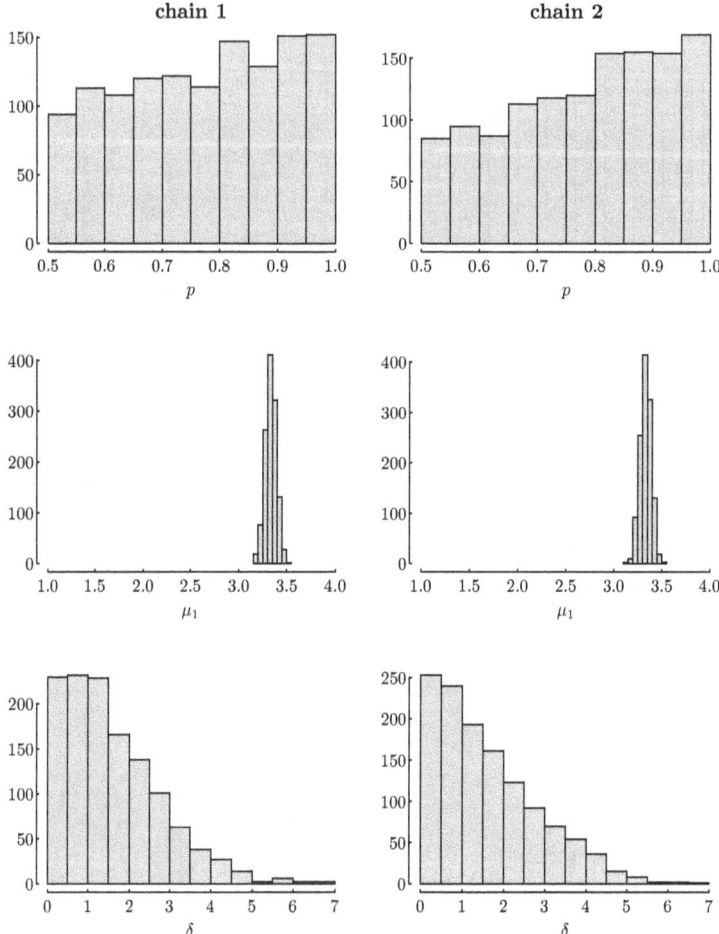

FIGURE 4.19: The identification problem is resolved with the addition limit of $p > 0.5$.

If we believe that the background concentration of lead in soil is the same in all sampling areas (perhaps because the limited spatial coverage of the study area), we should also prefer the hierarchical model estimated background concentration.

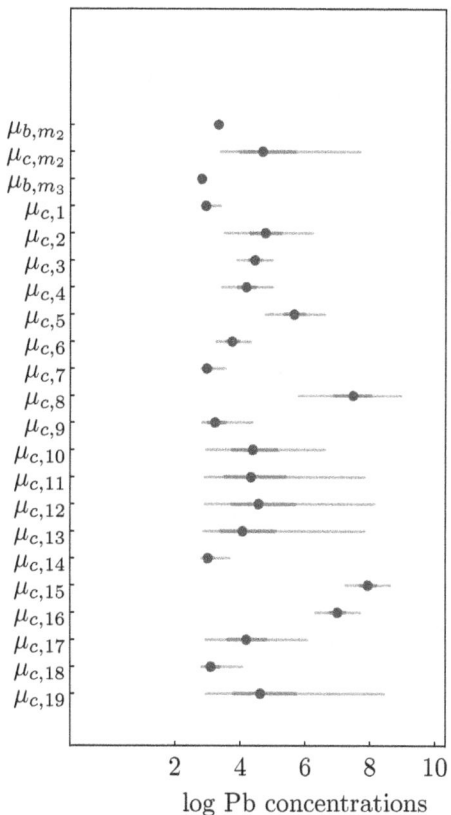

FIGURE 4.20: Estimated background and contaminated soil lead concentrations from model 2 $(\mu_{b,m_2}, \mu_{c,m_2})$ are compared to the same from model 3 $(\mu_{b,m_3}, \mu_{c,1:19})$.

4.6   Summary

The use of MCMC in Stan makes it possible to model more realistic models in a Bayesian analysis. In this chapter we showed our preferred workflow and a number of problems with normal response variables. As a model becomes more complicated, we discussed the need to have informative priors to overcome the identifiable problem. The identifiable problem will appear later in Chapters 5 and 6. We also showed the flexibility of using the `target +=` statement to specify the log-likelihood function in Stan.

Chapter 5

Population and Community: Count Variables

Ecology is the science of distribution and abundance of organisms. Distribution is about where and when an organism is present, and abundance is about the number of organisms of one or more species. Using occurrence data, we relate the presence of a species to variables of the surrounding environment to characterize the habitat of the species. Such occurrence data are often recorded as binary variables; an organism is either present or absent in a study site. When organizing occurrence data, we frequently count the number of presences in locations with similar environmental conditions. In environmental studies, we also use binary data to document the number of samples with concentrations of a pollutant exceeding a regulatory threshold and making management decisions accordingly. The abundance of a species and changes in abundance among a community of interacting species are studied using count variables as well. We use these count variables to study population dynamics and community structures.

A count variable is discrete and limited to be non-negative integers. The binomial and Poisson distributions are the most commonly used when analyzing count data, and are often used as the starting point. These distributions have only one parameter and are easy to work with computationally. They are often used as introductory examples in many Bayesian textbooks. Complications, however, often arise in field sampling and laboratory experiment processes, which make the binomial or Poisson distributions unable to model many important features of the data-generating process.

In this chapter, we introduce the basic count data models using binomial, Poisson, negative binomial, and multinomial distributions with examples from published papers. These distributions are rarely adequate in addressing variability in most ecological count data. The classical generalized linear models are often effective in standard applications. The value of using Bayesian inference is largely to accommodate increased complexity. As a result, we focus on such modifications, including over-dispersion and the inevitable imperfect detection associated with nearly all field and lab data-generating methods.

We start the chapter with a summary of the Poisson and negative binomial distributions and their connections, through a well-known example. We then discuss the classical generalized linear model using two examples. Using these examples, we present the variance components in a generalized linear model problem. We then introduce finite mixture models for imperfect detection problems.

5.1   Poisson and Negative Binomial Distributions

A 1943 paper on common probability distributions in biological science opened with the following sentence: "It is well known that distribution of a series of biological measurements usually conforms to one of three types" (binomial, normal, and Poisson) [Fisher et al., 1943]. The Poisson distribution is, perhaps, the most commonly used probability distribution for count variables. It has a probability distribution function with one parameter. Computationally, the Poisson distribution is quite easy. In the past, researchers often considered transformations that could leverage Poisson distribution for easy computation. For example, the multinomial-Poisson transformation allows the use of the Poisson distribution to model multinomial count variables [Baker, 1994, for example]. However, the Poisson distribution parameter (the rate parameter, λ) represents both the mean and the variance. In nearly all practical problems, a count variable's variance is most likely larger than its mean, a feature known as over-dispersion. As a result, when using the Poisson distribution, we often consider options to model the response variable variance that is larger than the mean. One approach of modeling the over-dispersion is using the Bayesian approach by assuming that the rate parameter λ has a gamma distribution. This idea is not exclusively Bayesian. For example, Fisher et al. [1943] used the same approach to extend the Poisson distribution. In the Bayesian context, the gamma distribution is the conjugate prior of the Poisson rate parameter (see Section 3.3), which means that the posterior distribution of the rate parameter is also a gamma distribution.

Suppose the count variable Y is a Poisson random variable with parameter λ, and the probability distribution is

$$\pi(Y = k) = \frac{\lambda^k e^{-\lambda}}{k!}. \tag{5.1}$$

When observing independent data $y_i, \cdots, y_n$, the likelihood function is

$$L = \prod_{i=1}^{n} \frac{\lambda^{y_i} e^{-\lambda}}{y_i!} \propto \lambda^{\sum_{i=1}^{n} y_i} e^{-n\lambda}.$$

Assuming the prior of λ is a gamma distribution with parameters α and β:

$$\pi(\lambda) = \frac{\beta^\alpha}{\Gamma(\alpha)} \lambda^{\alpha-1} e^{-\beta\lambda}.$$

The posterior distribution of λ is

$$\pi(\lambda \mid \boldsymbol{y}) \propto \lambda^{\alpha-1} e^{-\beta\lambda} \times \lambda^{\sum_{i=1}^{n} y_i} e^{-n\lambda} = \lambda^{\alpha+\sum_{i=1}^{n} y_i - 1} e^{-(\beta+n)\lambda}$$

which is a gamma distribution with parameters $\alpha + \sum_{i=1}^{n} y_i$ and $\beta + n$.

The negative binomial distribution is often used in ecological studies to model over-dispersed count data. In both classical and Bayesian statistics, the negative binomial distribution is seen as an extension of the Poisson distribution. Fisher et al. [1943] derived the negative binomial distribution as a natural extension of the Poisson distribution by using a χ^2 distribution to model the Poisson distribution parameter. Fisher's derivation is the same as in the Bayesian setting when we derive the predictive distribution of y when using the conjugate prior for λ (see equation (5.3)).

The negative binomial distribution has three different parameterizations. The initial definition of the distribution is through independent and identical Bernoulli trials (each with the same probability of success of p) as in the binomial distribution. In the binomial distribution, we consider the number of successes out of n trials as the random variable. In the negative binomial distribution, the random variable Y is the number of failures before r successes are achieved. As the last trial is the rth success, the probability of $Y = k$ can be derived through the binomial distribution:

$$\Pr(Y = k \mid r, p) = \binom{k + r - 1}{r - 1} p^r (1 - p)^k.$$

This parameterization is also known as the Pascal distribution. It is a generalization of the geometric distribution (when $r = 1$).

When the definition of r is extended to real values (not limited to integer values as in the Pascal distribution), the negative binomial is also known as the Pólya distribution. When r takes a real value, the binomial coefficient is extended to its real value definition through the gamma function:

$$\Pr(Y = k \mid r, p) = \frac{\Gamma(k + r)}{k! \Gamma(r)} p^r (1 - p)^k.$$

When the negative binomial distribution is used in the generalized linear model, we want to relate predictor variables to the mean of the distribution, which is $\mu = \frac{rp}{1-p}$. Hence, the distribution is reparameterized by replacing p with μ, that is, setting $p = \frac{r}{\mu+r}$ and $1 - p = \frac{\mu}{\mu+r}$, resulting in the third parameterization

$$\Pr(Y = k \mid r, \mu) = \frac{\Gamma(k + r)}{k! \Gamma(r)} \left(\frac{r}{\mu + r}\right)^r \left(\frac{\mu}{\mu + r}\right)^k. \tag{5.2}$$

Because the gamma distribution is the conjugate prior of the Poisson rate parameter, we also define the negative binomial through the gamma distribution parameter α and β, by setting $r = \alpha$ and $\mu = \alpha/\beta$:

$$\Pr(Y = k \mid \alpha, \beta) = \frac{\Gamma(\alpha + k)}{k! \Gamma(\alpha)} \left(\frac{\beta}{\beta + 1}\right)^\alpha \left(\frac{1}{\beta + 1}\right)^k$$

which is the predictive distribution of a Poisson random variable $Y = k$ with the prior of the rate parameter λ being gamma(α, β):

$$
\begin{aligned}
\Pr(Y = k) &= \int_\lambda \Pr(Y = k \mid \lambda)\pi(\lambda \mid \alpha, \beta)d\lambda \\
&= \int_\lambda \frac{\lambda^y e^{-\lambda}}{k!} \frac{\beta^\alpha}{\Gamma(\alpha)} \lambda^{\alpha-1} e^{-\beta\lambda} \\
&= \frac{\beta^\alpha}{\Gamma(\alpha)k!} \frac{\Gamma(\alpha+k)}{(\beta+1)^{\alpha+k}} \int_\lambda \frac{(\beta+1)^{\alpha+y}}{\Gamma(\alpha+k)} \lambda^{\alpha+k-1} e^{-(\beta+1)\lambda}d\lambda \\
&= \frac{\Gamma(\alpha+k)}{\Gamma(\alpha)k!} \left(\frac{\beta}{\beta+1}\right)^\alpha \left(\frac{1}{\beta+1}\right)^k.
\end{aligned}
\tag{5.3}
$$

Equation (5.3) is the same as the classical derivation presented in Fisher et al. [1943, page 54].

Because of the similarity between the gamma and the log-normal distributions, we often model the over-dispersion by modeling the Poisson rate parameter as a log-normal variable such that an over-dispersed Poisson regression problem can be set up as follows:

$$
\begin{aligned}
y &\sim Pois(\lambda) \\
\log(\lambda) &\sim N(\mu, \sigma^2).
\end{aligned}
\tag{5.4}
$$

Using this formulation, we can model the log-mean (μ) as a linear function of potential predictors.

A well-known example of an over-dispersed count variable problem was given by the fishery by-catch example in Hilborn and Mangel [1997]. In this example, the researchers wanted to analyze the observed number of seabird (albatross) by-catches in trawl fishing operations (fishing for squids) in order to design future by-catch observer programs, where official observers were placed in selected fishing boats to collect data. The objective of the analysis was to determine the adequate number of observers to obtain scientifically meaningful data. The data used were by-catches from 897 tows observed onboard five fishing vessels in one fishing season. Most tows did not accidentally catch birds in the net, while a small number of tows caught multiple birds. As a result, the observed variance far exceeded the observed mean, suggesting a Poisson model is not advisable. Hilborn and Mangel [1997] used the negative binomial to estimate the mean by-catch. We use the data to compare the three models discussed above: the Poisson model, negative binomial model, and the Poisson model using a conjugate prior. The over-dispersed Poisson model in equation (5.4) is designed for a generalized linear model problem, and hence not compared here.

In this example, the goal is to estimate the mean by-catch (average number of birds caught per tow). When using the Poisson model, the Poisson rate parameter is the mean. When using the negative binomial, the parameterization in equation (5.2) directly estimates the mean, and the over-dispersed Poisson model of equation (5.4) also uses the mean as a parameter. We compare the estimated means using three approaches: (1) assuming Poisson distribution using maximum likelihood, (2) assuming negative binomial using maximum likelihood, and (3) the Bayesian conjugate prior. To make the estimated means comparable, we use Stan for (1) and (2) by using non-informative priors.

Because of the large number of zeros, we can improve the model's speed by separately expressing the log-likelihood functions for zero counts and positive counts. When using the Poisson distribution, we use the Stan function `poisson_log_lpmf()` to specify the log-likelihood function. The Poisson model is the simplest:

```
#### Stan Code ####
## The Poisson model
Pois_bycatch <- "
    data{
        int<lower=1> n0; //number of 0's
        int<lower=1> np; //number of non-zero counts
        int<lower=1> yp[np];
    }
    parameters{
        real<lower=0> lambda;
    }
    model{
      target += n0*poisson_log_lpmf(0|log(lambda));
      target += poisson_log_lpmf(yp|log(lambda));
    }"
### End ###
```

The log probability mass function on the negative binomial model (equation (5.2)) is implemented in Stan function `neg_binomial_2_log_lpmf()`:

```
#### Stand Code ####
## Negative binomial model
NB_bycatch <- "
data{
        int<lower=1> n0; //number of 0's
        int<lower=1> np; //number of non-zero counts
        int<lower=1> yp[np];
    }
    parameters{
        real<lower=0> mu;
        real<lower=0> r;
    }
    model{
      mu ~ normal(0,5);
      r ~ normal(0,5);
      target += n0*neg_binomial_2_log_lpmf(0 | log(mu), r);
      target += neg_binomial_2_log_lpmf(yp | log(mu), r);
    }
"
### End ###
```

To compare the three approaches, we use MCMC samples of λ from the Poisson model and μ and r from the negative binomial model to replicate the observed data. That is, for each set of MCMC samples, we draw N random numbers from the Poisson or negative binomial with N being the sample size of the data ($N = 897$). For the Bayesian conjugate prior method, we impose a relatively vague prior on λ ($\lambda \sim gamma(0.01, 0.01)$), which leads to the posterior of λ being a gamma distribution with $\alpha = 250.01$ and $\beta = 897.01$, or $\lambda \mid y \sim gamma(250.01, 897.01)$. This process is known as posterior simulation. It is the process of drawing random numbers from the posterior predictive distribution, which is represented by an integral:

$$\pi(\tilde{y}) = \int_{\theta} \pi(\tilde{y} \mid \theta)\pi(\theta \mid Y)d\theta.$$

Using the MCMC samples of model parameters, we can approximate the integral numerically. Specifically for the Poisson model, we have 2500 MCMC samples of λ. For each random sample of λ, we draw the same number of Poisson random variates as the original data as a replicated sample. In this way, we have 2500 sets of replicated counts. For each replicate, we calculate the mean, standard deviation, and the percent of 0's. In other words, we simulated the model-predicted distribution of the mean, standard deviation, and the percent of 0. Comparing the model-predicted quantities to the respective observed values can give us a basis to judge the performance of the model.

The Poisson model and the conjugate prior model produced identical results (Figure 5.1). This outcome is expected, as in many simple models where informative priors are unavailable, the Bayesian and classical results coincide. In a way, the simulation we used for the Poisson model is exactly what is described in Fisher et al. [1943]. As long as we account for the uncertainty properly, the classical statistics result is nearly always similar to the respective Bayesian results with flat or non-informative priors.

The comparison shows that the Poisson model cannot account for the large number of zeros in the data and underestimates the standard deviation of the data. The negative binomial distribution can properly replicate these three statistics, which is the conclusion of Hilborn and Mangel [1997]. We will return to this example in Section 5.3.3.

5.2   Analysis of Variance/Deviance

The conventional use of ANOVA (including linear models) often achieves three goals: (1) exploratory analysis through partitioning the variance of a normal response variable among factor predictors (variance components), (2) testing sequentially nested models using F-test (hypothesis testing), and (3)

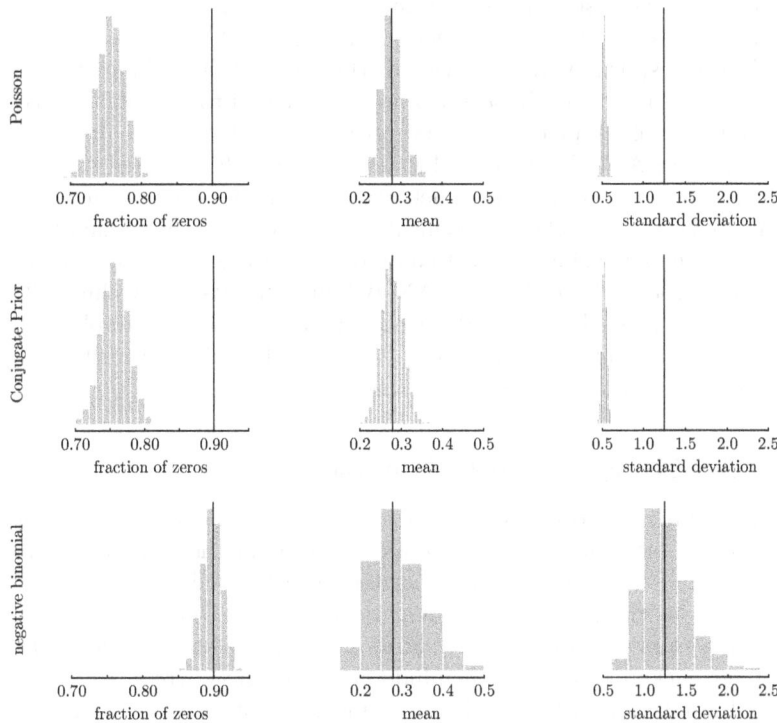

FIGURE 5.1: Fishery by-catch data were modeled using the Poisson and the negative binomial distributions. The Poisson model parameters were estimated using a "classical" method (top row, labeled as "Poisson") and the Bayesian method with non-informative gamma prior (middle row, "Conjugate Prior." The posterior simulation calculates the replicated fraction of 0s in the data (left column), the mean (middle column), and standard deviation (right column). The simulated statistics are shown in histograms and the observed statistics are shown by the vertical lines.

estimation of model coefficients and their standard errors (parameter estimation) [Gelman, 2005]. To simultaneously accomplish all three tasks, we have to limit the analysis to data with simple structures. When analyzing data with a complicated structure (e.g., unbalanced observational data) or non-normal response variable data, there may not be a single method that can achieve all three goals.

When analyzing count variables, the sum-of-squares calculus used in classical ANOVA (or the least-squares method in a linear model) is no longer appropriate. As a result, the partitioning of the response variable variance into variance components is impractical. We can, however, test sequentially nested models using the analysis of *deviance*. In R, we use the function **anova**, as in the linear regression model, to obtain a table of analysis of deviance. The table, however, does not represent a partitioning of the variance (nor deviance) in the response variable. Instead, the analysis of deviance table is a summary of a series of likelihood ratio tests, presented to resemble the traditional ANOVA table (replacing the sum-of-squares with deviance differences).

The Bayesian ANOVA, as introduced in Gelman [2005], uses the hierarchical computation to connect parameter estimation and the variance components in a natural way. The hierarchical computation method simplifies the adjustment when analyzing data with a more complicated structure. Qian and Shen [2007] introduced the Bayesian ANOVA first discussed in Gelman [2005] to readers of the journal *Ecology*. We use the Liverpool Moth example to illustrate the basic computation strategy and the Seedling Recruitment example to expand the method to more complicated data.

5.2.1   The Liverpool Moth Example

The experiment reported in Bishop [1972] demonstrated the evolution of the peppered moth (*Biston betularia*) in and around the city of Liverpool, England induced by air pollution associated with the Industrial Revolution. The peppered moth is a temperate nocturnal species. During the day, they rest in hiding from predators, mostly birds. Peppered moths are camouflaged against their backgrounds when they hide in the boughs of trees. Around Liverpool and north Wales, the moths are typically white with dark spots and patterns (hence peppered). The salt-and-pepper (light-colored) pattern effectively camouflaged them against the light-colored trees and lichens upon which they rested. The species *Biston betularia* has a melanic (dark) morph (form, appearance). Individuals of the melanic morph are mostly black. Because of the widespread pollution from burning coal during the Industrial Revolution in England, most lichens died out, so the trees became blackened by soot. As a result, the light-colored moths became visible to birds and became increasingly rare due to predation; whereas the dark morphed moths flourished because their color blended with the darkened tree trunks better. Bishop described an experiment to estimate survival rates using dead moths. He selected seven locations progressively farther away from the center of Liverpool (Sefton Park) to create a tree-trunk color gradient, from mostly soot-darkened tree trunks in Liverpool to light-colored tree trunks in the Welsh countryside. At each location, Bishop randomly selected eight trees to glue equal numbers of dark and light morphed previously frozen moths to these trees in life-like positions at heights between 0.5 and 2.5 meters. After 24 hours, he revisited these trees to record whether or not each of the moths was removed (presumably taken by birds).

The response variable is a binary response count variable: numbers of moths placed and moths taken. The predictor variables are (1) distance from Sefton Park and (2) morph of the moth. This is a typical binary regression example, where the response variable is modeled by the binomial distribution:

$$y_i \sim Bin(p_i, N_i) \tag{5.5}$$

where i is the index of observations, y_i is the number of moths removed, N_i is the number of moths placed, and p_i is the probability of a moth in the ith observation being removed. The distribution parameter p_i is linked to the linear function of the two predictors (morph of moth and distance from Sefton Park) through a logistic link function:

$$\log\left(\frac{p_i}{1 - p_i}\right) = \alpha + \beta_{m[i]} + \gamma_{m[i]} Dist_i \tag{5.6}$$

where $m[i]$ denotes that the ith observation is from morph m ($m = 1$ [dark] or 2 [light]). The parameter of interest is the slope γ_m representing the effect of distance along the tree trunk color gradient. The theory of evolution by natural selection suggests that the slope for dark morphed moths (γ_1) should be positive (increasingly more likely to be taken by birds) and the slope for light morphed moths (γ_2) should be negative (less likely to be taken by birds as tree trunk color gets lighter).

To accomplish the exploratory analysis goal, we want to know whether the probabilities of being removed depend on (1) the color of the moth (the morph effect), (2) the distance, and (3) the morph and distance interaction. When the total variance can be partitioned into the three components, we can at least qualitatively evaluate the relative contributions in place of a formal hypothesis test. The hierarchical computation method is to parameterize the model into batches, each representing a component [Gelman, 2005]. There are three batches in equation (5.6). The morph effect is represented by $\beta_{m[i]}$. To be able to estimate the parameters, they must be subjected to constraints. The constraint for the morph effect is $\sum_m \beta_m = 0$. The term $\gamma_{m[i]} Dist_i$ represents both the distance effect and the distance-morph interaction effect, which can be separated by setting $\gamma_m = \gamma_0 + \gamma_m$ and constraining $\sum_m \gamma_m = 0$. As a result, equation (5.6) becomes the sum of three batches (plus the overall mean):

$$\log\left(\frac{p_i}{1 - p_i}\right) = \beta_0 + \beta_{1m[i]} + \beta_2 Dist_i + \beta_{3m[i]} Dist_i \tag{5.7}$$

where β_0 is the overall average, β_{1m} is the morph effect (and $\sum_m \beta_{1m} = 0$), $\beta_2 Dist_i$ is the distance effect, and $\beta_{3m} Dist_i$ ($\sum_m \beta_{3m} = 0$) is the interaction effect. We can partition the variance in $\eta_i = \log\left(\frac{p_i}{1-p_i}\right)$ by calculating the component variances: $var(\eta_i) = var(\beta_{1m[i]}) + var(\beta_2 Dist_i) + var(\beta_{3m[i]} Dist_i)$. Gelman [2005] used the standard deviation of the constrained coefficients (finite population standard deviation) to represent the importance of each component. Implementation of the hierarchical computation using MCMC is straightforward (replacing the normal distribution function with a binomial distribution function). The variance component calculation can be included

directly in the Stan model code (as generated quantities) or calculated in R
from MCMC samples of β's. The basic Stan model is as follows:

```
#### R Code ####
## The Stan model
moth_var <- "
data{
  int n; //sample size
  int y[n]; //# of removed
  int NN[n]; //# of placed
  int nM;
  real D[n]; //distance
  int<lower=1> morph; //1=dark, 2=light
}
parameters{
  real beta0;
  real beta1[nM];
  real<lower=0, upper=5> sigma1;
  real beta2;
  real beta3[nM];
  real<lower=0, upper=5> sigma3;
}
model{
  real xb[n];
  beta1 ~ normal(0, sigma1);
  beta3 ~ normal(0, sigma3);
  for (i in 1:n)
    xb[i] = beta0+beta1[morph[i]]+beta2*D[i]+
            beta3[morph[i]]*D[i];
  y ~ binomial_logit(NN, xb);
}
"
### End ###
```

To calculate the variance components as part of the Stan model, we can
add the following code block to the model:

```
#### R Code ####
## the generated quantities block
"
generated quantities{
  real alpha0;
  real alpha1[nM];
  real alpha2;
  real alpha3[nM];
  real Int[n];
```

```
  real sM;
  real sD;
  real sInt;
  alpha0 = beta0 + mean(beta1[]);
  alpha2 = beta2 + mean(beta3[]);
  for (i in 1:nM){
    alpha1[i] = beta1[i]-mean(beta1[]);
    alpha3[i] = beta3[i]-mean(beta3[]);
  }
  for (i in 1:n)
    Int[i] <- alpha3[morph[i]]*D[i];
  sM = sd(alpha1[]);
  sD = abs(alpha2)*sd(D[]);
  sInt = sd(Int[]);
}
"
### End ###
```

As we did in Chapter 4, we use a function to organize input data, initial values, and the list of parameters to be monitored.

```
Input <- function(infile=moth, n.chains=nchains, vc=T){
    n <- dim(infile)[1]
    y <- infile$removed
    N <- infile$placed
    morph <- as.numeric(ordered(infile$morph))
    nM <- max(morph)
    Dist <- infile$distance
    data <- list(y=y, n=n, NN=N, nM=nM, morph=morph, D=Dist)
    inits <- list()
    for (i in 1:n.chains)
        inits[[i]] <- list(beta0=rnorm(1), beta1=rnorm(nM),
                           sigma1=runif(1), beta2=rnorm(1),
                           beta3=rnorm(nM), sigma3=runif(1))
    if (vc)
        paras <- c("alpha0", "alpha1", "alpha2", "alpha3",
                  "sM", "sD", "sInt", "beta0", "beta1",
                  "sigma1", "beta2", "beta3", "sigma3")
    else paras <- c("beta0", "beta1", "sigma1", "beta2",
                   "beta3", "sigma3")
    return(list(data=data, inits=inits, paras=paras,
               nchains=n.chains))
}
### End ###
```

To run the Stan model, we use the `rstan` function `stan_model` to compile the code and the function `sampling` to draw MCMC samples and use the function `extract` to extract the random samples. The name `extract` is also used by a function in package `tidyr`. If `tidyr` is loaded after loading `rstan`, we need to remember to use the `rstan` function by calling `rstan::extract`.

```
input.to.stan <- Input(vc=F)
fit <- stan_model(model_code=moth_var)
fit2keep <- sampling(fit, data = input.to.stan$data,
                     iter = niters, chains = nchains,
                     init=input.to.stan$inits,
                     pars=input.to.stan$paras, thin=nthin)
mothStanbeta0 <- rvsims(as.matrix(as.data.frame(
     rstan::extract(fit2keep, par="beta0", permuted=T))))
mothStanbeta1 <- rvsims(as.matrix(as.data.frame(
     rstan::extract(fit2keep, par="beta1", permuted=T))))
mothStanbeta2 <- rvsims(as.matrix(as.data.frame(
     rstan::extract(fit2keep, par="beta2", permuted=T))))
mothStanbeta3 <- rvsims(as.matrix(as.data.frame(
     rstan::extract(fit2keep, par="beta3", permuted=T))))
### End ###
```

In some cases, calculating the variance components outside of Stan may be computationally more efficient.

```
## calculate variance components
alpha0 <- mothStanbeta0 + mean(mothStanbeta1)
alpha2 <- mothStanbeta2 + mean(mothStanbeta3)
alpha1 <- mothStanbeta1[1]-mean(mothStanbeta1)
alpha1 <- c(alpha1, mothStanbeta1[2]-mean(mothStanbeta1))
alpha3 <- mothStanbeta3[1]-mean(mothStanbeta3)
alpha3 <- c(alpha3, mothStanbeta3[2]-mean(mothStanbeta3))

Int <- alpha3[input.to.stan$data$morph]*input.to.stan$data$D;
sM <- sd.rv(alpha1)
sD <- abs(alpha2)*sd(input.to.stan$data$D)
sInt <- sd.rv(Int)
## plotting variance components
vcomp <- c(sM, sD, sInt)
names(vcomp) <- c("Morph", "Distance", "Interaction")
par(mar=c(3, 5, 3, 1), las=1, mgp=c(1.25, 0.125,0), tck=0.01)
mlplot(vcomp, xlab="standard deviation", ylab="")
### End ###
```

We can present the variance components using an ANOVA-like graph comparing the estimated standard deviations of all components (Figure 5.2). The graph shows that the contributions from morph and the morph–distance inter-action are comparable, whereas the distance main effect is negligible. A strong morph–distance interaction effect indicates a significant difference in the distance slope between the dark and light morphs. We can show the difference by plotting the estimated slopes (Figure 5.3).

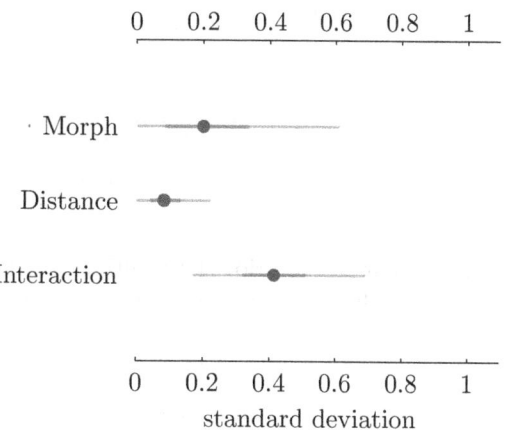

FIGURE 5.2: Estimated standard deviations of the morph, distance, and morph:distance interaction effects are shown in an ANOVA-like plot.

The factor variable (`morph`) has only two levels. As a result, computation of the variance component using finite standard deviation is unreliable. The classical generalized linear model is perhaps a computationally more effective method for this example, because the variance components were not essential in concluding that the probability of predation of the light morphed moths is decreasing and the probability that the dark morphed moths is increasing along the tree trunk color gradient. The generalized linear model (GLM) returns comparable results.

```
#### R Code & Output ####
> mothGLM <- glm(cbind(removed, placed-removed)~
  factor(morph)*distance,
>                  data=moth, family=binomial)
> display(mothGLM, 4)

glm(formula = cbind(removed, placed - removed) ~
    factor(morph) * distance, family = binomial,
    data = moth)
```

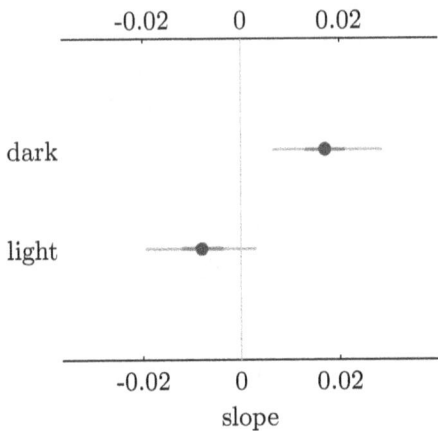

FIGURE 5.3: Estimated posterior distributions of distance slopes of the dark and light morphs show no overlap in their 95% credible intervals.

```
                                coef.est coef.se
(Intercept)                     -1.1290   0.1979
factor(morph)light               0.4113   0.2745
distance                         0.0185   0.0056
factor(morph)light:distance     -0.0278   0.0081
---
  n = 14, k = 4
  residual deviance = 13.2, null deviance = 35.4
  (difference = 22.2)
### End ###
```

The output shows the intercept (-1.1290) and slope (0.0185) of the dark morphed moths, and the difference in intercept (0.4113) and slope (-0.0278) between light morphed moths and dark morphed ones. As a comparison, we refit the model to present the estimated intercepts and slopes for the two moths.

```
#### R Output ####
glm(formula = cbind(removed, placed - removed) ~
                 factor(morph) *
                 distance - 1 - distance,
    family = binomial, data = moth)
                             coef.est coef.se
factor(morph)dark            -1.1290   0.1979
factor(morph)light           -0.7177   0.1902
```

```
factor(morph)dark:distance    0.0185    0.0056
factor(morph)light:distance  -0.0093    0.0058
---
  n = 14, k = 4
  residual deviance = 13.2, null deviance = 169.4 \
  (difference = 156.2)
### End ###
```

The Bayesian estimated marginal posterior distributions of the intercepts and slopes are:

```
#### R Output ####
## Intercepts
      name  mean   sd  2.5%   25%   50%   75% 97.5%
[1]   dark -1.08 0.19  -1.5 -1.21 -1.07 -0.94 -0.71
[2]  light -0.78 0.19  -1.1 -0.91 -0.78 -0.65 -0.42

## Slopes
      name   mean    sd   2.5%    25%    50%    75% 97.5%
[1]   dark  0.017 0.006  0.007  0.013  0.017  0.021 0.028
[2]  light -0.008 0.007 -0.020 -0.012 -0.008 -0.004 0.003
### End ###
```

The analysis of deviance table gives us the basis for the likelihood ratio test on a sequence of nested models.

```
> anova(mothGLM)
Analysis of Deviance Table

Model: binomial, link: logit

Response: cbind(removed, placed - removed)

Terms added sequentially (first to last)

                      Df Deviance Resid. Df Resid. Dev
NULL                                    13     35.385
factor(morph)          1   8.4494        12     26.936
distance               1   1.7745        11     25.161
factor(morph):distance 1  11.9315        10     13.230
### End ###
```

When comparing the null model (no predictor) and the model with morph, the change in deviance (-2log-likelihood) is 8.449. The null hypothesis of the first log-likelihood ratio test is that there is no morph effect. Under the null hypothesis, -2log-likelihood ratio (difference in the log-scale) is a χ^2 random variable. To test whether morph is a significant predictor, we use the difference in residual deviance ($35.385 - 26.936$) to calculate a p-value:

```
> 1-pchisq(8.4494, 1)
[1] 0.003651639
```

Adding `distance` to the model with `morph` as the only predictor results a decrease in deviance of 1.7745 ($p = 0.1828$), and adding the interaction term reduces the deviance by 11.9315 ($p = 0.00055$).

As in a linear regression problem, the use of the Bayesian inference is often computationally unappealing. The classical method for these standard models is effective. Often the problem of using the classical statistics methods is the over- and mis-use of hypothesis testing. We can avoid the p-value quagmire by emphasizing estimation and the magnitude (thereby practical implication) of the estimated quantities. Bayesian statistics focus on estimation. The Bayesian approach also allows us the flexibility of expanding the model beyond the confinement of a limited number of standard models in classical statistics. Our next example illustrates such an expansion.

5.2.2   The Seedling Recruitment Example

The unique topographic diversity in a mountainous area often leads to complicated environmental conditions due to varying levels of precipitation, temperature, and soil compositions. The complex physical structure, in turn, results in high levels of biodiversity and ecosystem complexity. Understanding how topography influences biological systems is the topic of a field known as mountain ecology. Topography often is the main factor influencing the abundance and distribution of organisms because of its impact on solar radiation, heat, moisture, soil, and fertility. Temperature tends to be lower in higher altitude locations, and precipitation distribution along a rising slope is likely uneven. Sunlight intensity on south-facing slopes is higher than that on north-facing slopes. As a result, topography and topography-induced ecological phenomena and processes are topics of mountain ecology.

In this example, we analyze data from an observational study intended to understand the effect of topography on seedling recruitment in a mixed evergreen–deciduous forest community in southwest China. The study reported in Shen [2002] included observations at several spatial scales. We use the data collected along a transect of 128 consecutive 5×5 m plots designed to understand the influence of topography. For example, how different types of trees are distributed along a gradient between the valley and the ridge top, after other environmental factors (e.g., light availability measured by canopy gap and soil fertility measured by soil organic carbon content) are controlled. The researchers counted the number of seedlings (with heights below 1 meter) in each plot (the response variable) and other related factors on seedling recruitment. A total of 49 species of seedlings were observed in the field and were classified into five types according to their status in the community: pioneer, early dominant, early companion, later dominant (including evergreen species), and tolerant [Shen et al., 2000]. Other physical and biological variables measured at the plot level included canopy gap (in %) and soil total organic carbon (TOC, %). The topography is represented by the variable "position," measured as the relative position along a hillside between valley (position = 1) and ridge (position = 5).

5.2.2.1 The Classical Generalized Linear Models

Using traditional model exploratory analyses based on the generalized linear model (assuming the seedling count following a Poisson distribution), we commonly determine whether a predictor variable is relevant or not based on various null hypothesis tests. These tests can yield confusing results. For example, the "main" effect of position using the model presented in Qian and Shen [2007] would be statistically significant using analysis of deviance. However, the estimated differences in intercept between different positions are not.

```
#### R Code ####
seedlingGLM <- glm(Numb ~ factor(type)*Total.C +
                         factor(type)*logit(Gap) +
                         factor(Position),
                  family=poisson, data=seedling)
#### R Output ####
> anova(seedlingGLM)
Analysis of Deviance Table
Model: poisson, link: log
Response: Numb
Terms added sequentially (first to last)
                          Df Deviance Resid. Df Resid. Dev
NULL                                      788      909.44
factor(type)              4   36.151     784      873.29
logit(Gap)               1   14.182     783      859.10
Total.C                  1    0.509     782      858.60
factor(Position)         4   20.463     778      838.13
factor(type):logit(Gap)  4   25.398     774      812.73
factor(type):Total.C     4   18.192     770      794.54
>
> display(seedlingGLM)
...
Total.C                   0.21      0.06
factor(Position)2        -0.16      0.12
factor(Position)3        -0.08      0.11
factor(Position)4         0.16      0.11
factor(Position)5         0.11      0.11
factor(type)2:logit(Gap) -0.39      0.25
...
### End ###
```

The analysis of deviance table shows that including position after type, gap, and soil organic carbon would further reduce the deviance by 20.463. The log-likelihood ratio test would return a p-value of 0.0004 (`1-pchisq(20.463,4)`). The estimated intercept differences between positions 2 through 5 and 1 are all not statistically different from 0. A direct test for the effect of position is to fit a second model without position and compare the two models using analysis of deviance:

```
#### R Code ####
seedlingGLM2 <- glm(Numb ~ factor(type)*Total.C +
                          factor(type)*logit(Gap),
                  family=poisson, data=seedling)
```

```
#### R Output ####
> anova(seedlingGLM2, seedlingGLM)
Analysis of Deviance Table

Model 1: Numb ~ factor(type)*logit(Gap)+factor(type)*Total.C
Model 2: Numb ~ factor(type)*logit(Gap)+factor(type)*Total.C
              + factor(Position)
  Resid. Df Resid. Dev Df Deviance
1       774    819.74
2       770    794.54  4   25.197
```

```
### End ###
```

In short, the classical statistical analysis suggests that topography represented by position is an important factor affecting seedling recruitment. However, the models used here are ambiguous on how topography influences recruitment. Although simply using a Bayesian computation method would not fundamentally change these models, the Bayesian emphasis on estimation may help to avoid ambiguity of conflicting hypothesis testing results. Furthermore, because we are not limited to the standard models implemented in R, we can extend the model to include relevant processes that must be ignored under classical statistics. In the rest of this example, we first implement the classical GLM in Stan and then expand the model to include over-dispersion and spatial auto-correlation.

5.2.2.2   Bayesian Implementation of GLM

Implementing a generalized linear model in Stan is similar to the Bayesian linear regression, except that the likelihood function is now based on binomial, Poisson, or other distribution from the exponential family. The models discussed in the previous section include two continuous predictor variables and two factor variables. The GLM models allow the slopes of the two continuous predictors to vary by one factor-predictor (tree type) and the intercept to vary by tree type and position. We can re-express the model as follows:

$$
\begin{aligned}
y_i &\sim Poisson(\lambda_i) \\
\log(\lambda_i) &= \beta_0 + \beta_{1j[i]} + \beta_{2k[i]} + \\
&\quad (\beta_3 + \delta_{3j[i]})C_{l[i]} + (\beta_4 + \delta_{4j[i]})logit(Gap_{l[i]})
\end{aligned}
\tag{5.8}
$$

where the index i represents observation, $j[i]$ indicates that the ith observation is for tree type j, $k[i]$ represents that the ith observation is at position k, and $l[i]$ represents the lth plot. The Stan model is very similar to the binomial model in the Liverpool moth example:

```
#### Stan Model ####
seedStan <- "
data{
  int n; //sample size
  int nt; //number of tree types
  int np; //number of positions
  int type[n];
  int position[n];
  int y[n];
  real soilC[n];
  real gap[n]; //logit of gap
}
parameters{
  real beta0;
  real beta1[nt];
  real beta2[np];
  real beta3;
  real delta3[nt];
  real beta4;
  real delta4[np];
  real<lower=0> sigma1;
  real<lower=0> sigma2;
  real<lower=0> sigma3;
  real<lower=0> sigma4;
}
model{
  real log_lambda[n];
  beta1 ~ normal(0, sigma1);
  beta2 ~ normal(0, sigma2);
  delta3 ~ normal(0, sigma3);
  delta4 ~ normal(0, sigma4);
  for (i in 1:n){
    log_lambda[i] = beta0 + beta1[type[i]] +
                    beta2[position[i]] +
                    (beta3+delta3[type[i]])*soilC[i] +
```

```
                   (beta4+delta4[type[i]])*gap[i];
  }
  y ~ poisson_log(log_lambda);
// or
// target += poisson_log_lupmf(y|log_lambda);
}
"
```

End

The variance component plot (Figure 5.4) shows that the uncertainty on type variance component is substantial.

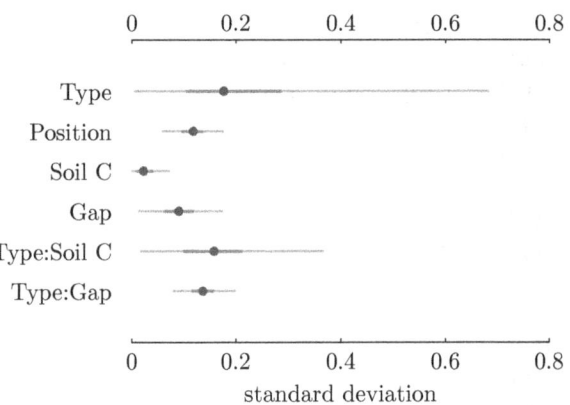

FIGURE 5.4: Estimated standard deviations of the tree type, topographic position, soil organic carbon, canopy gap, and two interaction effects are shown in an ANOVA-like plot.

One potential problem is that recruitment of different types of trees may vary by position. That is, there may be a type-position interaction. Including the interaction between type and position is equivalent to allowing the type effect to vary by position and the position effect to vary by type, or directly estimating the effect of the combined type-position variable:

$$\log(\lambda_i) = \beta_0 + \beta_{1,jk[i]} + (\beta_2 + \delta_{2j[i]})C_{l[i]} + (\beta_3 + \delta_{3j[i]})logit(Gap_{l[i]}) \quad (5.9)$$

Or, translating into Stan code:

Partial Stan Code
```
  for (i in 1:n){
    log_lambda[i] = beta0 + beta1[type_position[i]] +
      (beta2+delta2[type[i]])*soilC[i] +
      (beta3+delta3[type[i]])*gap[i];
```

```
}
### End ###
```

where $jk[i]$ indicates that observation i represents type j in position k, and we can create the `type_position` object by pasting `type` and `position` in R before passing to Stan:

```
type_position <- as.numeric(ordered(paste(type, position)))
```

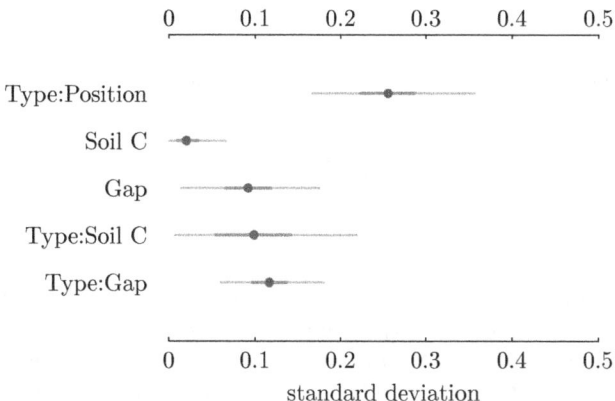

FIGURE 5.5: Estimated standard deviations of the tree-type:topographic-position interaction, soil organic carbon, canopy gap, and two interaction effects are shown in an ANOVA-like plot.

The variance component plot (Figure 5.5) suggests that the tree type and position interaction accounted for most of the seedling counts variation, which indicates that topography may shape the distribution of different types of trees. The estimated type position interaction effects (Figure 5.6) provide details that may lead to testable hypotheses. The relative abundances of the five types of trees show an opposite pattern between valley (position 1) and ridgetop (position 5). The valleys were mostly occupied by pioneer (type 1) and early dominant (type 2) species, with decreasing abundances for types 3 to 5 (companion, evergreen/late dominant, and tolerant species). On ridge tops, the order of abundances is reversed, where tolerant trees are the most abundant, followed by evergreen, companion, dominant, and pioneering species. However, different types of trees have their preferred positions. For example, although pioneer species is one of the most abundant types of trees, they are more abundant in mid-slope (position 3); Types 4 (late dominant, mostly evergreen species) and 5 (tolerant species) appear more on the ridge top (position 5).

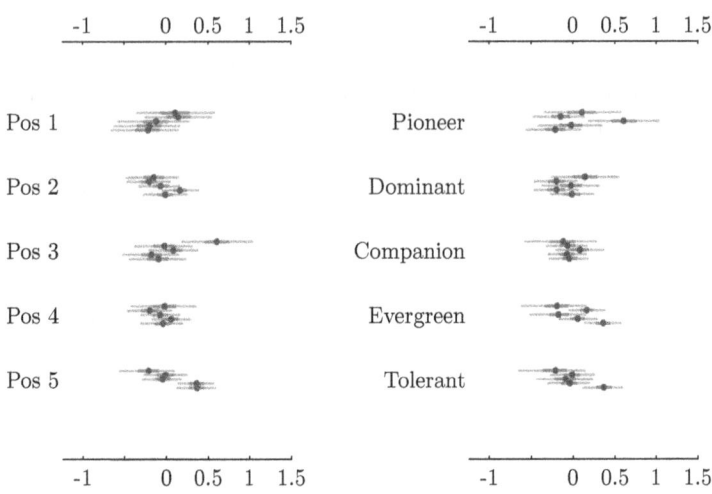

FIGURE 5.6: Estimated tree-type:position interaction effects are shown by positions (left) and by tree type (right). Each simplified boxplot represents a tree type (from top to bottom: pioneer, early dominant, companion, evergreen/late dominant, and tolerant) and position (from top to bottom 1:5). The dots are the estimated means, the dark thick lines are the mid-50% credible intervals, and the thin gray lines are the 95% credible intervals.

5.2.2.3   Over-dispersion

We mentioned that nearly all count variables are over-dispersed (Section 5.1) and one way to account for the extra variance in a Poisson model is to model the Poisson rate parameter as a gamma or log-normal random variable. For this example (a regression problem), we can add a model error term to equation (5.9):

$$\log(\lambda_i) = \beta_0 + \beta_{1,jk[i]} + (\beta_2 + \delta_{2j[i]})C_{l[i]} + (\beta_3 + \delta_{3j[i]})logit(Gap_{l[i]}) + \epsilon_i \quad (5.10)$$

where ϵ_i is assumed to be an independent normal random variable with mean 0 and a constant variance ($\epsilon_i \sim N(0, \sigma_e^2)$). As such the log rate parameter is a conditional normal random variable.

The variance component plot suggests that the over-dispersion (OD) is considerable (Figure 5.7). When using the classical GLM, we can use the option `family=quasipoisson` to account for the over-dispersion. This option assumes that the response variable variance is proportional to the mean (i.e., $\sigma^2 = \theta\mu$, where θ is known as the over-dispersion parameter), and a quasi-maximum likelihood estimator is used to estimate the Poisson model parameters and the over-dispersion parameter [Wedderburn, 1974]. When using

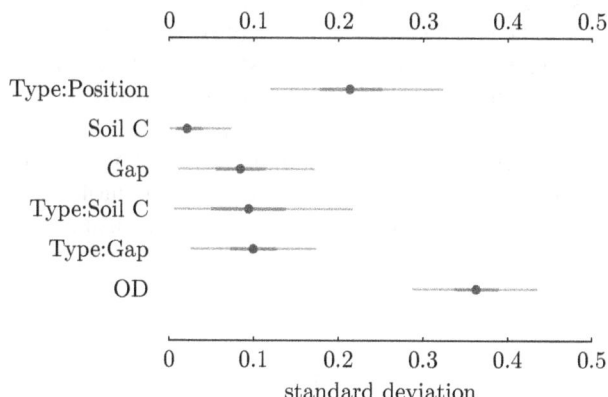

FIGURE 5.7: Estimated standard deviations of the tree type, topographic position, soil organic carbon, canopy gap, two interaction effects, model error (representing over-dispersion) are shown in an ANOVA-like plot.

the quasi-likelihood method, the probability distribution assumption about the response variable is no longer Poisson. The quasi-likelihood estimated mean model coefficients are the same as the estimated mean coefficients using `family=poisson`, but the quasi-Poisson estimated coefficient standard errors are the Poisson standard error times the square root of θ. The Bayesian estimated posterior distributions of coefficients using equation (5.10) are very close to the posterior distributions of the same coefficients estimated using equation (5.9) (Table 5.1).

We can use the posterior predictive simulation to demonstrate the over-dispersion phenomenon. For simplicity, we use models represented by equations (5.9) and (5.10) to replicate the observed seedling count in the data, and compare the observed standard deviation with standard deviations calculated from the replicated data.

Specifically, we use the predictor values in the data and the estimated posterior distributions of model coefficients. Each set of MCMC samples of model coefficients, combined with the predictive variable data, lead to one simulated λ (and σ_e). For each simulated λ (equation (5.9)), we draw one set of seedling counts from the Poisson distribution to replicate the observed data. For the over-dispersion model (equation (5.10)), each set of MCMC samples of model coefficients lead to a simulated log λ (without the error term) and a simulated σ_e. Using the simulated log λ and σ_e, we can draw a random sample of the Poisson distribution rate coefficient (from a log-normal distribution), which is then used to draw a replicated observed count from the Poisson distribution.

We replicated each observed seedling count using each of the 2500 sets of MCMC samples of model coefficients to obtain 2500 replicates of the observed seeding count data. For each set of replicates of $N = 789$ counts, we calculated their standard deviation (a total of 2500 standard deviations) to compare to the observed standard deviation. Without the over-dispersion term (ϵ_i) (i.e., using equation (5.9), the posterior simulated data standard deviation distribution was far smaller than the observed standard deviation, whereas the observed data standard deviation is near the 85th percentile of the simulated data standard deviation with the over-dispersion term (using equation (5.10), Figure 5.8).

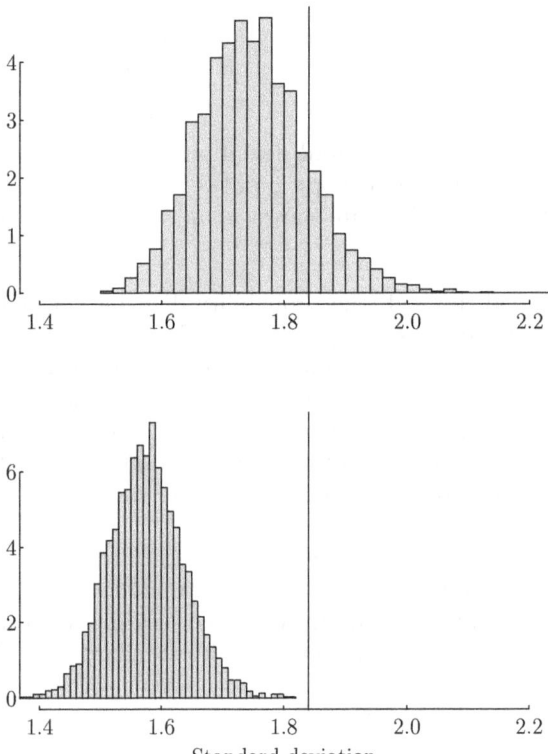

FIGURE 5.8: Posterior predictive simulation estimated seedling count standard deviations using the over-dispersed model (equation (5.10), top panel) and the Poisson model (equation (5.9), lower panel) are compared to the observed seedling count data standard deviation (the vertical lines).

5.2.2.4 Spatial Auto-correlation

In the over-dispersion model (equation (5.10)), the model errors ϵ_i are assumed to be independent. Because the seedling counts were made along a transect, the independence assumption is likely inappropriate. Plots close to each other are more likely to share similar environmental and other relevant conditions than plots far apart. As such, the spatial correlation in errors is likely. Because the sampling units are areal (plots), the commonly used method for modeling correlation due to spatial proximity is the conditional autoregressive (CAR) model [Besag et al., 1991]. Under CAR, we introduce a spatial random quantity ($\phi_i, l = 1, \cdots, N$) for each of the N areal sampling units (plots) and model the correlation among these random quantities based on their adjacency. Spatial adjacency is specified using an adjacency matrix $\boldsymbol{W}$ with diagonal elements $w_{ii} = 0$ and off-diagonal elements $w_{ij} = 1$ if i is a neighbor of j and $w_{ij} = 0$ otherwise. The joint distribution of $\boldsymbol{\phi} = (\phi_1, \cdots, \phi_N)'$ is:

$$\boldsymbol{\phi} \sim N\left(0, [\tau \boldsymbol{D}(\boldsymbol{I} - \alpha \boldsymbol{B})]^{-1}\right) \tag{5.11}$$

where τ is the spatial precision parameter (reciprocal of variance), $\boldsymbol{D} = \text{diag}(m_1, \cdots, m_n)$ is a diagonal matrix with the diagonal element m_i being the number of neighbors for plot i, $\boldsymbol{I}$ is an $n \times n$ identity matrix, α is a parameter controlling spatial dependence ($0 < \alpha < 1$), and $\boldsymbol{B} = \boldsymbol{D}^{-1}\boldsymbol{W}$ is the scaled adjacency matrix.

The spatial correlation is modeled by adding the spatial random quantity to the Poisson model:

$$\begin{aligned}
\log(\lambda_i) = \ & \beta_0 + \beta_{1jk[i]} + \\
& (\beta_2 + \delta_{2j[i]})C_{l[i]} + (\beta_3 + \delta_{3j[i]})logit(Gap_{l[i]}) + \\
& \phi_{l[i]}
\end{aligned} \tag{5.12}$$

The prior in equation (5.11) can be specified using the Stan function `multi_normal_prec`.

```
#### Stan Model ####
seedStanCar1 <- "
data{
   int n; //sample size
   int nt; //number of tree types
   int ntp; //number of type-position combinations
   int N; //number of plots
   int type[n];
   int typ_pos[n];
   int plot[n];
   int y[n];
   real soilC[n];
   real gap[n]; //logit of gap
   matrix<lower = 0, upper = 1>[N, N] W;
```

```
}
transformed data{
  vector[N] zeros;
  matrix<lower = 0>[N, N] D;
  {
    vector[N] W_rowsums;
    for (i in 1:N) {
      W_rowsums[i] = sum(W[i, ]);
    }
    D = diag_matrix(W_rowsums);
  }
  zeros = rep_vector(0, N);
}
parameters{
  real beta0;
  real beta1[ntp];
  real beta2;
  real delta2[nt];
  real beta3;
  real delta3[nt];
  real<lower=0> sigma[3];
  vector[N] phi;
  real<lower = 0> tau;
  real<lower = 0, upper = 1> alpha;
}
model{
  real log_lambda[n];
  sigma ~ normal(0, 2);
  beta0 ~ normal(0, 1);
  beta1 ~ normal(0, sigma[1]);
  beta2 ~ normal(0, 1);
  beta3 ~ normal(0, 1);
  delta2 ~ normal(0, sigma[2]);
  delta3 ~ normal(0, sigma[3]);
  phi ~ multi_normal_prec(zeros, tau * (D - alpha * W));
  tau ~ gamma(2, 2);
  for (i in 1:n){
    log_lambda[i] = beta0 + beta1[typ_pos[i]] +
                (beta2+delta2[type[i]])*soilC[i] +
                (beta3+delta3[type[i]])*gap[i] +
                phi[plot[i]];
  }
  y ~ poisson_log(log_lambda);
}
"
```

End

The model is excruciatingly slow because of the relatively high number of plots (125). The prior for ϕ is a 125×125 matrix. The log-probability density function of $p(\phi \mid \tau, \alpha)$ is:

$$\log(p(\phi \mid \tau, \alpha)) = -\frac{n}{2}\log(2\pi) + \frac{1}{2}\log(\det(\boldsymbol{W}^{-1})) - \frac{1}{2}\phi^T \boldsymbol{W}^{-1}\phi.$$

The inversion of the adjacency matrix $(\boldsymbol{W}^{-1})$ and the calculation of its determinant are very slow. The computational speed can be improved by using (1) a sparse representation of the inverse of the adjacency matrix $(\boldsymbol{W}^{-1})$ and (2) the proportional solution of $\det(\boldsymbol{W}^{-1})$ proposed by Jin et al. [2005]. In the case study developed by Max Joseph[1] a function `sparse_car_lpdf` is proposed based on these two improvements. The function is used to define the prior in the model block (replacing the function `multi_normal_prec`), along with a `transformed data` block to compute the eigenvalues of $D^{-\frac{1}{2}}WD^{-\frac{1}{2}}$) and generate a sparse representation for $\boldsymbol{W}$ (a two-column matrix where each row is an adjacency relationship between two sites). The Stan code included in our GitHub repository was based on the `function` and `transformed data` blocks from Max Joseph's GitHub repository. The sparse CAR model improved computation time by more than an order of magnitude over the multivariate normal prior model.

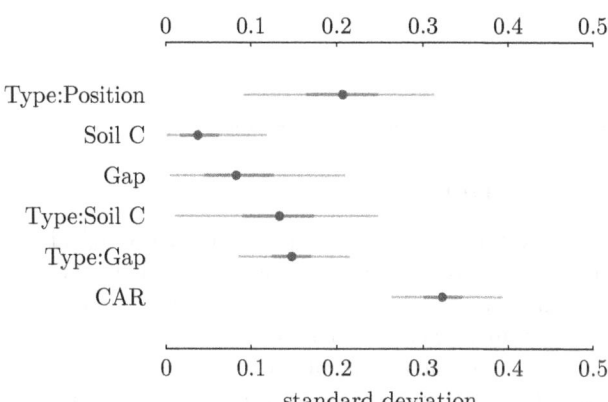

FIGURE 5.9: Variance components of the seedling recruitment model with spatial auto-correlation (CAR) are represented by the finite sample standard deviations of each component.

---

[1]`https://github.com/mbjoseph/CARstan`

The finite sample standard deviation of ϕ_i is used to represent the variance component of the spatial correlation (Figure 5.9). The variance component represented by the spatial autocorrelation is the largest among all batches, suggesting a significant over-dispersion. The inclusion of the spatial auto-correlation term results in slightly different parameter estimations (Table 5.1). But the general pattern of the type–position interaction did not change (Figure 5.10).

TABLE 5.1: A comparison of the estimated model coefficient posterior distributions (mean, standard deviation, and selected percentiles) from using equations (5.9), (5.10), and (5.12).

	mean	sd	2.5%	25%	50%	75%	97.5%
			equation (5.9)				
β_0	0.684	0.110	0.466	0.611	0.685	0.758	0.90
β_2	0.005	0.020	-0.033	-0.007	0.006	0.018	0.044
β_3	0.089	0.112	-0.142	0.036	0.089	0.143	0.313
			equation (5.10)				
β_0	0.616	0.114	0.389	0.541	0.614	0.692	0.849
β_2	0.005	0.021	-0.039	-0.008	0.005	0.019	0.047
β_3	0.083	0.097	-0.096	0.034	0.081	0.129	0.294
			equation (5.12)				
β_0	0.55	0.163	0.232	0.44	0.548	0.665	0.861
β_2	0.018	0.03	-0.037	-0.001	0.017	0.036	0.075
β_3	0.083	0.136	-0.192	0.012	0.08	0.155	0.357

5.3   Imperfect Detection

Imperfect detection is a common problem in ecological, environmental, epidemiological, and medical data analysis. In studying the distribution and abundance of organisms, ecologists visit study sites to collect specimens of the target organism. In most cases, we cannot guarantee that we can capture the organism when it is present at the site. In some cases, we may misidentify a specimen of a non-target organism as the target organism. If we fail to capture the target organism (reporting a 0) while the organism is present, the reported 0 (or a negative result) is a false negative. If we misidentify a non-target organism as the target organism while the target organism is absent, the reported 1 (or a positive result) is a false positive. In epidemiology, tests scientists use for detecting disease agents in individual patients are almost always imperfect. That is, false positives and false negatives are possible. Results from an imperfect test can be ambiguous, as a positive result may not always

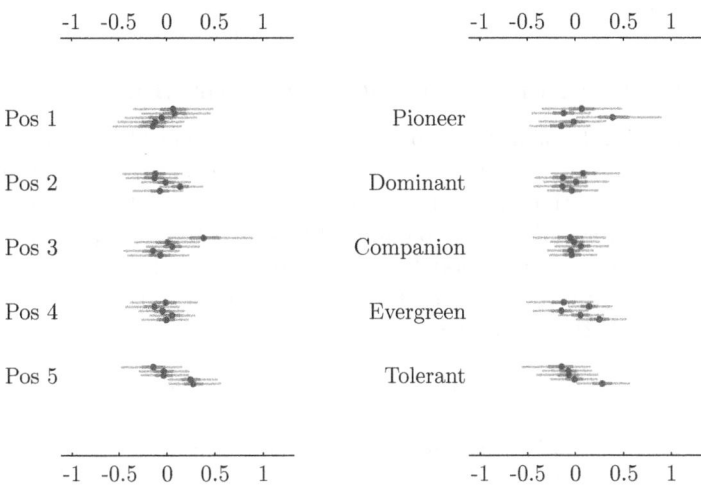

FIGURE 5.10: CAR model estimated tree-type:position interaction effects are shown by position (left) and by tree type (right). See Figure 5.6.

indicate the presence of the disease agent and vise versa. The imperfection poses challenges in data analysis because the data we have are a result of two random processes: one is the presence/absence of the target, and the other is the detection method. Observed count data are a combined result of the two processes. In many cases, the observed data alone do not have information to separate the effects of the two.

In this section, we discuss the imperfect detection problem. As in the snake fungal disease example (Section 1.1.1), data in an imperfect detection problem are the result of two separate processes – the presence/absence of the target and the positive/negative results of the detection method. The imperfection comes from the detection methods. In one type of problem, we want to estimate the population parameter of interest, for example, the prevalence of fungal disease in the snake population. In the other type of problem, we are only interested in the relative magnitude of the population parameter under different conditions, for example, the Gulf of Mexico hypoxia example (Section 4.2.2). When the absolute value of the population parameter (e.g., the prevalence of snake fungal disease in a particular population) is of interest, we noted that characterizing the error probabilities of the detection method is important because the observed data alone do not have information on both the population parameter of interest and the test method characteristics. When the relative value of the population parameter is of interest, we can ignore the method characteristics as long as the error probabilities are consistent throughout the study.

5.3.1   The Data Augmentation Algorithm

In a simple binary test problem (e.g., equation (1.4)), we have three parameters to describe the two random processes (see the snake fungal disease example in Section 1.1.1 on page 6): the disease prevalence θ (infected portion of the population), the probability of false positive f_p, and the probability of false negative f_n. The model used in that example is mathematically unidentifiable because the data and the binomial model contain information only on the probability of a positive observation

$$\Pr(+) = \theta(1 - f_n) + (1 - \theta)f_p. \tag{5.13}$$

As a result, θ and f_n, f_p cannot be uniquely determined without proper prior distributions for two of these three parameters. Without knowing the true status (in this case, whether a snake is infected or not) made the problem difficult. However, if the unknown status is explicitly specified as an unknown parameter (e.g., $z = 1$ for being infected and $z = 0$ otherwise), the joint likelihood function of y for a snake is the joint probability of y, z and parameters θ, f_p, and f_n in equation (1.4). The joint probability can be specified through the conditional probability formula

$$\pi(y, z, \theta, f_n, f_p) = \pi(y|z, f_p, f_n)\pi(z|\theta)\pi(f_p)\pi(f_n)\pi(\theta).$$

For a given observation, y takes value 0 (negative) or 1 (positive). The conditional probability of $y|z, f_p, f_n$ is readily available:

$$\begin{aligned}
\Pr(y = 1|z = 1, f_p, f_n) &= 1 - f_n \\
\Pr(y = 0|z = 1, f_p, f_n) &= f_n \\
\Pr(y = 1|z = 0, f_p, f_n) &= f_p \\
\Pr(y = 0|z = 0, f_p, f_n) &= 1 - f_p.
\end{aligned}$$

The probability of z given θ is $\Pr(z = 1|\theta) = \theta$ and $\Pr(z = 0|\theta) = 1 - \theta$. The variable z, representing the underlying true state, is known as a latent variable. Expanding the process from one snake to multiple snakes (e.g., $n = 20$ snakes and $y = 5$ were positive), we can introduce latent variables Z_1 representing the number of snakes that were infected and testing positive and Z_2 being the number of snakes that were infected and testing negative. The number of non-infected snakes is $n - Z_1 - Z_2$. The binomial modeling problem can be represented as in Table 5.2.

The problem is now a multinomial one. We have four possible outcomes:

- infected and positive (IP) with probability $\theta(1 - f_n)$,

- infected and negative (IN) with probability θf_n,

TABLE 5.2: A tabular representation of the relationship between the true state of tested subjects (infected or not infected) and their testing results (positive or negative) through the use of latent variables Z_1 and Z_2.

	Infected	Not infected	Sum
Positive	Z_1	$y - Z_1$	y
Negative	Z_2	$n - y - Z_2$	$n - y$
Sum	$Z_1 + Z_2$	$n - Z_1 - Z_2$	n

- not infected and positive (NiP) with probability $(1 - \theta)f_p$, and

- not infected and negative (NiN) with probability $(1 - \theta)(1 - f_p)$.

The likelihood function is

$$[\theta(1 - f_n)]^{Z_1}[\theta f_n]^{Z_2}[(1 - \theta)f_p]^{y-Z_1}[(1 - \theta)(1 - f_p)]^{n-y-Z_2}.$$

The three parameters θ, f_n, and f_p are probabilities, and we can use the beta distribution as their priors. Furthermore, the prevalence is about the snake population; while f_p and f_n are characteristics of the test, we can safely assume that θ is independent of f_p and f_n. False positives and false negatives often represent different aspects of a test. For example, a false negative is more likely related to the amount of virus on a snake's skin, while a false positive can be a result of a mismatch of the target DNA. As a result, we may also assume that f_p and f_n are independent of each other. Let the priors be

$$\begin{aligned} \theta &\sim beta(\alpha, \beta) \\ f_p &\sim beta(a_1, b_1) \\ f_n &\sim beta(a_2, b_2). \end{aligned} \qquad (5.14)$$

The joint posterior distribution of the three parameters is proportional to the prior in equation (5.14) and the likelihood function:

$$\theta^{\alpha-1}(1 - \theta)^{\beta-1}f_p^{a_1-1}(1 - f_p)^{b_1-1}f_n^{a_2-1}(1 - f_n)^{b_2-1}$$
$$[\theta(1 - f_n)]^{Z_1}[\theta f_n]^{Z_2}[(1 - \theta)f_p]^{y-Z_1}[(1 - \theta)(1 - f_p)]^{n-y-Z_2}.$$

This seemingly complicated distribution can be used to derive the full set of posterior conditional distributions of the three parameters and the two latent variables:

$$\begin{aligned} \pi(\theta \mid f_p, f_n, Z_1, Z_2, y, n) &\propto \theta^{\alpha+Z_1+Z_2-1}(1 - \theta)^{\beta+n-Z_1-Z_2-1} \\ \pi(f_p \mid \theta, f_n, Z_1, Z_2, y, n) &\propto f_p^{a_1+y-Z_1-1}(1 - f_p)^{b_1+n-y-Z_2-1} \\ \pi(f_n \mid \theta, f_p, Z_1, Z_2, y, n) &\propto f_n^{a_2+Z_2-1}(1 - f_n)^{b_2+Z_1-1} \\ \pi(Z_1 \mid Z_2, \theta, f_p, f_n, y, n) &\propto [\theta(1 - f_n)]^{Z_1}[(1 - \theta)f_p]^{y-Z_1} \\ \pi(Z_2 \mid Z_1, \theta, f_p, f_n, y, n) &\propto [\theta f_n]^{Z_2}[(1 - \theta)(1 - f_p)]^{n-y-Z_2} \end{aligned} \qquad (5.15)$$

That is, the conditional posterior of θ is a beta distribution with parameters $\alpha + Z_1 + Z_2$ and $\beta + y - Z1$:

$$\theta \mid f_p, f_n, Z_1, Z_2, y, n \sim beta(\alpha + Z_1 + Z_2, \beta + n - Z_1 - Z_2).$$

Likewise,

$$f_p \mid \theta, f_n, Z_1, Z_2, y, n \sim beta(a_1 + y - Z_1, b_1 + n - y - Z_2)$$

and

$$f_n \mid \theta, f_p, Z_1, Z_2, y, n \sim beta(a_2 + Z_2, b_2 + Z_1).$$

The conditional distribution of Z_1 is a binomial distribution:

$$Z_1 \mid Z_2, \theta, f_p, f_n, y, ns \sim binom(\phi_1, y),$$

where $\phi_1 = \frac{\theta(1-f_n)}{\theta(1-f_n)+(1-\theta)f_p}$. The conditional distribution of Z_2 is also a binomial distribution:

$$Z_2 \mid Z_1, \theta, f_p, f_n, y, n \sim binom(\phi_2, n - y),$$

where $\phi_2 = \frac{\theta f_n}{\theta f_n + (1-\theta)(1-f_p)}$.

With the full set of conditional densities, we can use the Gibbs sampler to sample θ, f_p, f_n and Z_1, Z_2 from their joint posterior distribution.

Similar Gibbs sampler algorithms for this type of problem can be found in the literature, especially in the 1990s and early 2000s. As we discussed earlier, the problem is mathematically unidentifiable unless two of the three priors in equation (5.14) are reasonably informative. The data augmentation algorithm does not change the basic mathematics that the likelihood function does not have the necessary information for simultaneously quantifying the three unknown probabilities. The Gibbs sampler algorithm is feasible only when proper priors for the three probabilities are available. We can use simulation to understand the characteristics of the method:

- Assuming θ, f_n, and f_p are known,

- the simulated number of infected x_1 is a binomial random variable ($x_1 \sim bin(N, \theta)$) and the number of not infected is $x_2 = N - x_1$,

- the true positives x_{p1} are from the x_1 infected ($x_{p1} \sim bin(x_1, 1 - f_n)$) and the number of false positives are from the x_2 uninfected ($x_{p2} \sim bin(x_2, f_p)$).

- The observed number of positives is $y_1 = x_{p1} + x_{p2}$ and the observed number of negatives is $y_2 = N - y_1$.

The simulated samples are then used to estimate the three parameters. This process is repeated many times, and each time we record the estimated means of these parameters.

```
#### R Code ####
rbin_imperfect <- function(n=10, N=100, theta=0.2,
                fp=0.1, fn=0.4){
## n: number of random samples
```

```
## N: total number tested
   InF <- rbinom(n, size=N, prob=theta)
      ##Infected
   InP <- rbinom(n, size=InF, prob=1-fn)
      ##Infected and positive
   NinF <- N-InF
      ##Not infected
   NiP <- rbinom(n, size=NinF, fp)
      ##Not infected and positive
   y1 <- InP+NiP
      ##positive, Y2=negative
   return(data.frame(Y1=y1, Y2=N-y1))
}
### End ###
```

Using the simulation method, we learned that the Gibbs sampler is fickle. In a simulation, we draw simulated data (number of positives and negatives) 50 times, and each time we used the latent variable method to estimate the three parameters. In the first simulation, nearly all 50 estimated mean parameter values missed their known true values (Figure 5.11). The estimated parameter values often have large variances. This result is expected because the data we have (numbers of positives and negatives) contain information on the probability of observing a positive result, which is $\Pr(+) = \theta(1-f_n)+(1-\theta)f_p$. We cannot properly identify the three parameters. For example, if $\theta = 0.2$, $f_p = 0.1$, and $f_n = 0.3$, we have $\Pr(+) = 0.22$. We can obtain the same $\Pr(+)$ if we set $\theta = 0.8$, $f_p = 0.01$, and $f_n = 0.7275$. The possible combinations of the three parameters that can lead to the same $\Pr(+)$ are countless. In a Gibbs sampler, this non-identifiability leads to poor mixing. That is, if we run multiple chains, each chain may be stuck to a particular combination of the three parameter values and may never mix with other chains. Without strong informative priors, we cannot uniquely identify the three parameters based on the data alone.

In general, the data augmentation method is to exploit the relatively simple task of specifying conditional probability densities when a latent variable is available. That is, the likelihood function (as a probability density) for any Bayesian computation problem ($\Pr(y \mid \theta)$) can be derived from its joint distribution with a latent variable Z:

$$\pi(y, Z \mid \theta) = \pi(Z \mid \theta)\pi(y \mid Z, \theta).$$

Because we can easily specify the two terms on the right-hand side, the likelihood function is then

$$\pi(y \mid \theta) = \int_Z \pi(Z \mid \theta)\pi(y \mid Z, \theta)dZ. \tag{5.16}$$

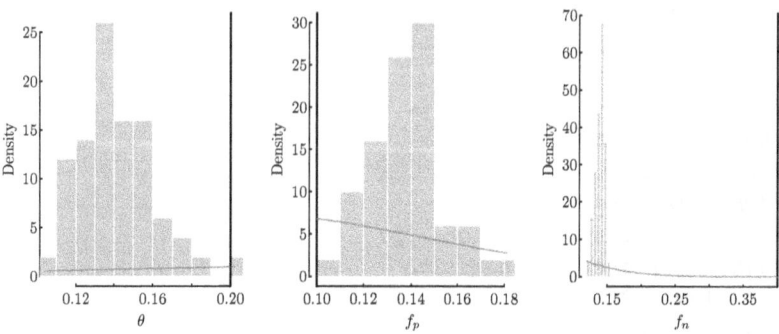

FIGURE 5.11: The Gibbs sampler implementation of the latent variable method failed to recover the known parameters used to generate the 50 sets of simulated data. The solid vertical lines show the true parameter values used to generate the data, and the histograms are the distributions of the 50 estimated mean values.

For categorical latent variables such as in our snake fungal disease example, the integral becomes the summation over all possible values of Z. See Tanner [1996] for more details of the data augmentation method.

Instead of using the Gibbs sampler as described in equation (5.15), we can derive the posterior using the data augmentation method:

1. The joint posterior of interest $p(\theta, f_p, f_n \mid Y_1, Y_2)$ is proportional to $p(\theta)p(f_p)p(f_n)p(Y_1, Y_2 \mid \theta, f_p, f_n)$.

2. The likelihood $p(Y_1, Y_2 \mid \theta, f_p, f_n)$ can be derived through the joint likelihood function of $Y_1, Y_2, Z = Z_1 + Z_2$, where Z is the latent variable (the unknown number of presences):

$$p(Y_1, Y_2, Z \mid \theta, f_p, f_n) = p(Z \mid \theta)p(Y_1, Y_2 \mid Z, f_p, f_n)$$

where $p(Z \mid \theta) \propto \theta^Z (1 - \theta)^{N-Z}$ and $p(Y_1, Y_2 \mid Z, f_p, f_n) = PP^{Y_1}(1 - PP)^{Y_2}$ and $PP = (Z(1 - f_n) + (N - Z)f_p)/N$. Hence,

$$p(Y_1, Y_2, Z \mid \theta, f_p, f_n) \propto \theta^Z (1 - \theta)^{N-Z} PP^{Y_1}(1 - PP)^{Y_2}.$$

Because Z can take values from 0 to N, the target likelihood function can be obtained by marginalizing out Z:

$$p(Y_1, Y_2 \mid \theta, f_p, f_n) \propto \sum_{Z=0}^{N} \theta^Z (1 - \theta)^{N-Z} PP^{Y_1}(1 - PP)^{Y_2}. \qquad (5.17)$$

Equation (5.17) can be used directly in Stan to specify the log-likelihood by using `target += lp`. The log-likelihood is

$$\log \left(\sum_{Z=0}^{N} \theta^Z (1 - \theta)^{N-Z} PP^{Y_1}(1 - PP)^{Y_2} \right)$$

which can be re-expressed as:

$$\log\left(\sum_{Z=0}^{N} e^{\log\left(\theta^Z (1-\theta)^{N-Z} PP^{Y_1}(1-PP)^{Y_2}\right)}\right)$$

so that the Stan function `log_sum_exp` can be used:

```
#### Partial Stan Code ####
model{
  //
  // insert priors for theta, fp and fn here
  //
  for (i in 1:n){
    int<lower=1> NN;
    real temp[NN+1];
    real PP;
    NN = Y1[i]+Y2[i];
    for (j in (1:(NN+1))){
      PP = ((1-fn)*(j-1)+fp*(NN-(j-1)))/NN;
      temp[j] = (j-1)*log(theta)+(NN-(j-1))*log(1-theta)+
                Y1[i]*log(PP)+Y2[i]*log(1-PP);
    }
    target += log_sum_exp(temp);
  }
}
### End ###
```

The function `log_sum_exp` uses a numerically efficient algorithm for avoiding overflow when calculating $\log \sum_{i=1}^{n} e^{x_i}$. In a mixture model problem, the log-likelihood is nearly always the log of the sum of two or more terms. The `log_sum_exp` function is usually a good option. In most cases, the elements of the summation are not directly expressed as exponential. We re-express individual elements as the exponential of log transformed elements.

Although marginalization does not resolve the non-identifiability problem, the implementation of the method in Stan allows quick diagnosis of the problem and meaningful exploration of how to solve the non-identifiability problem by exploring how to use prior information.

This binomial formulation, however, can be computationally inefficient when the total number of tests (N) is large. A more efficient way to construct the likelihood function is to treat each test as a Bernoulli trial. That is, for an observation with a total of $N_i = Y_{1i} + Y_{2i}$ tests, we derive the likelihood by multiplying the likelihood of the Y_{1i} positive results and the Y_{2i} negative results. Specifically, we use a latent variable z_{ij} for each test outcome y_{ij}. The value of y_{ij} is either 0 (negative) or 1 (positive), and the value of z_{ij} is also either 0 (not infected) or 1 (infected). The probability (likelihood) of observing y_{ij} is $p(y_{ij} \mid \theta, f_p, f_n)$, which can be derived through marginalizing the joint probability of y_{ij} and z_{ij}:

$$p(y_{ij}, z_{ij} \mid \theta, f_p, f_n) = p(z_{ij} \mid \theta)p(y_{ij} \mid z_{ij}, f_p, f_n).$$

Because z_{ij} takes values 0 or 1, the marginal likelihood is a sum of two terms:

$$
\begin{aligned}
p(y_{ij} \mid \theta, f_p, f_n) &= \sum_{z_{ij}=0}^{1} p(z_{ij} \mid \theta)p(y_{ij} \mid z_{ij}, f_p, f_n) \\
&= (1 - \theta)(f_p y_{ij} + (1 - f_p)(1 - y_{ij})) + \\
&\quad \theta((1 - f_n)y_{ij} + f_n(1 - y_{ij})).
\end{aligned}
$$

This likelihood is the sum of two terms, one for each of the two possible values of y_{ij}:

$$
\begin{aligned}
p(y_{ij} \mid \theta, f_p, f_n) &= (1 - \theta)(f_p y_{ij} + (1 - f_p)(1 - y_{ij})) + \\
&\quad \theta((1 - f_n)y_{ij} + f_n(1 - y_{ij})) \\
&= \begin{cases} (1 - \theta)f_p + \theta(1 - f_n), & \text{if } y_{ij} = 1 \\ (1 - \theta)(1 - f_p) + \theta f_n, & \text{if } y_{ij} = 0. \end{cases}
\end{aligned}
$$

For observation i, the likelihood is the product of N_i Bernoulli probabilities:

$$p(y_{i\cdot} \mid \theta, f_p, f_n) = \prod_{j=1}^{Y_{1i}} [(1 - \theta)f_p + \theta(1 - f_n)] \prod_{j=1}^{Y_{2i}} [(1 - \theta)(1 - f_p) + \theta f_n].$$

The log-likelihood is

$$
\begin{aligned}
\log(p(y_{i\cdot} \mid \theta, f_p, f_n)) &= \sum_{j=1}^{Y_{1i}} \log\left[(1 - \theta)f_p + \theta(1 - f_n)\right] + \\
&\quad \sum_{j=1}^{Y_{2i}} \log\left[(1 - \theta)(1 - f_p) + \theta f_n\right] \\
&= Y_{1i} \log\left[(1 - \theta)f_p + \theta(1 - f_n)\right] + \\
&\quad Y_{2i} \log\left[(1 - \theta)(1 - f_p) + \theta f_n\right] \\
&= Y_{1i} \log\left[e^{\log((1-\theta)f_p)} + e^{\log(\theta(1-f_n))}\right] + \\
&\quad Y_{2i} \log\left[e^{\log((1-\theta)(1-f_p))} + e^{\log(\theta f_n)}\right].
\end{aligned}
\tag{5.18}
$$

The Stan code is then:

```
#### Partial Stan Code ####
model{
  real temp1[2];
  real temp2[2];
  temp1[1] = log(1-theta)+log(fp);
  temp1[2] = log(theta)+log(1-fn);
  temp2[1] = log(1-theta)+log(1-fp);
  temp2[2] = log(theta)+log(fn);
  for (i in 1:n){
    target+=Y1[i]*log_sum_exp(temp1)+Y2[i]*log_sum_exp(temp2);
  }
}
### End ###
```

In addition to the reduced number of terms in the log-sum-exp function, the computation of the Bernoulli formulation (equation (5.18)) is simpler than the binomial formulation (equation (5.17)). However, if the goal is to estimate the prevalence (θ), we must have reasonably good priors for f_p and f_n. Because of the integration (equation (5.16)) over all possible values of the latent variable, the Stan implementation of the latent variable problem can effectively explore over the entire posterior distribution. As a result, we can easily use the resulting posterior samples to diagnose potential problems of the model.

5.3.2 Example: COVID-19 Testing in Ohio, USA

This is an example of imperfect detection. Because we have no definite knowledge of the test used in the early stage of the COVID pandemic, the reported numbers of positives and negatives cannot give us definite information on the true prevalence of the disease. Here, we use this example to illustrate the futility of estimating the prevalence of the disease without properly characterizing the testing method. This problem is especially ominous when the testing method is changing.

We use the reported daily COVID-19 test results during the early days (March to May 2020) of the COVID-19 pandemic in Ohio, USA, to illustrate the updating process. The daily tracking data were compiled by the COVIDTracking Project[2]. The test used for detecting the novel coronavirus (SARS-CoV-2) was a qPCR test that detects the presence of the viral DNA. As with all PCR tests, the test is imperfect. Furthermore, we do not have direct studies to quantify the test's false positive and false negative probabilities because SARS-CoV-2 is a novel virus. As a result, the public and, often, the medical professionals took a positive test result as a confirmation of infection of SARS-CoV-2. Because of this misconception, the initial reporting from many states in the U.S. was inconsistent. From March 5 to 15, 2020, the state of Ohio conducted very few tests and reported numbers of both positives and negatives. Media reports suggested that not all negative results were reported initially. As the number of tests increased, the state only reported the number of positive results from March 16 to 24. After March 25, Ohio resumed reporting both positive and negative test results. During this time, the number of daily tests increased from fewer than 200 to more than 2000. We used data from March 9, when the first positive was reported, to March 15 (the last day when both positives and negatives were reported) to estimate the three probabilities. Once the number of tests is in the thousands, the binomial distribution model is no longer computationally feasible. We use the Bernoulli formulation only.

The estimated posterior distributions are used to develop priors for the next phase, from March 26, when the state resumed reporting both positives and negatives, to May 30, when the state's "shelter-in-place" and "stay-safe-

---

[2]https://tinyurl.com/4zrm53p7

Ohio" orders were lifted. Again, the posterior distributions from the second phase were used as priors for the third phase, from the reopening of most businesses to the end of June when the number of positives reached new highs.

The goal of this example is to explore how to properly use the information other than the data to resolve the non-identifiability problem. Such exploration may not provide definite estimates of the three unknown parameters $(\theta, f_p, \text{ and } f_n)$. As a result, the goal of this example is to show that to properly analyze data from an imperfect test we need to (1) properly define the objective of the study (whether to estimate the prevalence or for disease diagnosis) and (2) use independent sources of information characterizing the quality of the test (f_p and f_n) and/or the population (θ). We first use a relatively diffuse prior for θ to show the divergent chains in the MCMC result. Based on what we learned during the COVID-19 pandemic, we experiment with limiting the ranges of $\theta, f_p,$ and f_n.

We used studies of similar tests during previous coronavirus outbreaks to derive our initial prior distributions for f_n and f_p. Several studies compared qPCR test results to later confirmed results of the presence/absence of coronavirus (SARS, MERS, H1N1) to establish the test's f_p and f_n [Alvarez-Martínez et al., 2006, Binsaeed et al., 2011, Rainer et al., 2004, Tham et al., 2012]. Based on these studies, we constructed our initial prior distributions for false positive ($beta(3, 23)$) and false negative ($beta(2, 22)$). The initial prior for θ was non-informative ($beta(1, 1)$).

5.3.2.1   Initial Testing

From March 9 to March 15, 2020, the numbers of tests performed in Ohio were low, given only to people with several known COVID-19 symptoms and confirmed exposure to the virus (e.g., direct contact with known COVID-19 patients and travel to countries with known outbreaks). As such, we expect that the prevalence (the fraction of population truly infected with COVID-19) in this highly selected population would be high. The estimated posterior mean of θ is 0.13, while the estimated posterior means of f_p and f_n (0.11 and 0.09) are the same as their respective prior means (Table 5.3).

The marginal distributions can be misleading when parameters are strongly correlated, as the MCMC samples are from the joint posterior distribution of the three parameters [Qian, 2012]. The pairwise scatter plots of the posterior samples show a negative correlation between θ and f_p, while f_n is largely independent of the other two parameters (Figure 5.12). The negative correlation is not expected because θ is a parameter about the population and f_p and f_n are characteristics of the qPCR test. The prevalence of COVID-19 in the population should not affect how the lab-based test would perform. The strong correlation is a sign of the non-identifiability issue we encountered when discussing the Gibbs sampler algorithm. Because the marginal posterior distribution of f_n is essentially the same as the prior, we either are not

TABLE 5.3: Numerical summaries (mean, standard deviation, and selected percentiles) of the marginal posterior distributions of θ, f_p, and f_n estimated separately for three periods characterized by, largely, the number of tests. Prior distribution for θ was $beta(1,1)$ (uniform between 0 and 1). Prior distributions for f_p and f_n were $beta(2,23)$ and $beta(2,22)$, respectively.

	mean	sd	2.5%	25%	50%	75%	97.5%
	Initial Period (low test numbers)						
θ	0.13	0.06	0.01	0.08	0.13	0.17	0.25
f_p	0.11	0.05	0.03	0.07	0.10	0.14	0.21
f_n	0.09	0.06	0.01	0.04	0.08	0.12	0.24
	Shelter-in-place (moderate test numbers)						
θ	0.04	0.02	0.00	0.02	0.03	0.05	0.08
f_p	0.06	0.02	0.02	0.04	0.06	0.08	0.09
f_n	0.09	0.06	0.01	0.04	0.07	0.12	0.23
	Reopening (high test numbers)						
θ	0.01	0.01	0.00	0.01	0.01	0.02	0.03
f_p	0.03	0.01	0.01	0.02	0.03	0.04	0.04
f_n	0.09	0.06	0.01	0.04	0.07	0.12	0.23

learning much about the three parameters from the data, or the qPCR test for SARS-CoV2 virus has similar error rates as tests for other coronaviruses.

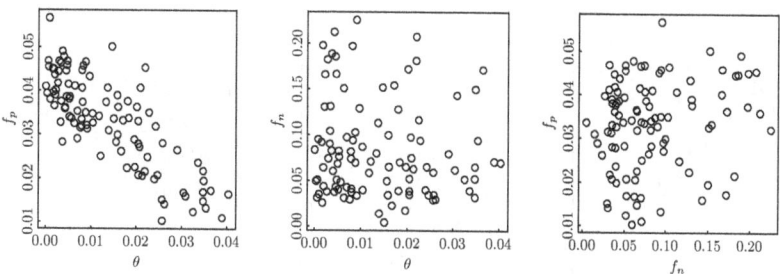

FIGURE 5.12: Pair-wise scatter plots of the MCMC samples from posterior distributions of prevalence (θ), false positive probability (f_p), and false negative probability (f_n) show a strong correlation between θ and f_p. The posterior distributions are based on initial testing data from March 9 to 15, 2020. During this time, the state's testing capacity was limited (less than 180 tests per day).

5.3.2.2 Shelter in Place and Reopening

With more tests and more days during the subsequent two periods, we see changes in the marginal posterior distributions of θ and f_p. The marginal posterior distribution of f_n stayed the same as the prior of f_n (Table 5.3). The correlation between θ and f_p in the joint posterior distribution of the three parameters is stronger (Figures 5.13 and 5.14), suggesting that increased sample sizes would not resolve the non-identifiability problem.

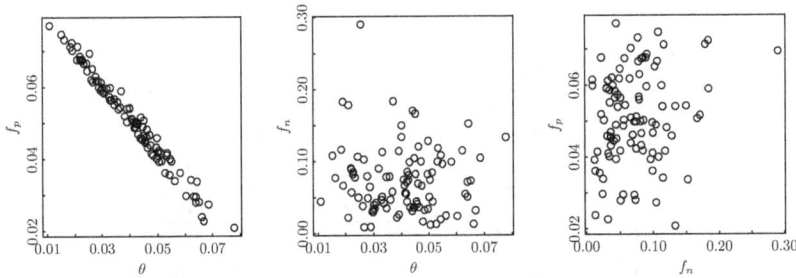

FIGURE 5.13: The estimated COVID-19 posterior distributions of prevalence (θ), false positive probability (f_p), and false negative probability (f_n) are shown by pair-wise scatter plots of MCMC samples from the joint posterior distribution of the three parameters. The posterior distribution is based on data collected from March 26 to May 30, 2020, when Ohio was under the shelter-in-place and stay-safe-Ohio orders. During this time, the state's testing capacity was greatly improved (increasing from near 1000 to over 20,000 tests per day).

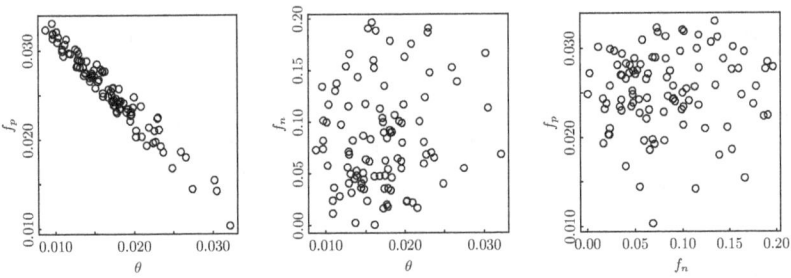

FIGURE 5.14: The estimated COVID-19 posterior distributions of prevalence (θ), false positive probability (f_p), and false negative probability (f_n) using data from May 31 to June 30, 2020, are shown by pair-wise scatter plots of MCMC samples from the joint posterior distribution. During this time, the state conducted from 30,000 to 50,000 tests per day.

The COVID-19 testing example illustrates the importance of properly documenting test characteristics. On the one hand, without reliable information about f_p and f_n of a binary test, testing data cannot be reliably used to estimate the prevalence of COVID-19, even with a large number of tests. As a result, testing has limited value as a tool for understanding the severity of the pandemic. On the other hand, individuals who were tested cannot reliably understand the meaning of a positive or negative result without a good estimate of the prevalence of the virus [Qian et al., 2020]. This ambiguity is not limited to the COVID-19 test; nearly all tests used in science are imperfect. Consequently, properly characterized f_p and f_n should be an important component of a test.

If a standard protocol is followed, we may reasonably assume that the two error probabilities are relatively stable. Assuming these error probabilities are constant, we can directly estimate the positive probability, which is a linear function of the prevalence (equation (5.13)).

5.3.2.3 Programming Notes

Additional limitations for the three parameters (θ, f_p, and f_n) must be imposed for the Stan model. When using $beta(1, 1)$ as the prior for θ, an additional limit on the range of θ is necessary because of the non-identifiability issue. In both simulated data and the COVID-19 testing data, we imposed range limits on all three parameters based on what we deem as appropriate. For example, we limit θ to be less than 0.5, as the prevalence of COVID-19 was unlikely to be more than 20% in the population during the early months of the pandemic. Furthermore, because both θ and $1 - \theta$ enter the formula of the probability of observing a positive result (equation (5.13)), we cannot properly identify all three parameters without some range limitation. For that reason, we also limit f_p and f_n to be less than 0.5, assuming that a test with more than a 50-50 chance of producing an erroneous result is faulty and should not have been approved for use by the government regulatory agency (an assumption unlikely to be true). The Bernoulli model Stan code is shown below.

```
#### Stan Model ####
## Stan model 3 through Bernoulli process
latent_Bern <- "
data{
  int<lower-1> n; // sample size
  int<lower=0> y1[n]; // number of positives
  int<lower=1> y2[n]; // number of negatives
  real alpha;
  real beta;
  real a1;
  real b1;
  real a2;
  real b2;
}
parameters{
  real<lower=0,upper=0.5> theta;
  real<lower=0,upper=0.5> fp;
```

```
  real<lower=0,upper=0.5> fn;
}
model{
  real temp1[2];
  real temp2[2];
  theta ~ beta(alpha, beta);
  fp ~ beta(a1, b1);
  fn ~ beta(a2, b2);
  temp1[1] = log(1-theta)+log(fp);
  temp1[2] = log(theta)+log(1-fn);
  temp2[1] = log(1-theta)+log(1-fp);
  temp2[2] = log(theta)+log(fn);
  for (i in 1:n){
    target+=y1[i]*log_sum_exp(temp1)+
            y2[i]*log_sum_exp(temp2);
  }
}
"

### End ###
```

We also used posterior samples of the three parameters to derive their prior (beta) distributions for sequential updating. For Ohio's COVID-19 testing data, the sequential updating did not change the model result.

```
#### R Code ####
## Beta method of moment
beta_mm <- function(x){
    mux <- mean(x)
    sigmax <- sd(x)
    alpha <- (mux*(mux*(1-mux)-sigmax^2))/sigmax^2
    beta <- alpha*(1-mux)/mux
    return(c(alpha, beta))
}


Bern_input <- function(Data=sim_data50, al=3, be=27,
                       a1=4, b1=16, a2=3, b2=7,
                       n.chains=nchains){
    n <- dim(Data)[1]
    y1 <- Data$Y1
    y2 <- Data$Y2
    data_in <- list(n=n, y1=y1, y2=y2, alpha=al, beta=be,
                    a1=a1, b1=b1, a2=a2, b2=b2)
    inits <- list()
    for (i in 1:n.chains)
        inits[[i]] <- list(theta=runif(1,0,0.5),
                           fp=runif(1,0.05,0.5),
```

```
                      fn=runif(1,0,0.5))
    paras <- c("theta","fp","fn")
    return(list(data=data_in, inits=inits, paras=paras,
            chains=n.chains))
}


stan_fit <- stan_model(model_code=latent_Bin)
input.to.stan <- Bin_input(Data=OhioInit, al=1, be=1,
                          a1=3, b1=23, a2=2, b2=22)
fit2keep <- sampling(stan_fit, data = input.to.stan$data,
                     init=input.to.stan$inits,
                     pars = input.to.stan$paras,
                     iter=niters, thin=nthin,
                     chains=input.to.stan$chains)
print(fit2keep)
pairs(fit2keep, pars=c("theta","fp","fn"))

theta_prior <- beta_mm(rstan::extract(fit2keep, pars="theta",
                               permuted=T)[[1]])
fp_prior <- beta_mm(rstan::extract(fit2keep, pars="fp",
                               permuted=T)[[1]])
fn_prior <- beta_mm(rstan::extract(fit2keep, pars="fn",
                               permuted=T)[[1]])
### End ###
```

5.3.3 Zero-Inflation

Zero-inflation is a specific kind of imperfect detection problem, typically associated with count data. A count variable is often modeled using one of the three distributions: Poisson, negative binomial (or over-dispersed Poisson), or binomial distributions. In these variants, the zero-inflation problem refers to the number of zeros in the response variable data in excess of the number expected by the assumed response variable distribution. For example, the probability of observing 0 under a Poisson distribution with parameter λ is $e^{-\lambda}$ if the model is appropriate. That is, we expect the proportion of zeros in the data should be close to $e^{-\lambda}$. As such, we often use simulation to diagnose zero-inflation. For example, Qian [2016] used "posterior" simulation in two Poisson regression examples where the generalized linear model is fit to the data, and the resulting model is used to generate replicates of the data. Frequencies of zeros in the model-generated replicates are compared to the observed fraction of zero in the data. In both examples, the observed fractions exceed the simulated frequencies. In both cases, we found the underlying reasons for observing the excess zeros in the data. In one example, the count variable is the number of individuals of an endangered bird species observed during repeated site visits. Because the number is recorded based on the number of distinct bird songs, the observed zeros can mean either that the bird was absent or that the bird was present but kept quiet during the survey. In the other example, the response variable is the detected numbers of a microorganism in drinking water samples. Although we use "concentration" to measure the level of microorganism contamination, the number of microorganisms in a water sample of a limited volume can be 0 by chance (an empty sample). As such, the lab detection process will always report a zero no matter what the actual concentration is. In the bird survey example, it is hard to estimate whether a 0 represents that birds were present but silent while being visited or that birds were absent from the site. As a result, the estimated λ represents the relative abundance of the target bird species if we can assume that the proportion of singing birds is relatively stable during the survey. In the drinking water example, we can use the unknown microorganism concentration to parameterize the likelihood of an empty sample. Let the unknown concentration be c; the expected number of microorganisms in a sample of volume v is $\lambda = vc$. We can assume that the number of microorganisms included in a random water sample y follows a Poisson distribution: $y \sim Poisson(\lambda)$. The probability that a given sample is an empty sample is then $e^{-\lambda}$. In short, a zero-inflated response variable is a result of two separate data-generating processes: a process of generating counts described by the assumed probability distribution (i.e., Poisson, negative binomial, or binomial) and a process of generating "true" 0 (e.g., an empty sample, birds absent). The excess number of zeros can be generated from one or both random processes. Therefore, the statistical modeling strategy is to use a mixture model to capture the two processes.

If, as done in Qian [2016], the observed count data are modeled using the Poisson model alone, we assume the number of birds that sang during the survey is a Poisson random variable and the estimated Poisson distribution mean (λ) is proportional to the number of song birds present at the study area. Using the estimated λ over time, we can make inferences on the population's temporal trend. When the mechanism of generating excess zeros is consistent, we underestimate the expected number of birds in the study area. If the estimated λ is a known (and constant) fraction of the number of the birds in the survey area, the underestimation is a constant fraction of the actual population size. Therefore, the estimated λ can be used to infer the population trend. In many situations, the distribution of individuals of a species is likely uneven. In fact, patchiness is almost always expected in animal distribution because of the fractured nature of the natural environment. As a result, the probability of no birds present is also an important variable in understanding the population distribution. In any case, the statistically estimated λ is often known as the "relative" population size. The true population size (the "absolute" population) is nearly always unknown.

For a zero-inflated Poisson response variable, we assume that the probability of drawing a "true" 0 is θ and the probability of drawing a Poisson random variate with parameter λ is $1 - \theta$. A true 0 represents the situation, for example, when the target bird was not at the site during the survey and the target microorganism was not captured in a water sample. A Poisson random variate can be 0 (e.g., when the bird kept quiet during the survey). The probability distribution function of the observed count data y is thus

$$\pi(y_i) = \begin{cases} \theta + (1 - \theta)Poisson(0 \mid \lambda) & \text{if } y_i = 0 \\ (1 - \theta)Poisson(y_i \mid \lambda) & \text{if } y_i > 0. \end{cases} \tag{5.19}$$

Because the bird count is based on their songs, the Poisson model parameter λ in equation (5.19) is the expected number of singing birds, presumably proportional to the total number of birds. In other words, the model estimates a relative population size even without the zero-inflation problem. As long as the survey followed the same protocol over time, we can infer the trend of the endangered population status.

In equation (5.19), an observed 0 is a mixture of true 0 and a Poisson 0. This probability distribution can be implemented in Stan using the "target" increment (`target +=`) method to specify the log-likelihood function. If there is no covariate, the likelihood function of the model in equation (5.19) can be grouped into zero and non-zero count parts:

$$L = \left[\theta + (1 - \theta)e^{-\lambda} \right]^{n_0} \times \prod_{i=1}^{n_p} (1 - \theta)\frac{\lambda^{y_i} e^{-\lambda}}{y_i!}$$

where n_0 is the number of 0 counts and n_p is the number of non-zero counts. The log-likelihood function is a sum of two terms

$$LL = n_0 \log \left[\theta + (1 - \theta)e^{-\lambda} \right] + \left(n_p \log(1 - \theta) + \sum_{i=1}^{n_p} \log \left(\frac{\lambda^{y_i} e^{-\lambda}}{y_i!} \right) \right)$$

which can be specified using two separate `target+=` statements in Stan:

```
model{
    target += n0*log_sum_exp(log(theta), log1m(theta)-lambda);
    for (j in 1:np)
      target += log1m(theta)+poisson_lpmf(yp[j] | lambda);
}
```

The second `target +=` statement can be vectorized to

```
target += np*log1m(theta)+poisson_lpmf(yp | lambda);
```

Lambert [1992] introduced a generalized linear model for a zero-inflated Poisson process. In the model, the Poisson distribution parameter (λ) and the probability of 0 (θ) are modeled as linear functions of predictor x and z using the appropriate link function:

$$\begin{aligned} \log(\lambda) &= X\beta \\ \text{logit}(\theta) &= Z\alpha. \end{aligned} \tag{5.20}$$

The GLM implementation allows us to incorporate factors that are known to influence the observation process to model the potential change in the population size (represented by λ) and the chance of observing a true zero.

Unlike the mixture model for imperfect test data we discussed earlier in this chapter, the zero-inflated Poisson model does not have the identifiability problem. That is, model parameters in a zero-inflated Poisson model (e.g., equation (5.19)) can be uniquely estimated [Li, 2012]. This is mostly because the model for non-zero counts is not a mixture, because we do not consider the possibility of imperfect detection. For example, we may misidentify the song of another species to be the song of the target species. If the error rate is a constant, we can quantify the Poisson distribution parameter as long as we have enough non-zero observations. The zero-inflation model estimated λ is, nevertheless, a relative population estimate.

5.3.3.1   Example: Simulated Data and ZIP Model

To illustrate the identifiability of the zero-inflated Poisson (ZIP) model, we start with a simulation, using data generated from the two underlying processes with known parameter values. The data simulation process consists of two sets of random numbers, one from a Bernoulli distribution and one from a Poisson distribution. We use the same method for posterior predictive simulation, replacing the known parameter values with MCMC samples of model parameters.

```
#### R Code ####
p <- 0.25
lambda <- 2.5
n <- 100
y <- rpois(n,lambda)*rbinom(n,1,p)
### End ###
```

We note that the Bernoulli parameter of $p = 0.25$ is the probability of observing 1, and the probability of observing 0 in the ZIP model should be $\theta = 1 - p = 0.75$. Using the vectorized version of the Stan model, the implementation is straightforward.

```
#### Stan Model ####
zip1 <- "
data{
    int<lower=1> n0;
    int<lower=1> np;
    int<lower=1> yp[np];
}
parameters{
    real<lower=0,upper=1> theta;
    real<lower=0> lambda;
}
```

```
model{
  theta ~ beta(1,1);
  lambda ~ normal(0,2.5);
  target += n0*log_sum_exp(log(theta),
                            log1m(theta)-lambda);
  target += np*log1m(theta);
  target += poisson_lpmf(yp|lambda);
}
"
```

End

The simulated count data are processed to organize the Stan model's input data, initial values, and the list of parameters to be monitored:

R Code
```
ZIP_in <- function(y, n.chains=nchains){
    n0 <- sum(y==0)
    np <- sum(y!=0)
    yp <- y[y!=0]
    data <- list(n0=n0, np=np, yp=yp)
    inits <- list()
    for (i in 1:n.chains)
        inits[[i]] <- list(theta=runif(1),
        lambda=abs(rnorm(1)))
    paras <- c("theta", "lambda")
    return(list(data=data, init=inits,
                para=paras, nchains=n.chains))
}
```
End

As we used default non-informative priors, the Bayesian estimated model parameters should be similar to the result from a maximum likelihood estimator.

R Code
```
packages(pscl)
mle_zip <- zeroinfl(y~1|1)
summary(mle_zip)$coef
```
End

The MLE estimated coefficients are presented in the default link function (log for Poisson and logit for binomial) space. We can show that both the Bayesian and the MLE are unbiased estimators using a simulation (Figure 5.15). We simulated the sampling distributions of these two estimators by estimating the known parameters using repeatedly generated zero-inflated count data.

```
nsims <- 1000
```

```
simulated <- matrix(rpois(n*nsims, lambda)*
                    rbinom(n*nsims, 1, theta),
                    ncol=n, nrow=nsims)

mle_sim <- t(apply(simulated, 1, FUN=function(x){
    temp <- zeroinfl(x~1|1)
    return(c(exp(temp$coef[[1]]),
             invlogit(temp$coef[[2]])))
}))

stan_sim <- matrix(0, nrow=nsims, ncol=2)
for (i in 1:nsims){
    print(paste(i, "of ", nsims))
    x <- rpois(n, lambda) * rbinom(n, 1, theta)
    input.to.stan <- ZIP_in(x)
    keep <- sampling(fit, data=input.to.stan$data,
                     init=input.to.stan$init,
                     pars=input.to.stan$para,
                     iter=niters,thin=nthin,
                     chains=input.to.stan$nchains,
                     show_messages=F, verbose=F)
    temp <- rstan::extract(keep, permuted=T)
    stan_sim[i,] <- c(mean(temp$theta),
                      mean(temp$lambda))
}
summary(stan_sim)
summary(mle_sim)
### End ###
```

5.3.3.2   Example: Seabird By-Catch Data

We now return to the fishery by-catch example in Section 5.1. Although the negative binomial model can adequately account for the large number of zeros (Figure 5.1), we must consider the possibility of zero-inflation. Seabird by-catch is only possible when seabirds are present during a trawling operation. Without further information from Hilborn and Mangel [1997], we proceed with the assumption that seabirds may be absent sometime, somewhere, or under certain conditions. This assumption suggests that some zeros in the data are "true zeroes." Under conditions that led to these true zeros, we would always observe 0. The statistical question is now whether we use the zero-inflated Poisson model or zero-inflated negative binomial model. If we use the Poisson distribution, we assume that observed larger-than-expected variance in the data is due largely to the excess number of zeros. If we choose the negative binomial distribution, we suggest that the data are over-dispersed even without zero-inflation.

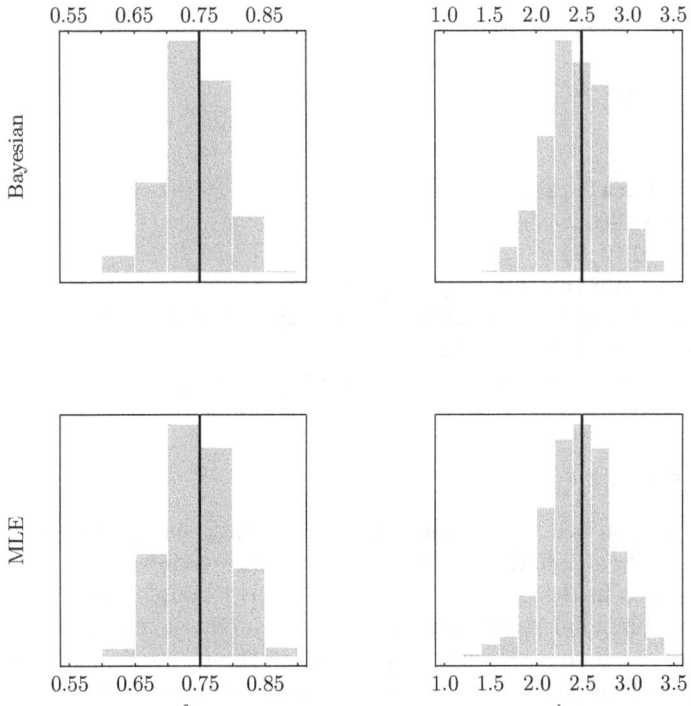

FIGURE 5.15: Estimated zero-inflated Poisson model parameters using both MLE and Bayesian methods (histograms) are compared to the true parameter values (dark black lines) used to generate the simulation data.

The implementation of the zero-inflated Poisson model is similar to the simulated data example in the previous sub-section. In fitting the negative binomial distribution, we simply replace Poisson log-probability mass function in the Stan code with the negative binomial one.

```
#### Stan Code ####
zinb_bycatch <-"
data{
  int<lower=1> n0;
  int<lower=1> np;
  int<lower=1> yp[np];
}
parameters{
  real<lower=0,upper=1> theta;
  real<lower=0> mu;
  real<lower=0> r;
```

```
}
transformed parameters{
  real eta;
  eta=log(mu);
}
model{
  theta ~ beta(1,1);
  mu ~ normal(0,5);
  r ~ normal(0,5);
  target += n0*log_sum_exp(log(theta),
    log1m(theta)+neg_binomial_2_log_lpmf(0|eta,r));
  target += np*log1m(theta) +
            neg_binomial_2_log_lpmf(yp | eta, r);
}
"
```

End

As in Section 5.1, we compare the two models using posterior predictive simulation. The simulation code is similar to the code we used to generate simulated data in the previous (simulated data) example: using the Poisson or negative binomial parameters to draw N random samples, multiplied by N Bernoulli random variates with probability of success $1 - \theta$. Both models can adequately account for the observed number of zeros and mean of the data (Figure 5.16). However, the Poisson model underestimates the standard deviation. In other words, we have one more piece of evidence to suggest that the data are over-dispersed.

Comparing the posterior predictive simulation of the negative binomial model (without zero-inflation) in Section 5.1 (Figure 5.1) and the zero-inflated negative binomial model, we find that these two models captured the data equally well, at least with respect to the three statistics we evaluated. If we are only interested in the abstract mathematics of the data distribution, we may conclude that these models are equivalent and the simpler one should be accepted as the better model. The famous Occam's razor, that is the simplest explanation is likely correct, would shave off the zero-inflation part from our model. Statistics is, however, not pure mathematics or logic. A statistical model should be compatible with the underlying data-generating process and the intended application. In this example, the data came from experiments intended to develop an effective observer program to better estimate the by-catch rate, such that regulators can provide guidelines or develop regulations to help the fishing industry in reducing by-catch. If by-catch is more likely under certain conditions, we want to identify these conditions so that the subsequent regulations can be better targeted. In other words, our knowledge of the field of application is an important consideration when using statistics. Specifically for this example, we should not stop at the negative binomial model. More information of the by-catch should be collected and used in

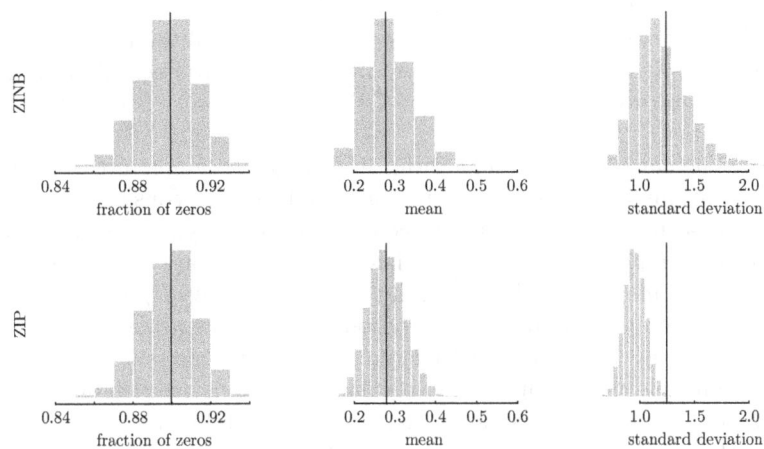

FIGURE 5.16: Fishery by-catch data were modeled using the zero-inflated Poisson (ZIP, bottom row) and the zero-inflated negative binomial (ZINB, top row) models. The posterior simulation calculates the replicated fraction of 0s in the data (left column), the mean (middle column) and standard deviation (right column) of the data. The simulated statistics are shown in histograms and the observed statistics are shown by the vertical lines.

developing a model that is more relevant to the underlying science or regulatory question.

5.3.3.3 Example: Estimating Sturgeon Population Trends

Atlantic sturgeons (*Acipenser oxyrinchus*) have long been over-exploited across their range [ASMFC, 2017], resulting in five distinct population segments (DPS) under the U.S. Endangered Species Act (as amended by U.S. Public Law 97-304). In this example, we are interested in the relative abundance of Hudson River juvenile Atlantic sturgeon through time as an index of recruitment and population recovery. Atlantic sturgeon reproduce in the major tributaries along the U.S. Eastern seaboard, including the Hudson River in New York State which is part of the endangered Mid-Atlantic Bight DPS. Young sturgeon remain in the brackish estuarine waters of the Hudson for several years before migrating back out to sea. As such, the juvenile life stage represents a consistently targetable portion of the population.

A standardized sampling protocol using gill nets within a fixed portion of the river during spring months (March and April) was developed to capture sturgeon and monitor abundance trends. A sample consists of fishing a gang of three gill nets on the bottom of the river for approximately two hours, retrieving those nets, and recording the number of sturgeon captured before returning them to the water. As a result, each sample consists of a count variable as well as an exposure variable (i.e., the length of time the nets were fished). The juvenile population is at low abundance resulting in many 0 and small catches, with few high catches. Additionally, environmental data (e.g., bottom temperature and salinity) and GPS location are recorded for each sample.

During the sample season and within the targeted sample area, environmental conditions fluctuate on a daily basis and are not consistent year-to-year. Temperature and salinity influence the susceptibility and availability of sturgeon to a temporally and spatially fixed survey. Fish are cold blooded, so metabolic rates and activity levels will increase with increasing temperatures. As fish move around more often, they become more susceptible to capture in gill nets set nearby [Hansson and Rudstam, 1995]. Juvenile sturgeon are sensitive to salinity levels, as their osmo-regulatory systems are still developing. Additionally, salinity levels influence the benthic invertebrate communities in the river, the sturgeons' main food source. Salinity levels can fluctuate within the targeted sample area as the salt-front (interface between fresh and salt water) migrates up and down river depending on river conditions such as tidal stage, discharge, and wind intensity and direction. As the salt-front moves farther away from the targeted sample area, the population core may also move, making the population less available to the survey. As a result, low abundance and variable habitat conditions have generated an over-dispersed count data set with a high proportion of 0's, while the source of zero-inflation remains unclear. Data were provided by the New York State Department of Environmental Conservation - Hudson and Delaware Marine Fisheries Unit[3].

The sturgeon data are over-dispersed. As a result, we use the negative binomial distribution to model the data. Specifically, we use the parameterization of equation (5.2), with a mean μ and an inverse over-dispersion parameter r. Equation (5.2) is represented by the Stan function `neg_binomial_2_lpmf`. The natural link functions for the mean μ and the probability of a 0 being a true zero (θ) (equation (5.20)) is used. In the Stan code, we can either define the negative binomial mean (i.e., $\mu = e^{X\beta}$, using Stan sampling function `y ~ neg_binomial_2(mu, r)`) or define the log mean (i.e., $\eta = \log(\mu) = X\beta$, using the sampling function `y ~ neg_binomial_2_log(eta, r)`.

Potential predictors are selected based on our understanding of the species. In the case of sturgeon, observed zeros are likely to come from two processes: susceptibility and availability. Susceptibility relates to the performance of the survey gear under varying conditions and can be expressed as the probability that sturgeon are captured given they are near the sample gear (detection probability $p_d = 1 - f_n$). In this case, gill nets are passive sampling gear, meaning they are fixed at one location and rely on fish movements to initiate encounters which result in capture. In this context, we would describe a zero generated by reduced susceptibility as a zero characterized by the negative binomial distribution (a false zero). We hypothesized that water temperatures,

---

[3]https://www.dec.ny.gov/animals/6945.html

which influence fish movement rates, would be a key variable in sturgeon susceptibility. Availability relates to sturgeon densities in the sample area. When sturgeon density is low, the probability of setting the net at a location with no fish presence increases, hence the probability of observing a 0 characterized by the Bernoulli distribution (true 0) increases; when sturgeon density is high the probability of true zero catches decreases. In this context, a zero catch represents the probability of sampling an unoccupied location within the targeted area which is characterized by the Bernoulli distribution, a true zero. Previous research has demonstrated juvenile sturgeon preferences for intermediate salinity near the salt-front [Niklitscheck and Secor, 2009, Allen et al., 2014]. We hypothesized that salt-front movement could bring fish in and out of the targeted sample area thus increasing or decreasing densities, catch rates, and the probability of zero catches. In addition, the relationship between sturgeon abundance and distance to the salt-front is nonlinear.

Based on these considerations, we propose a zero-inflated negative binomial model using temperature and distance to salt-front as predictors for both the abundance and the zero models. The model is similar to the zero inflated Poisson model of equations (5.19) and (5.20): (1) replacing the Poisson density in equation (5.19) with the negative binomial density and (2) using temperature as a predictor variable of θ (Z in equation (5.20)) and temperature and distance to salt-front as predictors of λ (X in equation (5.20)):

$$\begin{aligned}
\log(\lambda_{ij}) &= \beta_{0j} + \beta_1 Temp_{ij} + \beta_2 Dist_{ij} + \beta_3 \log(Dist_{ij}) + \text{offset}_{ij} \\
\text{logit}(\theta_{ij}) &= \alpha_0 + \alpha_1 Temp_{ij}
\end{aligned}$$

$$(5.21)$$

where the subscript ij represents the ith observation from the jth year, and "offset" is the effort (representing the sampling time of the gill net). The nonlinear relationship between λ and $Dist$ ($\log(\lambda) = \beta_0 + \beta_2 Dist + \beta_3 \log(Dist)$) resembles the log density of a gamma distribution (the gamma model). We explain this choice of the model in Section 5.3.3.4. To make the gamma model possible, we linearly transform the distance (`dist`) measured in kilometers:

R Code
```
Dist <- (dist-min(dist)+1)/max(dist)
```

Because the number of sturgeons captured is related to how long the gill net was soaked in water, we use the typical fishery study approach of evaluating "catch per unit effort" (CPUE) by including the time the net was in water as the "effort." In equation (5.21), "offset" is the logarithm of the effort. As such, the abundance model ($\beta_{0j} + \beta_1 Temp_{ij} + \beta_2 Dist_{ij} + \beta_3 \log(Dist_{ij})$) is the estimated expected log CPUE.

The goal of the study is to evaluate whether sturgeon abundance has changed over time. As such, we allowed the intercept to vary by year and assumed the year-specific intercepts are exchangeable. That is, we imposed a common prior:

$$\beta_{0j} \sim N\left(\mu_{b0}, \sigma_{\beta_0}\right). \tag{5.22}$$

Equation (5.22) is the Bayesian hierarchical model that will induce a shrinkage effect on the estimated model coefficients, help stabilize parameter estimates, and ultimately allow robust comparisons among years [Gelman et al., 2012], a key interest in the model.

As we did before, we group the data based on whether the observed count is zero or not and vectorize the Stan model:

```
### partial Stan Code ###
zinb1 <- "
data{
  int<lower=1> Np;      // number of positive counts
  int<lower=1> N0;
  int<lower=1> Ka;      // number of abundance model coefficients
  int<lower=0> Yp[Np];  // positive counts only
  matrix[Np, Ka] Xp;    // abundance model design matrix
  matrix[N0, Ka] X0;
  ...
}
parameters{
  ...
}
transformed parameters{
  vector[Np] eta_p;
  vector[N0] eta_0;
  vector[Np] lambda_p;
  vector[N0] lambda_0;
  vector[Np] zi_p;
  vector[N0] zi_0;
  vector[Np] theta_p;
  vector[N0] theta_0;
  for (i in 1:Np){
    eta_p[i] = b0[yearP[i]]+ Xp[i] * beta + offsetP[i];
    zi_p[i]  = alpha[1] + Zp[i] * alpha[2];
  }
  for (i in 1:N0){
    eta_0[i] = b0[year0[i]]+ X0[i] * beta + offset0[i];
    zi_0[i]  = alpha[1] + Z0[i] * alpha[2];
  }
  lambda_p = exp(eta_p);
  theta_p = inv_logit(zi_p);
  lambda_0 = exp(eta_0);
  theta_0 = inv_logit(zi_0);
}
model {
  // priors
```

```
tau_b ~ normal(0,5);
mu_b ~ normal(0,5);
b0 ~ normal(mu_b, tau_b);
beta ~ normal(0,5);
alpha ~ normal(0,5);
target += gamma_lpdf(phi | 0.01, 0.01);

// likelihood
for(i in 1:N0){
  target += log_sum_exp(log(theta_0[i]),
            log1m(theta_0[i]) +
                neg_binomial_2_log_lpmf(0 | eta_0[i], phi));
  }
  target += log1m(theta_p) +
            neg_binomial_2_log_lpmf(Yp | eta_p, phi);
}
"
```

End

The model results show the strong influence of both temperature and distance to the salt-front on sturgeon catches from the standardized survey (Figure 5.17).

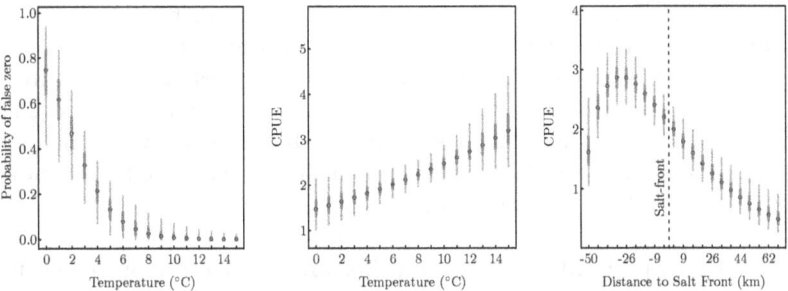

FIGURE 5.17: Estimated probability of a true zero is negatively related to water temperature (left panel), indicating a lower probability of capturing juvenile Atlantic sturgeon (*Acipenser oxyrinchus*) at low temperatures. The catch-per-unit-effort (CPUE) is positively related to temperature (middle panel). The CPUE is a unimodal and asymmetric function of the distance to the salt-front (right panel) with higher CPUE in higher salinity waters below the salt-front (negative values).

The probability of encountering a true zero decreases substantially as temperature increases, likely due to increased activity and susceptibility. We also see an increase in the catch rates associated with increased temperature, which is also likely related to increased activity levels and redistribution of over-wintering sturgeon. The dome-shaped relationship, achieved by including the "gamma" model of the distance to the salt-front, shows that the highest sturgeon densities occur approximately 32 km below the salt-front in moderate salinity waters. Finally, the magnitude of the inverse dispersion parameter ($r = 1.1$) also indicates a certain degree of over-dispersion, which is not uncommon for fisheries catch data as many unknown factors contribute to the success and magnitude of an individual sample.

As in all fisheries analysis, the model estimated abundance is relative abundance. This is because the sampling method records only the number of sturgeon caught and there is no practical means to quantify the (conditional) probability of capturing a fish when it is present. In most fisheries studies, we use a standard sampling method, which implies a constant detection probability (the conditional probability of capturing a fish when the fish is present). Because the detection probability is unknown, the estimated abundance, most commonly expressed as CPUE, represents a relative abundance. That is, the true (or absolute) abundance is likely proportional to the estimated relative abundance. In this example, the main interest was to evaluate the temporal trend of the population size. Although we used the term "true 0" in this example, we know that sturgeons use the sampled habitat. A true 0 only suggests the absence of sturgeon in the vicinity of the gill net at the time of sampling. As a result, to evaluate the temporal trend of the sturgeon population in the area, we work solely with the negative binomial portion of the model (the abundance model) moving forward. Using the abundance model, the previously recorded false zeros are replaced with predictions based on positive catch relationships with temperature and distance to the salt-front. To control for the variance in fish abundance due to changes in temperature and distance to the salt-front, we compare the model-estimated expected CPUE at a given temperature and distance to the salt-front. When we fit the model, we centered all predictors. As a result, we can simply compare the abundance model intercept (β_{0j} in equation (5.21)) (Figure 5.18).

5.3.3.4   Example: Effects of Urbanization on Stream Ecosystems

This example is based on data from Qian and Cuffney [2014]. We use this example to extend the zero-inflated Poisson model using the Bayesian hierarchical modeling (BHM) approach to combine data from multiple related sources. The general background of the study is introduced in Section 1.4.2 (page 16).

In this example, we expand the zero-inflated Poisson (ZIP) model to model multiple count responses using the Bayesian hierarchical model (BHM), using taxon abundance data of mayfly (Ephemeroptera), stonefly (Plecoptera), and caddis fly (Trichoptera) (collectively known as EPT taxa) from the 30 watersheds in the Boston, Massachusetts metropolitan area as an example. We focus on the interpretation of model coefficients, including the

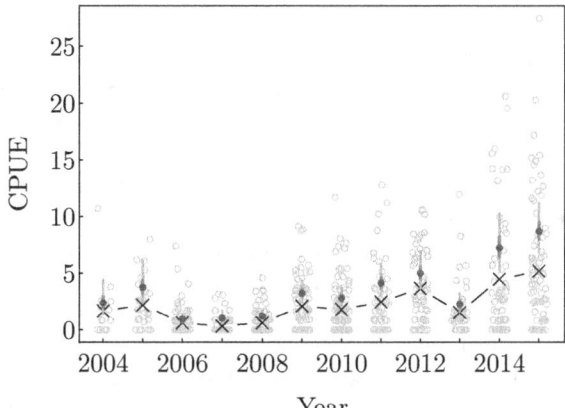

FIGURE 5.18: Estimated annual expected sturgeon population (in CPUE, dots) is compared to the CPUE calculated based on the catch data (crosses).

hyper-parameters. By comparing results from the other eight regions, we discuss the hierarchical structure based on spatial scales.

Taxa included in the example occurred in at least two of the 30 watersheds in each region. Counts of benthic macroinvertebrates were expressed as density (no./m^2) and urban intensity was represented by % developed land (National Land Cover Database or NLCD class 2). Responses of EPT taxa were modeled because EPT taxa are known to be sensitive to pollution and are the basis of many biological indicators of water quality [Barbour et al., 1999]. Watersheds in the nine metropolitan areas were selected to represent the urban gradient.

Because EPT taxa are known to be sensitive to pollution, we expect that some of them would disappear in stream with high levels of urbanization in the watersheds. In other words, not all taxa exist in all streams. As a result, counts of taxa are potentially zero-inflated. If we are interested in modeling the response of an individual taxon to increased urbanization in a watershed, we should consider both the response in abundance and the response in the probability of disappearance of the taxon, that is, using a zero-inflated model.

Instead of using a generalized linear model formulation for the Poisson model (equation (5.20)), Qian and Cuffney [2014] proposed to use a unimodal function to model the changes in taxon density along the urban gradient (the abundance model):

$$\log(\lambda) = \beta_0 + \beta_1 x + \beta_2 \log(x) \tag{5.23}$$

where x is the % developed land in the watershed. The right-hand side of equation (5.23) is proportional to the log density function of the gamma distribution. Using this formulation, we have the flexibility of modeling the abundance along the urban gradient as a monotonically decreasing curve (for pollution-sensitive taxa), a unimodal curve (moderately tolerant taxa), and a monotonically increasing curve (tolerant taxa). This formulation is based on ecological observations that taxon abundance along an environmental gradient often can be approximated by a unimodal curve, where a taxon has its "optimal" value along the gradient at the point where the abundance of the taxon is the largest and a range (tolerance) within which the taxon is likely found [Whittaker, 1956, 1967]. Such behavior was first observed in studies of diatom response to acidification (along a pH gradient) and a bell-shaped normal distribution density function was developed (the Gaussian model, Gauch and Whittaker [1972]). The normal density function is symmetric, which fits the response along a pH gradient well. When the environmental variable is nutrient concentration or other non-toxic measures, symmetric response is often unrealistic. The biological response to low nutrient (limiting growth) and high nutrient (limiting by competition) are unlikely to be the same. Oksanen and Minchin [2002] recognized the limitation of the Gaussian model and proposed two asymmetric alternatives using data from several vascular plant species along an altitude gradient on the Mt. Field Plateau in Tasmania, Australia. The first alternative is the beta model, a function proportional to the rescaled beta distribution density function. The second alternative is the Huisman-Olff-Fresco (HOF) model ($\log(\lambda) = \beta_0 - \log[1 + exp(\beta_1 + \beta_2 x)] - \log[1 + exp(\beta_3 - \beta_4 x)$, [Huisman et al., 1993]). Although both alternatives are mathematically flexible, they require at least 5 non-zero observations to quantify the abundance model. The model in equation (5.23) (the gamma model) was shown to outperform these alternatives in a simulation by Qian and Pan [2006], as long as constraining $\beta_1 > 0$ and $\beta_2 > -1$.

As in the previous example, observed zeros can be a result of sampling error (the target taxon was present but not caught) and true 0 (the target taxon was absent due to the unsuitable environmental conditions of the site). The probability of a true 0 (θ) is modeled using a logistic model:

$$\log\left(\frac{\theta}{1 - \theta}\right) = \alpha_0 + \alpha_1 \text{logit}(x). \tag{5.24}$$

We used the logit transformed % developed land so that the data points are more evenly distributed along the x-axis. This formulation is compatible with the knowledge that EPT taxa are known to be sensitive to pollution associated with urbanization. The probability of their absence increases with the level of urbanization.

Taxon-specific Models

For a single taxon, the Stan model can be written similarly as the model without co-variate on page 187 by grouping the data of zero counts and positive counts separately:

```
zip2 <- "
data{
  int<lower=1> n0;
  int<lower=1> np;
  int<lower=0> yp[np];
  vector[np] xp;
  vector[n0] x0;
}
parameters{
  real alpha0;
  real<lower=0> alpha1;
  real beta0;
  real<lower=0> beta1;
  real<lower=-1> beta2;
}
transformed parameters{
  vector[n0] theta0;
  vector[n0] lambda0;
  vector[np] theta1;
  vector[np] lambda1;
  theta0  = inv_logit(alpha0+alpha1*logit(x0/100));
  lambda0 = exp(beta0-beta1*x0 + beta2*log(x0));
  theta1  = inv_logit(alpha0+alpha1*logit(xp/100));
  lambda1 = exp(beta0-beta1*xp + beta2*log(xp));
}
model{
  for (i in 1:n0){
    target += log_sum_exp(log(theta0[i]),
                log1m(theta0[i])-lambda0[i]);
  }
  target += log1m(theta1);
  target += poisson_lpmf(yp|lambda1);
}
"
```

End

We note that in the line `target += log1m(theta1)`, the number of 0 observations (n0) is not included, compared to the code for the simulated data example on page 187. This change is made because `theta1` here is a vector (hence the sum of all elements of the vector), whereas `theta` in the code on page 187 is a scalar.

To illustrate the gamma model, we fit the model to data from three taxa. These three taxa were selected to represent three representative types of EPT taxa.

1. Taxon *Serratella serrata* has a very low theoretical tolerance to pollution (pollution-sensitive taxa) and was detected mostly in watersheds with very low levels of urbanization. We use this taxon to represent the cases where the abundance model is monotonically decreasing and the zero model has a rapid change in slope (Figure 5.19(a)).

2. Taxon *Acentrella turbida* is theoretically moderately tolerant, but very rare in the Boston study area. In the EUSE study, *Acentrella turbida* was detected only in two watersheds. We use this taxon as an example of cases with very few positive counts (the moderate tolerance suggests a unimodal abundance model). With only two positive counts, the fitted model is unidentifiable because there can be multiple unimodal curves going through the two data points and the origin (Figure 5.19(b)) with different combinations of the three coefficients. The non-identifiability is reflected in the strong correlation among the three coefficients (shown by using `pairs(fit2keep, pars=c("beta0","beta1"))`).

3. Taxon *Baetis flavistriga* is moderately tolerant and is a common taxon in the Boston study area (detected in nearly all watersheds). The abundance of non-zero observations made the gamma model robust (Figure 5.19(c)).

As in a generalized linear model, a ZIP model is limited by the available data. When the number of positive counts is small, the Poisson model can be ill-defined or non-identifiable. Similarly, the binary part of the model can also be non-identifiable if zeros and non-zero counts are perfectly separated along the predictor variable [Gelman and Hill, 2007].

Scientists in the EUSE project were interested in using EPT taxa as an indicator of the overall environmental quality. They often use the richness weighted tolerance (or RichTOL) as a summary indicator. RichTOL is the weighted average of the theoretical tolerance values for taxa represented in the sample. The tolerance value of each taxon is weighted by the observed abundance. Each taxon has only one theoretical tolerance value, whereas a taxon's tolerance to pollution can be influenced by other natural factors. For example, taxon *Acentrella turbida* is theoretically moderately tolerant, but it is a rare species in the Boston region. When compared to the main pollution gradient (represented by the urbanization gradient), this taxon behaves like a sensitive one. It occurred only in two sites with low urban development. For this reason, Qian and Cuffney [2014] proposed a model-based alternative indicator: representing the tolerance of a taxon by the predictor variable value that resulted in a probability of true-zero of 0.5. Because the environmental gradient (% developed land) is a measure of stress to a taxon, they call this indicator the taxon's stress-tolerance 50 (or ST50). This indicator can be derived from the fitted model: $\text{logit}(0.5) = \alpha_0 + \alpha_1 x$, where x is the logit transformed % developed land corresponding to the probability of disappearance of 0.5 (i.e., ST50). Measured in the fraction of developed land use in the

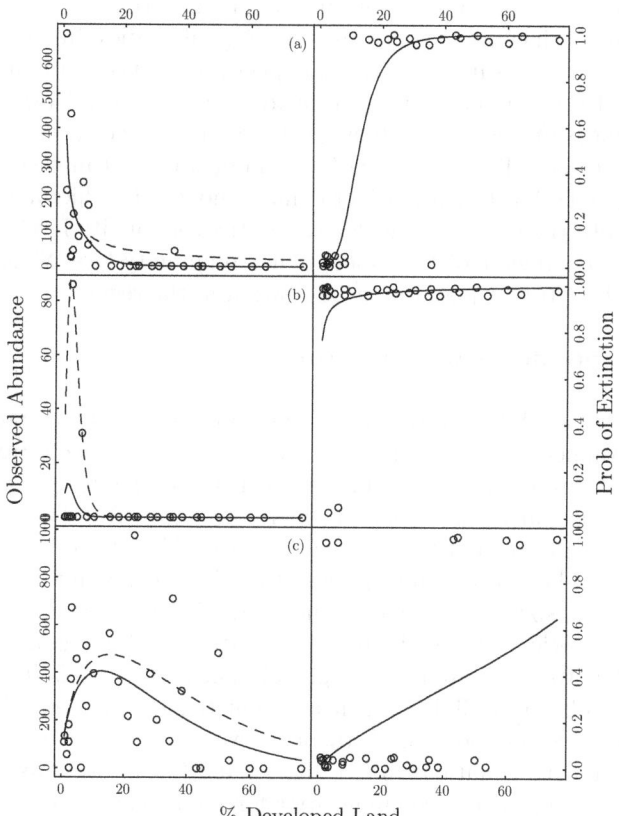

FIGURE 5.19: Taxon-specific zero-inflated Poisson models of three taxa representing three typical types of data. *Serratella serrata* (first row) is a sensitive taxon, *Acentrella turbida* is a moderately sensitive, but rare, taxon, and *Baetis flavistriga* is a common taxon. The dashed lines in the left column represent the gamma model (equation (5.23)), the expected abundance when the taxon does exist. The solid lines in the left panel represent the expected mean abundance (the dashed line multiplied by 1 minus probability of extinction). The right column shows the probability of extinction as a function of the predictor (% developed land).

watershed, the indicator is

$$ST50 = \frac{e^{-\alpha_0/\alpha_1}}{1 + e^{-\alpha_0/\alpha_1}} = \frac{1}{1 + e^{\alpha_0/\alpha_1}}.$$

When urban intensity is at ST50, the taxon has a probability of disappearance of 0.5. As a result, we can view ST50 as a measure of a species' response (or sensitivity) to a specific stressor, instead of a generic measure of a species' tolerance (i.e., RichTOL) used in stream-ecological studies. In stream ecology, we aggregate the measure of individual species tolerances to pollution (e.g., RichTOL) into a community-level measure of collective tolerance. Such an aggregated measure serves as a biological measure of the stream's ecological condition. Because ST50 is a model-based indicator, we can easily aggregate the taxon-specific ST50 using a hierarchical model. The hierarchical model can return both the taxon-specific ST50 and the community-level ST50 based on the hyper-parameter of the model. The community-level ST50 is then a measure of the stress imposed by urbanization in the region.

Region-specific Hierarchical Models

Ecologists use EPT taxa richness as a community-level indicator for evaluating environmental quality. In many states in the U.S., EPT taxa richness and RichTOL are often used as biological metrics for stream water quality assessment [Barbour et al., 1999]. We mentioned that RichTOL is a generic metric not directly related to a specific stressor. Also, EPT taxa richness is often a crude indicator as many species in the EPT community perform similar functions. A species sensitive to one stressor can be replaced by another less-sensitive species. The model-based indicator ST50 is region-specific and taxon-specific. To aggregate it to a regional indicator of the EPT community, we model all observed EPT taxa in a region together under a hierarchical structure. That is, we model each taxon as we did for the three taxa in the Boston region using equations (5.19), (5.23), and (5.24), and linking all models together by imposing a common prior for model coefficients for all taxa. To simplify the model, we first assume that taxon-specific model coefficients, $\theta_j = \{\beta_{0j}, \beta_{1j}, \beta_{2j}, \alpha_{0j},$ and, $\alpha_{1j}\}$, are exchangeable among regions. Specifically,

$$\begin{pmatrix} \beta_{0j} \\ \beta_{1j} \\ \beta_{2j} \end{pmatrix} \sim MVN \left(\begin{pmatrix} \mu_{\beta_0} \\ \mu_{\beta_1} \\ \mu_{\beta_2} \end{pmatrix}, \Sigma_\beta \right) \tag{5.25}$$

and

$$\begin{pmatrix} \alpha_{0j} \\ \alpha_{1j} \end{pmatrix} \sim MVN \left(\begin{pmatrix} \mu_{\alpha_0} \\ \mu_{\alpha_1} \end{pmatrix}, \Sigma_\alpha \right). \tag{5.26}$$

Follow the suggestions of Gelman and Hill [2007], we first assume that these coefficients are a priori independent, that is, $\theta_j \sim N(\mu_\theta, \sigma_\theta^2)$. This is the model presented by Qian and Cuffney [2014]. The Stan model can be modified from the individual taxon model (`zip2` on page 199) by linking all taxa together using a taxon-indicator:

```
zip3 <- "
data{
  int<lower=1> nsp;
```

```
  int<lower=1> n0;
  int<lower=1> np;
  int<lower=0> yp[np];
  vector[np] xp;
  vector[n0] x0;
  int<lower=0> TX0[n0];
  int<lower=0> TXp[np];
}
parameters{
  vector[nsp] alpha0;
  vector<lower=0>[nsp] alpha1;
  real a0;
  real a1;
  vector[nsp] beta0;
  real b0;
  vector<lower=0>[nsp] beta1;
  real<lower=0> b1;
  vector<lower=-1>[nsp] beta2;
  real<lower=-1> b2;
  real<lower=0> sigma[5];
}
transformed parameters{
  vector[n0] theta0;
  vector[n0] lambda0;
  vector[np] theta1;
  vector[np] lambda1;
  for (i in 1:n0){
    theta0[i] = inv_logit(alpha0[TX0[i]]+
                          alpha1[TX0[i]]*
                          logit(x0[i]/100));
    lambda0[i] = exp(beta0[TX0[i]]-beta1[TX0[i]]*x0[i] +
                 beta2[TX0[i]]*log(x0[i]));
  }
  for (i in 1:np){
    theta1[i] = inv_logit(alpha0[TXp[i]]+
                          alpha1[TXp[i]]*
                          logit(xp[i]/100));
    lambda1[i] = exp(beta0[TXp[i]]-beta1[TXp[i]]*xp[i] +
                 beta2[TXp[i]]*log(xp[i]));
  }
}
model{
  beta0 ~ normal(b0, sigma[1]);
  beta1 ~ normal(b1, sigma[2]);
  beta2 ~ normal(b2, sigma[3]);
```

```
    alpha0 ~ normal(a0, sigma[4]);
    alpha1 ~ normal(a1, sigma[5]);
    for (i in 1:n0){
      target += log_sum_exp(log(theta0[i]),
              log1m(theta0[i])-lambda0[i]);
    }
    target += log1m(theta1);
    target += poisson_lpmf(yp|lambda1);
}
"
```

End

At the regional scale, we can also define the ST50 using the hyper-parameters:

$$ST50_R = \frac{100}{1 + e^{\mu_{\alpha_0}/\mu_{\alpha_1}}},$$

which is an aggregated community-level stressor-specific tolerance indicator. Literally, the indicator represents the average watershed developed land-use as a fraction of the total watershed area at which the mean probability of extinction of individual taxa is 0.5. The higher the $ST50_R$ is, the more tolerant the EPT community is in the region.

Cross-region Comparison

We make two comparisons. First, model coefficients (and ST50s) for individual taxa estimated from using an individual taxon model can be contrasted to the same estimated from the regional hierarchical model. This comparison illustrates the shrinkage effect of the hierarchical model. By modeling all EPT taxa together using a hierarchical model, model coefficients (and ST50s) for an individual taxa shrink toward the overall center (the hyper-parameters, Figure 5.20). Shrinking the magnitude of estimated coefficients is always an effective strategy to reduce estimation uncertainty as the definition of estimation error is that the estimated coefficient is either too large or too small compared to the true value. As such, shrinking toward the overall center of coefficients of all taxa in the region has a high probability of reducing estimation error.

Second, across the six low antecedent agriculture land use regions (ATL, BOS, BIR, POR, RAL, and SLC), we compare the regional ST50 ($ST50_R$'s) to illustrate the effectiveness of the community-level indicator to represent the level of stress imposed by urbanization. The comparison is focused on the six regions because the other three regions (DEN, DFW, and MGB) represent regions with high antecedent agriculture land use, another type of human activity that is known to have adverse impacts on stream ecosystems. As such, the effects of urbanization on stream ecosystems are dependent on the ecosystem conditions before the watershed was urbanized. When urban expansion happened in previously undeveloped watersheds, urbanization represents a

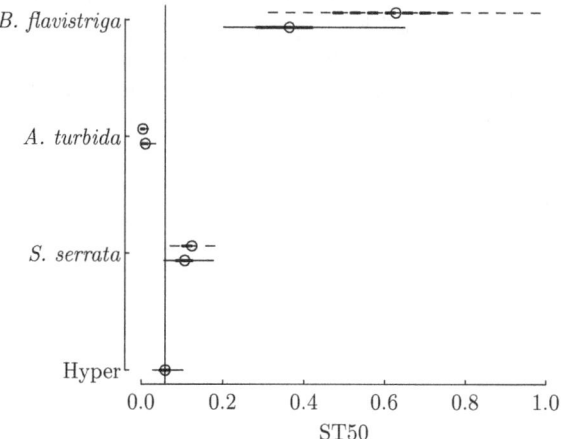

FIGURE 5.20: Species-specific ST50s estimated by taxon-specific ZIP models of three taxa shown in Figure 5.19 (dashed lines) are compared to the same estimated by the hierarchical model (solid lines). The amount of shrinkage toward the hyper-parameter-based ST50 ($ST50_R$, labeled as "Hyper") depends on the level of uncertainty in the specific-specific estimates and the distance to $ST50_R$.

drastic change to stream ecosystems. But when urban development replaces existing agriculture land, the impact on stream ecosystems may not be as drastic. The lack of response to urbanization is reflected in the high-levels of estimation uncertainty in model coefficients (and in ST50, Figure 5.21). In previous analyses of the EUSE data (e.g., Qian [2016], Qian et al. [2010]), we have noted that many univariate metrics do not or only slightly vary as a function of % developed land in these three regions with high levels of antecedent agriculture land use. In these three regions, we found a smaller number of EPT taxa and almost none of them respond to changes in urbanization. For the six regions with low antecedent agriculture land use, the responses of many univariate metrics to % developed land also vary. The among-region variation was often explained by the variation of annual average temperature and precipitation among the regions. The six regions, however, also have two contrasting patterns of urbanization distribution. The % developed land in RAL was nearly uniformly distributed and the SLC distribution was skewed high (more watersheds with a high percentage of developed lands) whereas the same distributions for the other four regions were skewed low (more watersheds with low urban development, Figure 1.6). The region-specific community-level ST50s show 3 clusters (Figure 5.21). The three regions with high antecedent agriculture land use show little response to urbanization, where the estimated ST50s are centered near 0 and with a large estimation uncertainty (EPT taxa in these three regions were largely unresponsive to watershed urbanization). Although we normally regard EPT species as sensitive to pollution, this study showed that some of the EPT species are quite tolerant. ST50s of RAL and SLC are higher than the other four regions. As we noted that ST50 is a stress-specific indicator, this pattern is expected.

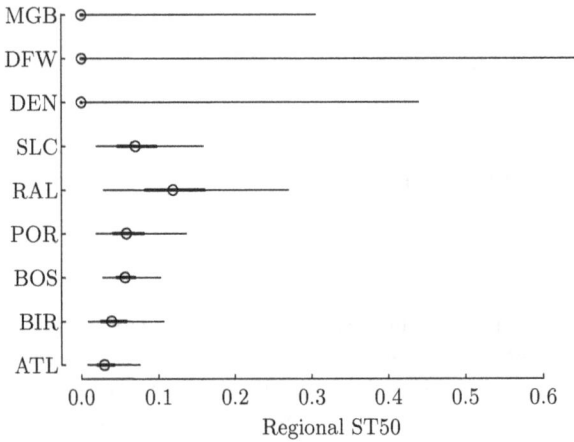

FIGURE 5.21: The hierarchical model estimated regional-level ST50s ($ST50_R$).

5.4   Multinomial Count Data

Many ecological problems can be described as multinomial problems. In stream ecology, we often use benthic macroinvertebrates to form indicators of ecosystem conditions. For example, the relative abundance of macroinvertebrates belonging to the three relatively pollution-sensitive "flies" groups, the orders Ephemoptera (mayflies), Plectoptera (stoneflies), and Trichoptera (caddisflies), are often used to form bio-indicators of stream conditions. More generally, species of macroinvertebrates have been classified based on their tolerance to pollution and the relative abundances of various tolerance groups in a macroinvertebrates sample are often used as an indicator of a river's ecological condition. In studying behavior of animals, ecologists also classify certain aspects of behavior into a limited number of categories. Observations of such studies are often in the form of compositions: numbers of occurrences of different groups. For example, numbers of macroinvertebrates belonging to various tolerance groups in a sample and number of observed behaviors in different behavior groups. Measures of richness, abundance, and composition of taxa or aggregations of taxa traits (i.e., assemblage metrics) are commonly used to describe responses or expected conditions. These measures are all based on counts of individual species (or taxa). Consequently, analyses of composition data in ecological and environmental studies are generally about distributions of count variables. We used the Poisson distribution to describe count data (e.g., species richness), and binomial distribution to model presence/absence data (e.g., COVID-19 testing data). In this section, we describe the multinomial model as a generalization to the binomial model to study composition data.

We explore the multinomial response variable model through three examples. The first example is developed based on a study of insect oviposition behavior in evolutionary ecology. The data for this example includes observed number of eggs laid by a species of wasp. This species of wasp is an insect parasitoid, which lays eggs in or on the eggs, larvae, pupae, or adults of other insects. The number of eggs they laid in each host is known as the clutch size. Some parasitoids are used for biological control of insect pests in orchards and other agricultural settings. On the one hand, the number of eggs laid in a host can affect the survival and fitness of the offspring. The ecological hypothesis is that the clutch size is evolved to produce the maximum number of offspring from each host that are fit to further propagate the population. Too many eggs will lead to competition among offspring for the limited resource (reducing the fitness of offspring), too few eggs constitutes a waste of the resource. On the other hand, the number of eggs a parasitoid lays in a single host can be affected by other factors. It takes time and effort for a parasitoid to find a host and then locate suitable spots on the host to lay eggs. Laying too few eggs would cost the parasitoid time and energy. Hilborn and Mangel [1997] used data from an observational study of a number of wasps to learn whether the clutch size is also a function of numbers of eggs each insect carried (egg complements).

The second example was derived from the EUSE example. In the EUSE example, we commented that counts of macroinvertebrates were often capped at a manageable number, for example, 300 or 500. As a result, ecologists often view the relative abundances (individual species counts as fractions of the total number) as the more relevant statistics. The limit of sampling methods made the use of relative abundances more informative. Furthermore, ecologists also view relative abundances of species in a community as a result of ecological conditions of the ecosystem, which shape the interaction among these species (e.g., competition, predation, and habitat and resources availability). In ecological literature, relative abundances of species in a community are often known as biological assemblages. In statistics literature, we often call them compositional data. Compositional data or biological assemblages are commonly used to assess ecological conditions [Barbour et al., 1999, Davies and Jackson, 2006] and to quantify the effects of anthropogenic disturbances in streams [Brown et al., 2009, Walsh et al., 2001, Kennen and Ayers, 2002,

Roy et al., 2003, Barbour and Paul, 2010]. Although the observed data are counts of individual species, the appropriate statistical model for these counts is the multinomial distribution and the parameters of the multinomial distribution describes the relative abundance as probabilities of observing each species in a random sample. These probabilities form a unit simplex (summing to 1). In the EUSE example, benthic macroinvertebrate data (counts for each taxon expressed as no./m^2) were stored in matrix format with rows representing sampling sites and columns representing taxa. An additional column contained the urban intensity value (% developed land) for each site. To analyze data of the assemblage as multinomial data, the response variables are the taxa count variables and the predictor variable is % developed land.

The multinomial distribution is a generalization of the binomial distribution (the probability distribution of the number of "successes" in n independent Bernoulli trials). In the context of species composition data, an independent Bernoulli trial is the process of identifying the species of a sample, and a trial is a "success" if that a given sample is identified to be a group of interest. For example, we may characterize each species of macroinvertebrates based on their tolerance to pollution and group them into "tolerant" and "sensitive" two groups. A Bernoulli trial is the process of classifying individual observations into success (e.g., belonging to the tolerant group) or failure (belonging to the sensitive group). The statistical model to describe the randomness of the process is the binomial distribution of the number of successes (x) in n trials:

$$x \sim binom(\pi, n) \tag{5.27}$$

where π is the probability of success representing the mean of the Bernoulli distribution (or fraction of tolerant species). Statistical models for response variables with binomial distribution is the logistic regression, where the probability of success π (after logit transformation) is modeled as a linear function of one or more predictors. The logit transformation of π is $logit(\pi) = \log\left(\frac{\pi}{1-\pi}\right)$, the log odds of the trial is a success. We can use π_1 as the probability of success (e.g., an individual belonging to the tolerant group) and use π_2 as the probability of failure (an individual belonging to the sensitive group). Because there are two possible outcomes, π_1 and π_2 sum to 1 (i.e., $\pi_1 = 1 - \pi_2$, only one free parameter). The logit transformation of π_1 can be expressed as

$$\log\left(\frac{\pi_1}{\pi_2}\right),$$

the logarithm of the probability ratio of the one over the other. A statistical assumption of the model is that both π_1 and π_2 are strictly positive, implying, for example, that there are always individuals belonging to the tolerant group in a given location. When π_1 is small, the chance of observing 0 intolerant taxa in a sample is high. In other words, an observed 0 in a sample does not imply that tolerant taxa do not exist, rather that the chance of seeing an individual belonging to the tolerant group is low. The commonly used empirical relative abundance represents an estimate of the true relative abundance, which is subject to estimation uncertainty. To properly account for the uncertainty in the data, the GLM should be used with a proper probabilistic assumption on the raw count data.

When the outcome is multinomial (more than two possible categories, e.g., more than two species groups), the response variable is a vector of more than two count variables, each represents the observed counts of one category. If there are k species groups, we need k probabilities $(\pi_1, \cdots, \pi_k)$ to describe the composition. The k probabilities form a simplex, that is $\sum_{i=1}^{k} \pi_i = 1$. The logit transformation under a multinomial distribution is a set of $k-1$ log odds ratios:

$$
\begin{aligned}
\mathrm{logit}(\pi_2) &= \log\left(\frac{\pi_2}{\pi_1}\right) \\
\mathrm{logit}(\pi_3) &= \log\left(\frac{\pi_3}{\pi_1}\right) \\
&\cdots \\
\mathrm{logit}(\pi_k) &= \log\left(\frac{\pi_k}{\pi_1}\right).
\end{aligned}
\tag{5.28}
$$

We call the first category a reference category. As in all applications of the generalized linear models, we define a multinomial regression model in two steps.

First, a distributional assumption is made on the response variable. In analyzing composition data, the response variables $Y = \{y_1, \cdots, y_k\}$, the observed number of occurrences, are assumed to be from a multinomial distribution:

$$
Y \sim multinomial(\pi, N)
\tag{5.29}
$$

where $N = \sum_{j=1}^{k} y_j$ is the observed total abundance and $\pi = \{\pi_1, \cdots, \pi_k\}$, the variable of interest in a multinomial distribution problem, is the vector of relative abundances (with constraint $\sum_{j=1}^{k} \pi_j = 1$).

Second, the mean of each relative abundance is linked to a linear function of the predictors through a link function. In the multinomial case, the mean variable is the simplex of relative abundances π. Because these probabilities sum to one, only $k - 1$ sets of free parameters need to be estimated. Setting π_1 as the baseline, the probability of occurrence is linked to the predictors through the generalized logit transformation:

$$
\begin{aligned}
\log(\pi_2/\pi_1) &= \boldsymbol{X\beta_2} \\
\log(\pi_3/\pi_1) &= \boldsymbol{X\beta_3} \\
&\cdots \\
\log(\pi_k/\pi_1) &= \boldsymbol{X\beta_k}
\end{aligned}
\tag{5.30}
$$

where $\boldsymbol{X\beta_j}$ represents a linear function of predictor variables, or $X\beta_j = \beta_{j0} +$

$\beta_{j1}x_1 + \cdots + \beta_{jp}x_p$. Because $\sum_{j=1}^{k} \pi_j = 1$, we have

$$\pi_1 \;=\; \frac{1}{1+\sum_{j=2}^{k} e^{X\beta_j}}$$

$$\pi_2 \;=\; \frac{e^{X\beta_2}}{1+\sum_{j=2}^{k} e^{X\beta_j}}$$

$$\cdots$$

$$\pi_k \;=\; \frac{e^{X\beta_k}}{1+\sum_{j=2}^{k} e^{X\beta_j}}.$$

Alternatively, we can set $\boldsymbol{\beta_1} = 0$ and $\boldsymbol{\eta_j} = \boldsymbol{X\beta_j}$ for $j = 1, \cdots, k$, and the probability formula is simplified to be:

$$\pi_j = \frac{e^{\eta_j}}{\sum_{i=1}^{k} e^{\eta_i}}. \tag{5.31}$$

Efficient maximum likelihood estimators of the multinomial regression model are widely available. For example, the R function `multinom` from the R package `nnet` in the VR bundle [Venables and Ripley, 2002] is a well documented package with extensive references and examples. The multinomial distribution is also part of the Stan software. In most applications of multinomial data analysis, the classical generalized linear model implementation is sufficient. We illustrate the use of function `multinom` using data from the insect oviposition and EUSE examples, followed by a missing data problem where Bayesian implementation is necessary.

5.4.1   The Insect Oviposition Example

The data reported in Hilborn and Mangel [1997] are the number of clutches of different sizes laid by insects carrying different numbers of eggs (egg complements). The egg complement varied from 4 to 23 and there were only four observed clutch sizes (1 through 4) (Table 6.1 in Hilborn and Mangel [1997]). Hilborn and Mangel [1997] dismissed a simple analysis of the data (regressing the average clutch sizes against the respective egg complements, showing a positive correlation between average clutch size and egg complement) and discussed how to confront four alternative models of fixed clutch sizes (i.e., assuming clutch size is one of the four values, 1:4). Their approach of calculating the sum of squared differences between the observed clutch sizes and the assumed fixed clutch size led them to conclude that the models of fixed clutch size of 2 and 3 are comparable and better supported by the data than the other two models. To understand the role of the egg complement on the clutch size, they proposed a threshold model to describe the relationship between clutch size ($c_1 = 2$ and $c_2 = 3$) and egg complement (e): when $e \leq e_1$, $c = c_1$ and when $e > e_1$, $c = c_2$. They calculated the sum of squared values for all possible values of e_1 (between 4 and 23) to determine the optimal "switching value" (between 7 and 10). In a sentence, the model predicts a clutch size of 2 when the insect carries 8 or fewer eggs and 3 otherwise.

The clutch size is limited to four values. From a data analysis perspective, we are more interested in the relative likelihood of clutch sizes. Specifically, we want to be able to use the probability of the clutch size being $k = 1 : 4$ to describe our uncertainty in predicting the clutch size as a function of the egg complement. The response variable of the study is a vector of four count variables: number of clutches with the four possible sizes: y_1, y_2, y_3, y_4. What we want to know is the probability of having the clutch size in one of the four categories: p_1, p_2, p_3, p_4. Because there are only four possibilities, these probability values must sum to unity: $p_1 + p_2 + p_3 + p_4 = 1$. Statistically, we can model the response variable using a multinomial distribution:

$$\{y_1, y_2, y_3, y_4\} \sim multinomial(p_1, p_2, p_3, p_4, N)$$

where $N = y_1 + y_2 + y_3 + y_4$ is the observed total number of clutches, and we can fit a generalized linear model using the R function `multinom`. As with most statistical software, the function `multinom` will return the estimated model coefficients (β's in equation (5.30)). These coefficients describe changes in the log ratios of probability of occurrence of a given group over the probability of occurrence of the reference group. The relationship between the probability of occurrence and the predictor (x, egg complement) is nonlinear. Consequently, the statistical significance test associated with model coefficients is related to specific conditions and should not be interpreted as in a linear model situation. The estimated coefficients should always be converted to the relative abundances as in equation 5.31 and the model results presented graphically for interpretation. The choice of reference group is mathematically inconsequential and different software may have a different default reference group. The R function `multinom` uses the left most column of the group matrix as the reference group.

As the multinomial regression is a multivariate model, the response variable in R model formula is a matrix of counts:

```
#### R Code ####
## Data -- the insect oviposition behavior (Ecological Detective)
oviposition <- data.frame(
        complement=4:23,
        one=c(0,0,1,1,0,0,0,0,0,1,rep(0,10)),
        two=c(2,5,11,5,2,1,4,3,1,2,0,3,2,2,0,0,0,1,0,0),
        three=c(1,1,3,1,1,0,3,4,6,4,3,4,6,4,2,6,2,1,0,1),
        four=c(rep(0,5),1,rep(0,4),1,rep(0,9))
        )
oviposition <- oviposition[-19,] ## removing the row with all 0s

## multinomial model (glm)
ovi_M1 <- multinom(as.matrix(oviposition[,-1])~complement,
                data=oviposition)
summary(ovi_M1, corr=F)
### End ###
```

Because the multinomial model coefficients are difficult to interpret, we always transform the fitted model to report the estimated probability of occurrences.

```
#### R Code ####
beta <- coef(ovi_M1)
X   <- cbind(1, 4:23)
n.grps <- 4
Xb <- matrix(0, nrow=dim(X)[1], ncol=n.grps-1)
for (i in 1:(n.grps-1)) Xb[,i] <- X%*% beta[i,]

denomsum <- apply(exp(Xb), 1, sum)
PP <- matrix(0, nrow=dim(X)[1], ncol=n.grps)
PP[,1] <- 1/(1+denomsum)
for (i in 2:n.grps) PP[,i] <- exp(Xb[,i-1])/(1+denomsum)
### End ###
```

To compare the estimated probability of occurrence, we calculate the relative frequency of each clutch size in each observation:

```
#### R Code ####
dataP <- t(apply(oviposition[,-1], 1,
                 function(x) return(x/sum(x))))
```

The multinomial model that estimated probabilities of observing different clutch sizes showed: (1) the probabilities of observing clutch sizes of 1 and 4 are very small and do not appear to respond to egg complements, (2) the probability of observing a clutch size of 2 (and 3) decreases (increases) as the egg complement increases (Figure 5.22). Compared to the threshold model described in Hilborn and Mangel [1997], the multinomial model describes the pattern shown in the data better. An abrupt threshold where the clutch size changes from 2 to 3 is not apparent in the data.

One obvious drawback of using the maximum likelihood estimator is the difficulty in translating the estimation uncertainty represented in the standard errors of model coefficients to the uncertainty in the estimated probabilities. When using the Bayesian approach, we estimate the posterior distributions of model coefficients and estimation uncertainty can be directly represented in the posterior distributions of the probabilities of presence. Implementation of the multinomial model in Stan is straightforward as shown in the Stan manual:

```
#### Stan Model ####
multN <- "
data {
  int<lower = 2> K;
  int<lower = 1> N;
  int<lower = 1> D;
```

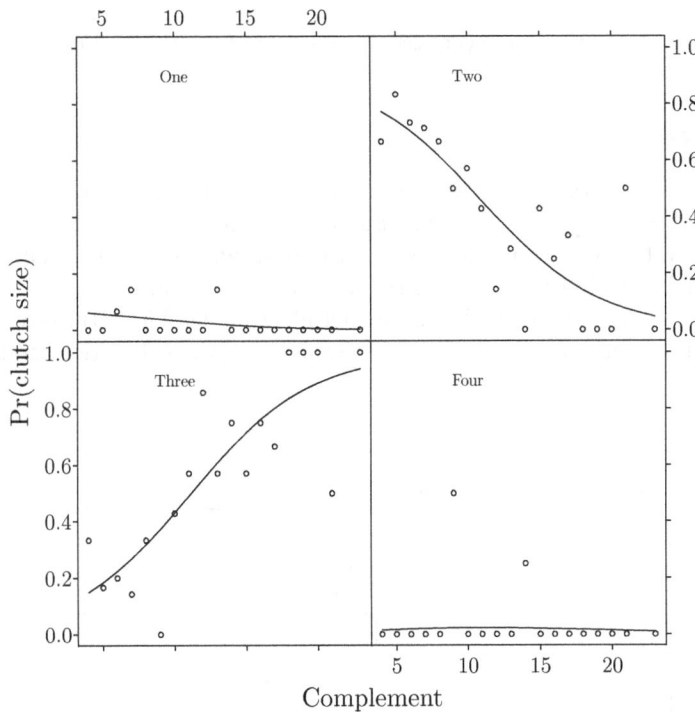

FIGURE 5.22: Multinomial regression estimated probabilities of observing four clutch sizes as a function of egg complements (solid lines) are compared to the respective observed relative frequencies (open circles).

```
  int y[N, K];
  matrix[N, D] x;
}
transformed data {
  row_vector[D] zeros = rep_row_vector(0, D);
}
parameters {
  matrix[K - 1, D] beta_raw;
}
transformed parameters {
  matrix[K,D] beta;
  beta = append_row(beta_raw, zeros);
}
model {
  matrix[N, K] x_beta = x * beta';
```

```
  to_vector(beta) ~ normal(0, 5);
  for (n in 1:N)
    y[n, ] ~ multinomial(softmax(to_vector(x_beta[n,])));
}
"
```

End

Here the function `softmax` transforms a vector x into a simplex: $\mathtt{softmax}(\mathtt{x}) = e^x / \sum_{k=1}^{K} e^{x_k}$. As `softmax` takes vectors as input, the `for` loop is needed. In the Stan code, we use the `transformed data` and `transformed parameter` blocks to create the matrix of model coefficients, with the last row being 0 (i.e., $\boldsymbol{\beta}_K = 0$) to make the model identifiable. The estimated mean probabilities from Stan are similar to the same using the R function `multinom` (Figure 5.23).

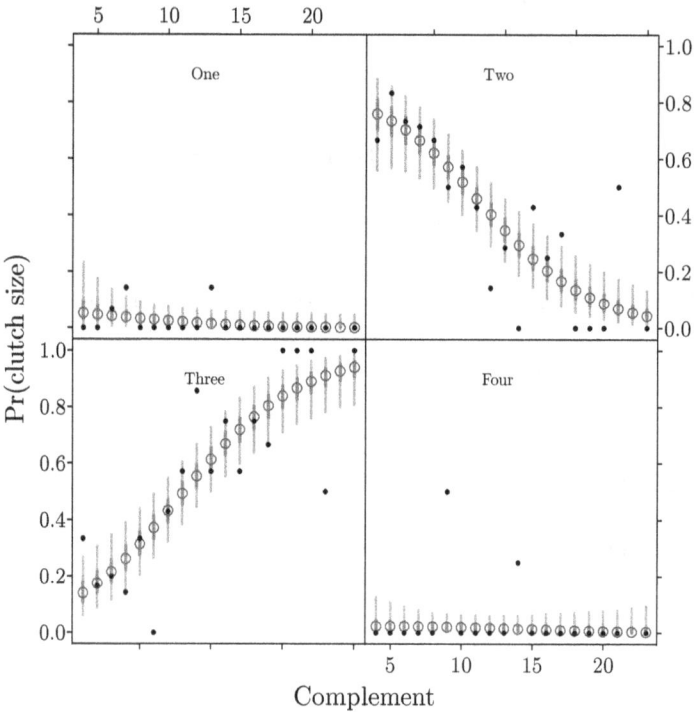

FIGURE 5.23: Bayesian multinomial regression estimated probabilities of observing four clutch sizes as a function of egg complements (simplified boxplots) are compared to the respective observed relative frequencies (solid circles).

5.4.2 The EUSE Example – Multinomial Logistic Regression

In this example, we group the EPT taxa collected from the Boston region into four groups based on their tolerance to pollution. For example, Qian et al. [2012] used four tolerance groups: sensitive, moderate-tolerant, tolerant, and unknown. Just as in the insect oviposition example, the response variable is a vector of four count variables $(y_{sen}, y_{mod}, y_{tol}, y_{unk})$, which are linked to the parameters of interest (relative abundances) through the multinomial distribution with four probabilities $(\pi_{sen}, \pi_{mod}, \pi_{tol}, \pi_{unk})$ to represent the relative abundances.

$$\{y_{sen}, y_{mod}, y_{tol}, y_{unk}\} \sim multinomial(\pi_{sen}, \pi_{mod}, \pi_{tol}, \pi_{unk}, N)$$

where $N = y_{sen} + y_{mod} + y_{tol} + y_{unk}$ is the observed total count. The four relative abundances form a unit simplex (i.e., $\pi_{sen} + \pi_{mod} + \pi_{tol} + \pi_{unk} = 1$).

The R code used in this example is nearly identical to the R code in the oviposition behavior example. Like the oviposition behavior example, the multinomial regression cannot properly convey the estimation uncertainty in the parameters of interest, in this case, the estimated relative abundances (Figure 5.24).

When using early MCMC programs (e.g., WinBUGS), we often read that computation of a multinomial model can be simplified when using the multinomial-Poisson transformation [Baker, 1994]. Agresti [2010] showed that when considering count data from a multinomial distribution as independent Poisson random variates, the joint distribution function conditional on the total count being the observed total is the same as the multinomial likelihood function. Spiegelhalter et al. [1996] showed that a logistic multinomial model (equation (5.30)) is equivalent to modeling each count variable as an independent Poisson random variable:

$$y_{ij} \sim Pois(\lambda_{ij}) \tag{5.32}$$

and

$$\log(\lambda_{ij}) = \mu_i + \boldsymbol{X_i\beta_j} \tag{5.33}$$

where μ_i is given a locally uniform prior distribution and $\boldsymbol{X_i\beta_j} = \beta_{0j} + \beta_{1j}x_{i1} + \cdots + \beta_{Kj}x_{iK}$ represent the linear model. When using BUGS, the multinomial-Poisson transformation can speed up the computation. In Stan, this transformation is not necessary because we can directly use the target increment (`target +=`) statement to specify the likelihood function, which is

$$\prod_{i=1}^{I} \frac{e^{\sum_{j=1}^{K} y_{ij} \boldsymbol{X_i\beta_j}}}{\left[\sum_{j=1}^{K} e^{\boldsymbol{X_i\beta_j}}\right]^{n_i}}.$$

The log-likelihood is

$$\sum_{i=1}^{I} \sum_{j=1}^{K} y_{ij} \boldsymbol{X_i\beta_j'} - n_i \log\left(\sum_{j=1}^{K} e^{\boldsymbol{X_i\beta_j}}\right).$$

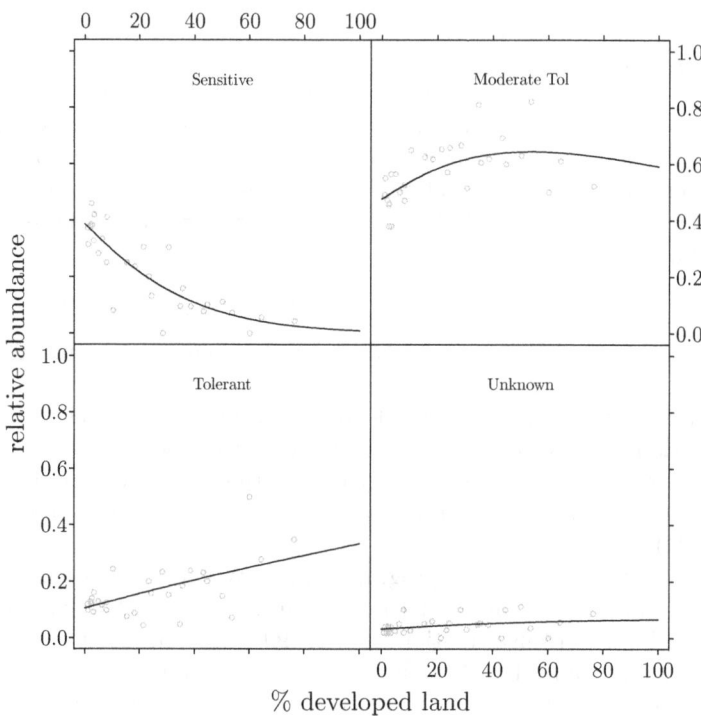

FIGURE 5.24: Multinomial regression estimated probabilities of presence (solid lines) of four groups of macroinvertebrates as a function of % developed land are compared to the respective observed relative abundances.

This likelihood function can be expressed in Stan using:

```
### Partial Stan code ###
model{
    matrix[N, K] x_beta = x * beta';
    matrix[N, K] yx_beta = y * x_beta';
    for (i in 1:N){
        target+=sum(yx_beta[i,])-sum(y[i,])*log_sum_exp(x_beta[i,]);
    }
}
### End ###
```

A `for` loop is needed because the function `log_sum_exp`, as with the function `softmax`, accepts vectors as input.

The Bayesian model estimated relative abundances of the four groups of EPT taxa are identical as the MLE estimates (Figure 5.25). Although the readily available estimation uncertainty on the estimated relative abundances is an obvious benefit of the Bayesian method, the classical simulation-based method [Qian, 2016] can approximate the estimation uncertainty equally well [Qian and Cuffney, 2014]. One advantage of using the Bayesian model (and the explicit expression of the log-likelihood function) is in a missing data problem – estimating a missing predictor variable (x) value, as in the ELISA example in Chapter 4 (Section 4.3.2).

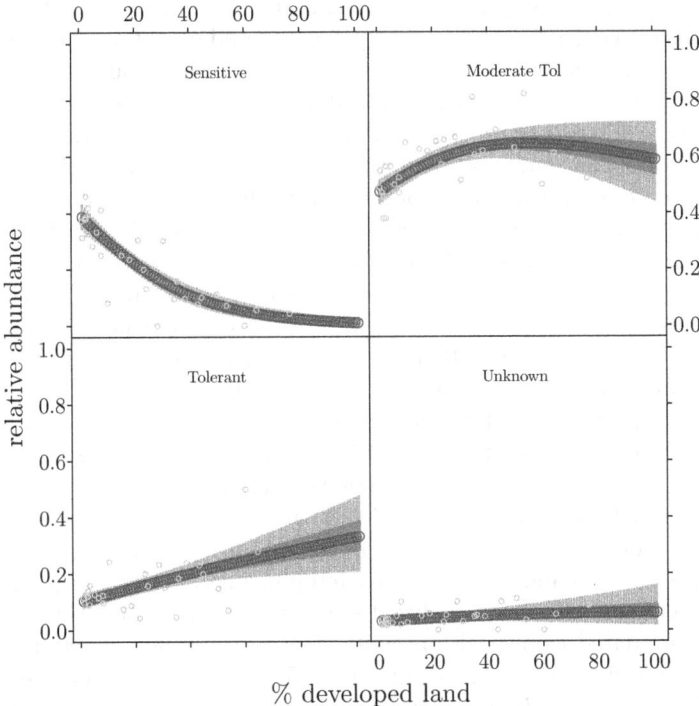

FIGURE 5.25: Bayesian multinomial regression estimated probabilities of presence (solid lines) of four groups of macroinvertebrates as a function of % developed land are compared to the respective observed relative abundances.

5.4.3 The Everglades Example – A Missing Data Problem

In this example, we illustrate the use of species composition data for reconstructing historical (or missing) environmental variable values. The data we used are from various studies in the Everglades conducted in the 1990s [Cooper et al., 2008, 1999, Jensen et al., 1999, Pan et al., 2000]. Qian and Pan [2006] summarized the data from some of these studies and implemented the Bayesian multinomial model using the multinomial-Poisson transformation under WinBUGS. In the rest of this section, we introduce the Everglades experiment and the objectives of collecting the data, as well as the ecological basis of inferring missing environmental conditions using species composition data. The statistical method we used is similar to the nonlinear regression problem we discussed in Section 4.3.2, where chemical measurements were estimated as missing predictor variable values. See Section 1.4.3 for general information of the Everglades study.

Data for this example were collected from the Everglades wetlands with an objective of estimating the "background" (or pre-human perturbation) soil phosphorus concentration. Learning the background condition is the first step of developing a science-based Everglades restoration plan, similar to estimating soil background concentrations of lead and mercury in Section 4.5. As part of the effort, soil samples were taken in the Everglades to reconstruct historical soil phosphorus concentrations through diatom species composition.

Data used in this study were collected from the Water Conservation Area - 2A (WCA2A) in the northern Everglades. WCA2A is a 547 km^2 diked marsh with a mosaic of sawgrass (*Cladium jamaicense* Crantz) prairies and open water sloughs. It has been receiving agricultural runoff from the north for decades. As a result, a north to south phosphorus gradient has established [Craft and Richardson, 1993, Reddy et al., 1993, Urban et al., 1993].

The diatom species composition data were collected from WCA2A in 1996 [Cooper et al., 2008]. The data set includes surface sediment and soil samples from 31 sites covering most area in WCA2A, as well as three soil cores, one collected in the phosphorus-enriched northern area of WCA2A and the other two at two southerly locations in WCA2A, areas that are not visibly affected by nutrient enrichment at the time. Both the surface samples and the soil core samples were analyzed for diatoms and pollen, and total phosphorus. The collected peat soil cores were analyzed at every 2 cm interval of the cores. The samples were dated using ^{210}Pb activity (within the range of 100–150 years) and ^{137}Cs activity for recent sediment (~35 years). There were 90 diatom species that can be positively identified in the data set. Cooper et al. [1999] and Jensen et al. [1999] studied the changes in diatom and pollen assemblages using the same data set.

The most commonly used method for environmental reconstruction at the time was the generalized linear model based correspondence analysis. The basic form of the model is the Gaussian model, where the expected value of either counts of abundance or present/absent data is modeled as a quadratic function of the environmental variable:

$$\eta(\mu_y) = \beta_0 + \beta_1 x + \beta_2 x^2$$

where μ_y is the expectation of the response (expected number for abundance data or the frequency of occurrence for present/absent data), η is a link function (for abundance data modeled as from a Poisson distribution $\eta(\mu_y) = \log(\mu_y)$ and for present/absent data modeled as from a binomial distribution $\eta(\mu_y) = \text{logit}(p_y))$, x is the environmental variable, and $\beta_0, \beta_1, \beta_2$ are the regression model coefficients. Because the quadratic model is proportional to the log of the normal distribution density function, the model is known as the Gaussian model. The peak of the response is called the optimum (reached at $u_x = -\beta_1/(2\beta_2)$) and the quantity resembling the normal distribution standard deviation is called the tolerance of a species ($tol = 1/\sqrt{-2\beta_2}$). The modeling process includes a regression step and a calibration step. The regression step is to fit independent generalized linear models for individual species. The fitted model is used, in the calibration step, to predict the environmental variable with known species count data. With multiple species and each with a different response curve, the unknown environmental variable x is estimated using the maximum likelihood estimator, assuming the estimated model coefficients as known constants and species are independent of each other.

Qian and Pan [2006] argued that the Gaussian model is unlikely to hold for environmental disturbances represented by the changes in phosphorus concentration, based on the concept of subsidy-stress [Odum et al., 1979]. A unimodal asymmetric response pattern is more reasonable. After comparing several asymmetric alternatives to the Gaussian model, Qian and Pan [2006] concluded that the gamma model (see Section 5.3.3) is the most appropriate for this problem. The model is the same as in equations (5.29) and (5.30), with the linear model $\boldsymbol{X}\boldsymbol{\beta}_j$ represented by the gamma model:

$$\boldsymbol{X}\boldsymbol{\beta}_j = \beta_{0j} - \beta_{1j}x_i + \beta_{2j}\log(x_i). \tag{5.34}$$

By separating the surface sediment soil data (with known soil TP concentrations) and soil core data (with TP unknown), we create two separate target += increment statements (see page 216) in Stan:

```
#### Partial Stan Code ####
transformed parameters{
...
  for (i in 1:N1)
    for (j in 1:K){
      xbeta1[i,j] = beta0[j]-beta1[j]*x[i]+
                    beta2[j]*log(x[i]);
      yxbeta1[i,j] =y1[i,j]*xbeta1[i,j];
  }
  for (i in 1:N2)
    for (j in 1:K){
      xbeta2[i,j] = beta0[j]-beta1[j]*x_miss[i]+
                    beta2[j]*log(x_miss[i]);
      yxbeta2[i,j] =y2[i,j]*xbeta2[i,j];
  }
}
model {
```

```
for (i in 1:N1){
  target += sum(yxbeta1[i,]) -
          sum(y1[i,])*log_sum_exp(xbeta1[i,]);
}
for (i in 1:N2){
  target += sum(yxbeta2[i,]) -
          sum(y2[i,])*log_sum_exp(xbeta2[i,]);
}
}
"
```

End

It is reasonable to assume that the missing TP values are within the range of known soil TP in WCA2A. We plot the estimated missing (historical) soil TP concentrations against the estimated dates (years) when the sediment layers were deposited based on ^{210}Pb or ^{137}Cs activities to evaluate the model performance. The estimated soil TP concentrations were relatively stable for the soil layers dated as before 1940s (Figure 5.26). After 1940s, the estimated TP concentrations from the soil core taken from the nutrient-enriched site increased steadily over time, while the estimated TP concentrations from the two sites not impacted by agriculture runoff showed a slight decreasing trend over time. The stable TP levels prior to large-scale development and settlement (started in the 1950s) is reasonable and the increasing trend in soil TP in the nutrient enriched site is also expected. The decreasing temporal trend in the two sites not impacted by agriculture runoff is unexpected, perhaps because of the many other elements in the water altered by agriculture runoff that may also change diatom species composition.

Separately, we evaluated the model by using the Jackknife simulation, fitting the same model by removing one TP value from the 31 surface soil sample data and letting the model estimate the set-aside value as a missing value. The model-estimated missing values are qualitatively comparable to the known values (Figure 5.27). As agriculture and other human activities led to many changes in the environment, in addition to increased phosphorus concentration in water and soil, the species composition model based on present-day soil data is unlikely to accurately capture the response of the diatom community to changing phosphorus levels. Reconstructing historical environmental conditions based on how present-day organisms respond to changes in one environmental variable is always associated with a certain level of uncertainty.

We examined the estimated model coefficients, especially the two slopes (β_{1j} and β_{2j} in equation (5.34)). The generalized linear model for a multinomial problem is linear on the logistic transformed distribution parameters. The parameters of interest, the probabilities or relative abundances, are not a linear function of the environmental variable. As we see in the EUSE example (Section 5.4.2), the estimated relative abundances are unimodal and asymmetric. For this example, we refit the model using the linear function of TP (and log TP) (equation (5.30)). The estimated missing soil TP values from

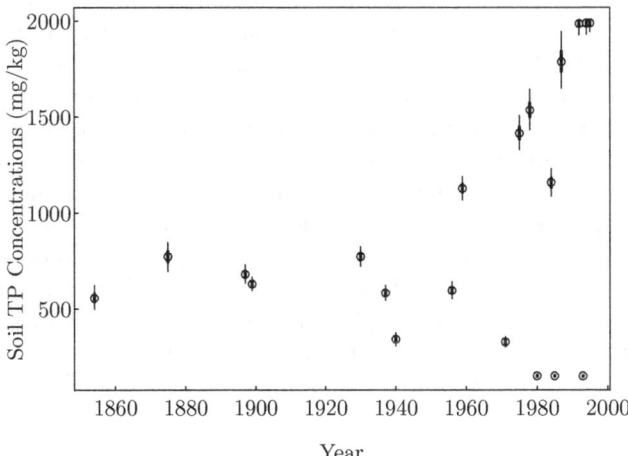

FIGURE 5.26: Multinomial model-estimated historical soil total phosphorus (TP) concentration.

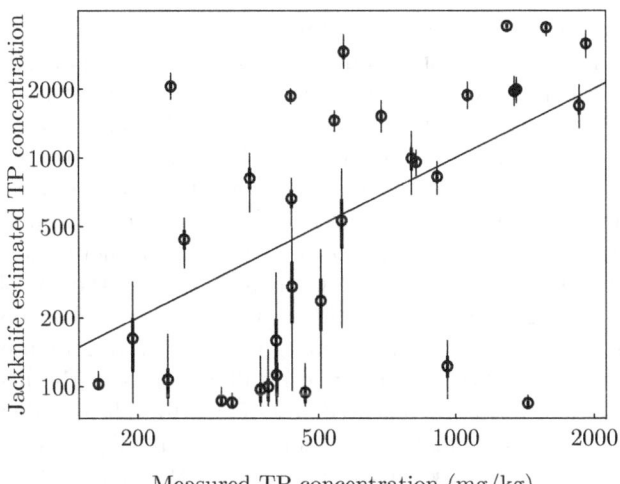

FIGURE 5.27: Jackknife simulation as an assessment of the multinomial model for estimating missing historical soil total phosphorus (TP) concentrations in the Everglades.

both linear models are comparable to the estimates from the gamma model. The Jackknife simulations for the two alternative linear models are similar to the gamma model results. The linear model is simpler and easier to work with.

There is no reason for using the gamma model in a multinomial model for this problem. The confusion stemmed from the multinomial-Poisson transformation (equations (5.32) and (5.33)), where counts of each species are modeled as independent Poisson variables (equation (5.32)). However, to achieve the equivalency in the likelihood function between the multinomial model and the independent Poisson models, these Poisson models must be conditional on the sum of these count variables having the observed total counts. The condition is achieved by adding a locally uniform variable μ_i (equation (5.33)). Although the transformation is mathematically effective, the Poisson models in this case do not have the physical meaning (how the abundance of a species change along the gradient) we imply when justifying the use of a unimodal response curve. The physical interpretation is, however, sound in the EUSE example (Section 5.3.3), where the zero-inflated Poisson model was used for individual species.

5.5   Summary

Count data are the most common type of data in ecology, the study of the abundance and distribution of organisms. Imperfect detection is an inevitable problem ecologists face. As we demonstrated in this chapter, statistical models for such data are always complicated and nuanced, because of the identification problem largely due to independent information on the rates of false positive and false negative. When such independent information is not available, we compensate by collecting data using a consistent sampling method to ensure these rates are relatively constant. As a result, models for such data can only provide estimates of relative population size. In the COVID-19 test data example, we highlight the need of knowing the rates of false positive and false negative of the test. Without knowing these two rates, a patient cannot properly interpret a positive or negative result in terms of the likelihood of infection without requiring a repeated test. For public health departments, test results from a large number of tests cannot be readily used to estimate the prevalence of the disease in the population. When the Gibbs sampler first appeared, many in the field believed that the data augmentation method would allow us to simultaneously estimate the two rates and the prevalence. In the COVID-19 example, we demonstrated that the data augmentation method cannot avoid the identification problem. Our example showed that the MCMC samples of the rate of false positive and prevalence are highly correlated. How we define the prior of the false negative rate does not influence the model performance. Although the example is about a virus test, the result can shed light on many ecological studies. In the EUSE example, a zero in the data can be a false negative and an identified individual could be a false positive because of mis-identification. In biology, taxonomy mis-identification has long been recognized as a serious problem [Vink et al., 2012]. But in many studies, misidentification may not be explicitly acknowledged. We have discussed the imperfect detection problem in a binomial model problem; the solution to the problem depends on knowing the rates of false positive and false negative. We have not seen how the imperfect detection problem can be properly addressed in a multinomial modeling problem.

In this chapter, we used the `target +=` increment statement frequently. Because of the capability of explicitly including the log-likelihood in Stan code, we can often improve computational efficiency by simplifying the likelihood function as we did in the data augmentation section (Section 5.3.1) (integrating out the augmented variable). In the Everglades example, we used the likelihood function of the multinomial model directly to bypass the multinomial-Poisson transformation. The resulting code is simpler and helped us understand the transformation better. With many efficient mathematical functions available in Stan, we should always consider explicitly expressing the likelihood function before coding.

Chapter 6

Hierarchical Modeling and Aggregation

We have mentioned the term "exchangeable" many times in previous chapters without fully exploring its meanings. In statistics, the concept is defined in terms of a joint probability distribution of variables $\{X_1, \cdots, X_k\}$. The random variables $\{X_1, \cdots, X_k\}$ are exchangeable if their joint distribution $\pi(X_1, \cdots, X_k)$ is invariant with respect to the order of the sequence. That is, if $\{X_1, X_2, X_3, X_4, X_5\}$ are exchangeable, the joint distribution of $\{X_1, X_2, X_3, X_4, X_5\}$ is the same as the joint distribution of $\{X_5, X_2, X_4, X_3, X_1\}$ or the joint distributions of any other permutations of the five random variables. The concept is closely related to the concept of "independently, identically distributed" (i.i.d.) random variables used in both classical and Bayesian statistics. The assumption that observations are from i.i.d. random variables is the basis for nearly all maximum likelihood based estimation methods. In the Neuse River example in Section 3.2, we use data from multiple sampling events in a year to estimate the mean nutrient concentrations. The basis of the method is to assume that each concentration value is a random sample from a random variable. In this case, the random variable represents the distribution of the nutrient concentration in a given sampling event. The i.i.d. assumption imposed on the data implies that data from the same year are generated from random variables with the same underlying distribution. Because of the i.i.d. assumption, we can express the joint distribution as the product of the densities of these observations (the likelihood function). The joint distribution (likelihood function) is invariant to the order of observations. The i.i.d. assumption is the basis for aggregating random samples to estimate distribution parameters. In this chapter, we discuss the exchangeable assumption on random variables at a conceptual level and explore the use of the exchangeable assumption as an organization principle when analyzing (and aggregating) data from multiple sources. As in previous chapters, we explore the concept using examples.

6.1   Aggregation in Science and Management

In exploring the use of multilevel modeling in ecological studies, Qian et al. [2010] stated that "ecosystem processes involve interactions at multiple scales, where processes at one temporal or spatial scale (e.g., a watershed) interact with processes at another scale (e.g., regional patterns in temperature and precipitation)," and "understanding the interplay between fine and broader-scale patterns and processes is key to understanding ecosystem dynamics." There, they used two examples to illustrate the use of multilevel or hierarchical modeling for properly combining data from multiple sources/regions, where measurements of fine-scale variables (within a source/region) are mixed with measurements from coarse-scale variables (across source/region). In one example (the EUSE example) initial studies analyzed data from different regions separately and the regional differences in the same ecological relationship raised questions. In the other example (soil N_2O emission), the initial analysis attempted to combine data from different sources to understand the effect of fertilizer application on soil N_2O emission. The apparent non-association between soil N_2O emission and nitrogen fertilizer application when analyzing the combined data from multiple studies was contradicted by conclusions of many studies represented in the combined data. In the EUSE example, Qian et al. [2010] showed that differences among regional models can be explained by the varying regional patterns in weather and land use. That is, the regional variation in the watershed scale (fine scale) summary of how stream ecosystems respond to watershed urbanization can be explained by the variations in regional scale (coarse scale) weather and land use patterns. Within each region, weather and historical land use patterns are relatively stable among watersheds. As a result, these regional scale patterns are statistically unrelated to the changes in stream ecosystem indicators. In the soil N_2O emission example, the apparent contradiction is a result of variation in soil organic carbon content among individual studies. Soil organic contents are relatively stable within individual studies. Just as regional-level weather and land use patterns in the EUSE example, study-level soil organic content cannot be statistically related to changes in N_2O emissions from different study plots within a study site. In both cases, the regional-/study-level patterns determine the region-/study-level model coefficients. Coefficients of the statistical model fit to data from a region or study are summaries of region-level/study-specific data. In other words, region- or study-specific model coefficients represent regional/study aggregation of watershed/plot data.

In a way, the two examples in Qian et al. [2010] are illustrations of how the statistical phenomenon known as Simpson's paradox [Simpson, 1951] plays out in ecological research. The correlation between soil N_2O emission and fertilizer application at plot-level within a study is likely positive, but the correlation is close to 0 when combining data from all studies. In both examples, regional-/study-level data should be aggregated based on the proper hierarchical structure. These two examples used relatively simple and small data. But the approach of properly analyzing data from multiple sources (cross-sectional data) has the same underlying principles. In a later study, Qian et al. [2019] discussed the implications of Simpson's paradox on lake eutrophication research.

Likewise, proper aggregation is an important consideration in environmental management and policy development. Qian et al. [2004b] and Wu et al. [2011] are examples of summarizing statistical results in different spatial and/or organizational aggregations to meet regulatory and management needs. These two examples are related to drinking water safety regulation and policies in the U.S. and China. Qian et al. [2004b] reported how data analysis and model results are aggregated into drinking water system categories based on regulatory needs in the U.S. Wu et al. [2011] explored the proper classifications for source waters of drinking water systems to support regulatory rule-making in China.

The U.S. drinking water safety regulations developed by the U.S. Environmental Protection Agency under the U.S. Safe Drinking Water Act (SDWA) require a cyclic review of all drinking water systems in the country and reporting of the frequency or number of drinking water systems with mean contaminant concentrations exceeding the maximum contaminant level (MCL), the maximum contaminant concentration that is deemed safe and allowable in drinking water [U.S. EPA, 2003]. In reporting the frequencies of certain contaminants, the EPA divided drinking water systems in the country into 10 size and source-water type categories based on whether the source water is surface water or groundwater and the size of population served by the system (e.g., ≤ 500, 501–3300, 3301–10000, 10001–50000, and >50000). Source water type often determines the likelihood of contamination by various pollutants. The population served by a system is often the basis for the legally mandated cost-benefit analysis when modification of MCL is proposed for a contaminant. In a typical SDWA compliance assessment, water quality data (measured concentrations of regulated contaminants) from all drinking water systems are compiled and analyzed to produce an aggregated summary of frequencies of drinking water systems with mean concentrations above MCLs. Such aggregated results provide a clear picture of the country's drinking water safety status and can be used as the basis for proposing changes of existing regulations (e.g., reducing the MCL of a regulated chemical or adding a chemical to the regulated contaminant list). The drinking water compliance assessment is a statistical problem because (1) only a limited number of water samples are available from selected drinking water systems and (2) only a small fraction of contaminant concentration measurements are above the respective chemical analytic method detection limits (MDLs).

Under the Chinese Environmental Quality Standards for Surface Water (GB 3838-2002), waters in China are classified into five functional grades using the "single factor method." Under this method, each source water is first classified into pollutant-specific grades based on each regulated pollutant. The functional grade of the water is the worst (highest grade) single pollutant grade of the water. This simple and clear classification method is, however, less informative because it cannot specify the extent and degree of a specific contaminant occurrence at the national level. In summarizing the results of the first national census of centralized source waters in 2006, Wu et al. [2011] explored three approaches for stratifying source waters:

1. Stratification based on administrative boundaries: source waters are first stratified by province, waters within a province are stratified by city/region, and source waters within a city/region are considered exchangeable. This stratification puts emphasis on local management.

2. Stratification based on hydrographical relations in China: waters in China are classified into ten class 1 water resource divisions, each represents watersheds of a large river basin. Subwatersheds are further divided into class 2 water resources divisions. Waters within a class 2 division are considered exchangeable because of their close hydrologic relations.

3. Stratification based on source water type and size (population served). China's source waters are classified into four types (reservoir, lake, stream, and groundwater) and four size categories ($\leq$10000, 10001–50000, 50001–200000, and >200000 population served). Waters within each of the 16 type-size groups are assumed exchangeable. This stratification was intended to support the Chinese government's effort in developing management requirements for different sizes of source waters.

In the U.S. SDWC cyclic review, the target was treated drinking water. As such, each source water type and system size category is likely represented by drinking water systems that are relatively homogeneous. The source water type represents the potential sources of pollution and the system size indicates potential differences in regulatory requirement. The review of the Chinese drinking water source water survey data was aimed at establishing such relatively homogeneous groups to aid future rule-making process. The basic principles of properly organizing and analyzing data can be summarized by the roles of what Fisher called *subjective ignorance* and *objective knowledge* [Fisher, 1956].

6.2   Subjective Ignorance and Objective Knowledge

Statistical analysis starts with sorting out what we know and what we do not know. What we know is the basis for model formulation and knowing what we do not know can help us decide the proper computational method.

For example, when evaluating the water quality compliance status of a water body, we collect water samples to measure concentrations of the water quality constituent of interest. Based on empirical and theoretical knowledge [Ott, 1995, e.g.,], we know that the distribution of concentration values can be approximated by the log-normal distribution. As a result, we analyze the log transformed concentration values to take the analytical advantage of the normal distribution. In addition to the log-normality assumption, we also know that measured concentration values from water samples can be considered random samples (they were collected from the same pre-selected locations on a predetermined schedule). As a result, we consider these samples as representative of the water body of interest. We are, however, ignorant about the relative magnitudes of each observation: we know that the next observation is almost surely different from the previous one, but we do not know the nature of the difference. The combination of the objective knowledge (concentration is a log-normal random variable) and subjective ignorance (individual concentration values are independent of each other) is the basis for pooling all concentration values and using the maximum likelihood estimator to estimate the distribution parameters. The roles of subjective ignorance and objective knowledge are often obvious in many situations and, therefore, not explicitly recognized. In more complicated situations, especially when analyzing data from multiple sources across multiple spatial/temporal scales, properly sorting out these two is the important first step of analyzing such data.

The independence assumption is an expression of subjective ignorance. Without it, we cannot pool data points together to construct the likelihood function. The statistical formal definition of subjective ignorance is the concept of exchangeable units. The n units $\{X_1, X_2, \cdots, X_n\}$ are exchangeable if the joint probability distribution $p(X_1, X_2, \cdots, X_n)$ is invariant under permutation of the units. The independence assumption is a special case of the exchangeable assumption, where the units are individual observations. For example, we may have n water samples from the same lake taken in different days, and the sequence when the samples were taken is inconsequential if we have no other information to indicate that sample from one day is more likely to have a higher or lower concentration value than samples from another days. When applied to the statistical method, we explicitly use the independence assumption to formulate the likelihood function as the product of densities of individual concentration values. The order of data points does not affect the resulting likelihood function. Our objective knowledge (data are all TP concentration values that can be approximated by the log-normal distribution) and subjective ignorance (we do not know which value would be higher in advance) allow us to combine these values for analysis.

In an ANOVA problem (e.g., the seaweed grazer example in Chapter 4) the measured response variable values are grouped by treatments. Within each treatment, we assume that the response variable measurements are independent of each other. In conducting an ANOVA test, we want to learn whether the treatment means are different. As a result, measurements from one treatment are potentially not independent (or exchangeable) from measurements from a different treatment. The alternative hypothesis of an ANOVA test suggests that not all treatment means are the same, which is the same as suggesting that the treatment means are likely different but we do not know how they are different. When we analyze the data using ANOVA, how we order the treatments is of no consequence. In other words, we assume that treatment means are exchangeable. The independence assumption (measurements within a treatment are exchangeable) suggests that we can calculate treatment averages (MLE of treatment means) separately. The exchangeable assumption with respect to treatment means allows us to use the resulting treatment averages to calculate the overall mean and the among-treatment variance. In this case, separating what we know and what we don't know allows us to determine how to aggregate the data and in what order.

Subjective ignorance and objective knowledge together determine how we set up a statistical model. In analyzing the nutrient concentration data in Section 3.2, we use the subjective knowledge to set up the model: the log nutrient concentration (y) is a normal random variable: $y_i \sim N(\mu, \sigma^2)$, and the subjective ignorance to develop the parameter estimation method: the likelihood function of observing $y_1, \cdots, y_n$ is the product of the density functions of the data: $L = \prod_{i=1}^{n} \frac{1}{\sqrt{2\pi}\sigma} e^{-\frac{(y_i - \mu)^2}{2\sigma^2}}$, which serves as the basis for both the classical maximum likelihood estimator and the Bayesian estimator. In a one-way ANOVA problem, we set up the statistical model in the same way: the independence assumption about the observations within each treatment is the basis for the first-level model $y_{ij} \sim N(\theta_j, \sigma^2)$, and the exchangeable assumption about treatment means gives us the second-level model $\theta_j \sim N(\mu, \tau^2)$.

All examples we used so far can be described in this general framework of statistical modeling: aggregating data into unit(s) of underlying patterns (summarizing what we know) and a unit of noise (what we don't know). We use the unit(s) representing underlying patterns to learn about the subject under study and to make statistical inference. As a result, how to aggregate (at what level) depends on the objectives of the study and how the data were generated. In the Neuse River example (Section 4.4), we initially interpreted the problem as to find the underlying mean concentrations of chlorophyll *a* and total nitrogen. Accordingly, the Bayesian updating routine we used systematically updated the estimated means every time we had new data. When we later revisited the problem, we made a different interpretation of the Clean Water Act and concluded that environmental standard compliance assessment should be based on underlying annual means. As a result, we have several units (years) representing the underlying patterns (how annual means changing over time) and each associated with a characterization of the noise (within-year and among-year variances). The seaweed recovery and Gulf of Mexico hypoxia examples in Chapter 4 are other examples where the number of units of aggregation was decided by scientific hypotheses and how the data were collected. When predictor variables are available, the unit representing the underlying pattern is represented by a linear or nonlinear function. The specific form of the function is often unknown and decided based on a series of exploratory analyses. In the PCB in fish example, the process of establishing the mean function is an iterative model-fitting, model-checking using residuals, and model-revision as illustrated in Qian [2016, Chapter 5]. The empirical approach of a linear regression analysis is often the exploratory data analysis of a statistical modeling problem. Such analyses often result in a better understanding of the underlying pattern. In other cases, the mean function is known and the modeling task is to estimate model parameter(s). In the ELISA example (Section 4.3.2.1), we use the four-parameter logistic function to characterize the standard curve. In both cases, the process of fitting a statistical model is a process of aggregating data into units that convey information at different levels of aggregation.

In the EUSE example in Chapter 5, we fit a zero-inflated Poisson model to data from individual species. These models aggregate data of individual species from multiple sampling locations to summarize how each species responded to changes in watershed urbanization (individual observations to species) in a given region. We then fit a regional Bayesian hierarchical model to model data from all species in the EPT group. The hierarchical models included hyper-parameters that represent the community-level mean and variance. As such the region-specific hierarchical model represents two levels of aggregation: from individual observations to species response, and from species response to community-level characteristics. The ST50 index derived from hyper-parameters becomes the community-level indicator of the general environment in a region. A species can appear in many regions, but how the species respond to environmental changes induced by urbanization may also depend on factors other than watershed urbanization level, such as different levels of competition due to different weather conditions. Many species in the EPT community may have similar ecological functions. Consequently, they may be more common in one region but not the other. As a result, aggregated summaries of a community are often more meaningful in ecological study and in environmental management.

In this chapter, we illustrate the use of the exchangeable units (sub-populations) concept to properly analyzing large cross-sectional data. We discuss the Bayesian hierarchical modeling approach as a natural tool for data aggregation at multiple levels through several examples. All examples are presented first with a conceptual description of what we know and what we don't know, followed by the quantification of the conceptual description using Bayesian hierarchical models.

6.3   Stein's Paradox and Bayesian Hierarchical Model

Lindley and Novick [1981] used the concept of exchangeable units to explain Simpson's paradox, a well-discussed topic in social and political sciences. The paradoxical results are often a consequence of similar results derived from non-exchangeable units. An early case of Simpson's paradox was the graduate admission paradox of the University of California at Berkeley [Bickel et al., 1975], where the campus-wide aggregated graduate admission rate showed a bias against female applicants, whereas disaggregated data showed neutral or favorable rates toward female applicants in most departments. More recently, the apparent switch of allegiance of the two major U.S. political parties (blue states, favoring the Democratic Party, are more affluent than red states, favoring the Republican Party) was contradicted by data showing that wealthy people are more likely to vote for Republican candidates [Gelman, 2009]. There are numerous statistical studies on the topic of Stein's Paradox. We find the concept of exchangeable units is especially valuable for understanding the paradoxical phenomenon and deriving proper analysis methods.

Although the concepts of exchangeable units [Lindley and Novick, 1981, e.g.,] and sub-populations [Fisher, 1956] have long been accepted in statistics literature as the basic principle for developing proper statistical models, the importance of these concepts has not been appreciated in many applied fields. In limnology, combining data from multiple lakes has been a practice since the late 1960s and early 1970s [Vollenweider, 1968, Dillon and Rigler, 1974]. When Dillon and Rigler [1974] published their study using reported sample averages from a combination of 46 North American lakes, lake years, and segments of lakes to estimate a simple (log-log) linear regression model relating log chlorophyll a (Chla) concentration to log total phosphorus (TP) concentration, the intention was to quantify the nutrient and primary productivity relationship among lakes. Numerous subsequent papers applied similar regression approaches using data from individual lakes and compared their estimated equations to the equation obtained by Dillon and Rigler [1974]. Such practice was questioned almost immediately after it was advocated [Jones and Bachmann, 1976, e.g.,] and continuously questioned by additional authors in following years [Malve and Qian, 2006, Wagner et al., 2011, e.g.,]. However, combining data from multiple lakes is still promoted [Pollard et al., 2018] and applied for developing regulations intended for individual lakes [Yuan and Pollard, 2015].

Suppose that we have TP (representing the level of eutrophication) and Chla (summarizing the primary productivity) data as shown in Figure 6.1. Initially, we want to analyze Chla data separately to understand the distribution of Chla across these lakes. We assume log-normality of concentration variables, that is,

$$\log(Chla_{ij}) \sim N(\theta_j, \sigma^2).$$

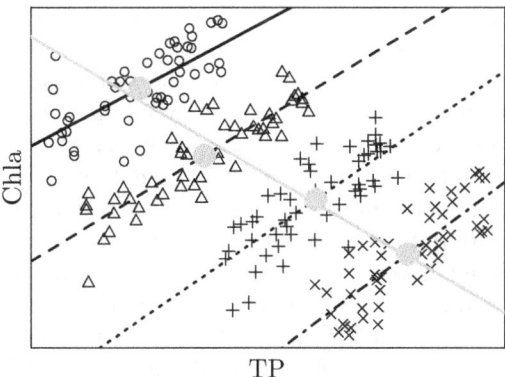

FIGURE 6.1: Four hypothetical lakes and their *Chal* and *TP* relationship (from Qian et al. [2019], Figure 1). Gray dots are lake means and black symbols are lake-specific observations.

This is because we know that lakes are different and combining data across different lakes can be misleading. In some large lakes, we may have reasons not to combine data from different parts of a lake. For example, western Lake Erie, part of the Laurentian Great Lakes, is eutrophic and experiences frequent nuisance algal blooms, while eastern Lake Erie is closer to oligotrophic. Chla concentrations from western Lake Erie are almost always higher than the samples taken on the same day in eastern Lake Erie. As a result, in classical statistics, we estimate the mean θ_j using the sample average of $\log(Chla_{ij})$ for lake (or lake segment) j (the maximum likelihood estimator). This estimator is the best estimator (unbiased and least variable) if only data from lake (or lake segment) j are available. When using Bayesian statistics, we must supply a prior distribution for the unknown parameter θ_j. If we have no other information to distinguish one lake from another with respect to θ_j (i.e., θ_j's are exchangeable *á priori*), we are compelled to use the same prior for all θ_js (e.g., $\theta_j \sim N(\mu, \tau^2)$). If we use non-informative priors for μ and τ^2, we cannot estimate them using data from one lake. The posterior distribution of μ, τ^2 can only be estimated with data from multiple lakes. Using the hierarchical approach to analyze data from multiple lakes such as the hypothetical ones in Figure 6.1 summarizes what we termed as organizing a model based on what we know (log-normality of Chla concentration in individual lakes) and what we don't know (how the mean concentrations vary among lakes).

The hierarchical modeling described in the previous paragraph is the empirical Bayes approach for analyzing large parallel data. Compared to the sample averages, the empirical Bayes estimated lake means $\hat{\theta}_j$ are shifted closer toward the overall mean μ. This effect is known as the shrinkage effect, that is, the range of $\hat{\theta}_j$s is narrower than the range of the corresponding sample averages. In a way, by using the same prior for all lakes, we partially combine the data from all lakes to estimate their respective means. This empirical Bayes approach is similar to the James-Stein estimator in classical statistics, which showed that shrinking of the sample averages toward the overall mean can improve the overall accuracy [Stein, 1956, James and Stein, 1961]. The James-Stein estimator is also known as Stein's paradox. It is a paradox because the best estimator for a single data set (e.g., sample average as the best estimator of the mean concentration of one lake) is no longer admissible when there are data for estimating multiple parameters simultaneously (data from multiple lakes). Efron and Morris [1977] summarized Stein's paradox in statistics and explained its improved overall estimation accuracy from an empirical Bayes angle. Efron [1978] stated that the Bayesian estimator of a population mean is always better than the maximum likelihood estimator when a proper (and informative) prior is available. This is largely because the informative prior provides additional information about the parameter we want to estimate. When we say that a sample average is an estimate with error, we mean that the sample average is either above or below the (unknown) true mean. When using a "proper" prior, we have reason to believe that the population mean is likely near the prior mean. The Bayesian estimator is a weighted average of sample average and prior mean. That is, the Bayesian estimated mean is "pushed" closer to the prior mean than the sample average is. The amount of push is decided by the relative information (variances) in the data and in the prior. When no prior information about the population mean is available, the Bayesian estimator is reduced to the maximum likelihood estimator. When data from multiple populations are available, the multiple sample averages provide some information on the likely distribution of the means. The James-Stein estimator and the empirical Bayes estimator explicitly use the mean of these individual sample averages to adjust the estimates of individual means. When data from multiple populations (lakes) are available, we have information in the form of multiple sample averages. The overall mean of these averages represents a reasonable guess of the mean for the next similar population, and the variation among the averages provides an estimate of the uncertainty about the mean. The closer the observed individual averages are to one another, the more confident we are that the next population would also have a mean in close proximity of the observed overall mean. As a result, we can use the observed sample averages to estimate a prior distribution of the mean of an unobserved population. The Bayesian hierarchical model

$$
\begin{aligned}
y_{ij} &\sim N(\theta_j, \sigma^2) \\
\theta_j &\sim N(\mu, \tau^2)
\end{aligned}
\tag{6.1}
$$

is a generalization of the James-Stein estimator when non-informative priors are used for μ, σ^2, and τ^2. The Bayesian hierarchical modeling framework should also be viewed as a practical way to derive a prior distribution for parameters of the population that are not represented in the current data. In other words, we can view the hyper-distribution $N(\mu, \tau^2)$ as the distribution of all exchangeable lake means.

We are able to use the hierarchical model of equation (6.1) when we only have Chla data. Although we know that lakes are different, without additional information, we can only assume that lake means of Chla concentrations are different but otherwise uncertain. In other words, we assume that lakes are exchangeable with respect to their means of log Chla concentration.

When we have information about the average nutrient concentration for each lake, our limnological knowledge informs us that lakes with higher nutrient levels are likely to have higher Chla concentrations. Knowing lake mean TP concentrations made the model of equation (6.1) untenable. Lake mean Chla concentrations are no longer exchangeable (although Chla concentration observations within a given lake are still exchangeable, or i.i.d.). We may assume that lake mean log Chla can be predicted by the mean log TP ($\mu_{TP,j}$):

$$\theta_j \sim N(\alpha_0 + \alpha_1 \mu_{TP,j}, \tau^2)$$

which is similar to the soil N_2O emission example, where emission of N_2O from control plots is proportional to soil organic carbon content. This is essentially the model fit to lake means of Chla and TP (Figure 6.1, gray line and dots). We can re-express the model as

$$\theta_j = \alpha_0 + \alpha_1 \mu_{TP,j} + \epsilon_j$$

and the model implies that we assume ϵ_j's are exchangeable, specifically, $\epsilon_j \sim N(0, \tau^2)$.

When we have paired observations of Chla and TP concentrations, the observed Chla concentrations are no longer i.i.d. Given the observed TP concentrations, we can use a regression model to predict Chla concentration. For example, the log-log linear regression is commonly used in limnology literature:

$$\log(Chla_{ij}) \sim N(\beta_{0j} + \beta_{1j} \log(TP_{ij}), \sigma^2). \tag{6.2}$$

Each lake has its own regression coefficients β_{0j} and β_{1j}. Without additional information on factors related to these coefficients, we can assume that these coefficients (equation (6.2)) from the lakes in question are exchangeable.

$$\begin{pmatrix} \beta_{0j} \\ \beta_{1j} \end{pmatrix} \sim MVN \left\{ \begin{pmatrix} \mu_{\beta_0} \\ \mu_{\beta_1} \end{pmatrix}, \Sigma \right\}. \tag{6.3}$$

If the lake in question is included in the data, we can directly use the lake-specific model for inference. The hierarchical model provides lake-specific estimates (i.e., β_{0j} and β_{1j}). Because we do not have additional information about these lakes, we use a common prior for the lake-specific model coefficients. By combining equations (6.2) and (6.3), we estimate lake-specific coefficients for all lakes, as well as the "hyper-parameters" μ_{β_0} and μ_{β_1} together. These hierarchical model estimated lake-specific coefficient values (β_{0j} and β_{1j}) are closer to the respective hyper-parameters μ_{β_0} and μ_{β_1} than the respective coefficients estimated separately using data from individual lakes.

If the lake of interest is not included in the analysis, the lake-specific regression models would provide useful information about model coefficients (e.g., the likely values and ranges). If we consider the lakes included in the data as a representative sample of all lakes of concern, these hyper-parameters summarize the information we have about the Chla-TP relationship for a generic lake (which means that a lake that is exchangeable with the lakes in the data used for develop the hierarchical model). A reasonable use of the hierarchical model in equations (6.2) and (6.3) is to use the posterior distribution of μ_{β_0} and μ_{β_1} as the prior for a lake not included in the data.

Many simple examples of Simpson's paradox can be explained by the imbalance of sample sizes of sub-populations (e.g., the Berkeley graduate admission paradox). Pearl et al. [2016] proposed a more general explanation of Simpson's paradox, that the paradoxical phenomenon is a result of one or more "hidden" causal factors that also affect the outcome. This is in line with the concept of "group-level" predictors such as the study-level soil organic carbon content and regional average temperature and precipitation in the two examples in Qian et al. [2010]. When such hidden causal factors can be identified, incorporating them into our models often leads to improved understanding of the relationship under study. An example presented by Tang et al. [2019] showed that the variation of the Chla-TP relation among lakes in eastern China can be predicted by watershed soil iron content in regions where the lakes were located. When such hidden factors are unavailable (as in most data analysis and modeling problems using historical data), we can rely on the exchangeable units concept to properly structure the data analysis so that the intended applications of the resulting models can be explicitly incorporated. In a way, the problem of Simpson's paradox should be addressed by Stein's paradox. In the rest of this chapter, we use examples to show the use of the hierarchical modeling approach to analyze data from multiple spatial, temporal, and organizational levels.

6.4   Examples

We use eight examples to illustrate the use of BHM. These examples represent several types of data and data structure. The first two examples (Example 1 and Example 2) are for analyzing univariate data. In the first example (Section 6.4.1), setting the TP environmental standard for the Everglades, we used data on ecological responses of various ecological indicators to this common pollutant to develop a parameter to represent the ecosystem-level response and use it as the basis for setting the environmental standard. The hierarchical modeling approach aggregates indicators representing different aspects of an ecosystem to represent the ecosystem-level response to elevated nutrient levels. While the first example illustrates how to aggregate from group-level parameters to hyper-parameters to represent the distribution of group-level parameters, the second example (Section 6.4.2) shows how the hyper-parameters can be properly used to improve group-level parameter estimation. We use these two examples to discuss how a hierarchical modeling approach can improve the process of setting and assessing the compliance of an environmental standard. In the second example, we emphasize that the shrinkage effect of the hierarchical model can improve the overall accuracy in the compliance assessment process. The next two examples (Examples 3 and 4) are about regression problems. More specifically, how to use multilevel regressions to combine data from multiple sources. Data from these examples are from Qian [2016] and Tang et al. [2019] (Example 3 in Section 6.4.3), DuFour et al. [2019, 2021] (Example 4 in Section 6.4.4). The next three examples are related to drinking water safety compliance assessment. Examples 5 and 6 used heavily censored data. In the U.S. Safe Drinking Water Act compliance assessment (Example 5 in Section 6.4.5.1), the goal was to estimate the proportions of drinking water systems that are out of compliance in the 10 source-water and size-based categories. In the source-water quality assessment example (Example 6 in Section 6.4.5.2), we are interested in evaluating the most effective ways of grouping source waters into categories. As we are interested in using the Bayesian hierarchical model for routine assessment, the best way to group these waters is that source waters within a group are exchangeable. The last drinking water related example is a mixture distribution example (Example 7 in Section 6.4.5.3), where the goal is to evaluate the status of contamination of a harmful microbe in the U.S. drinking water systems. In Example 7, we describe the mixture model methods and an effective computation strategy. We conclude the chapter with another example (Example 8), which improperly combined data and reached a questionable conclusion.

Because we normally use non-informative priors for the hyper-parameters (e.g., μ and τ^2 in equation (6.1)), we can often use the maximum likelihood estimator of the multilevel model (or mixed effect model) as implemented in the R package lme4. In these examples, we use lme4 for problems that fit the standard forms of the multilevel model and use Stan for situations that cannot be easily implemented using classical statistical methods (e.g., censored observations, mixture of two probability models). We often use lmer or glmer as a shortcut to explore different model forms. Once a proper model is selected, we code the model in Stan for better quantifying model coefficients, especially variance variables.

6.4.1   Example 1: Setting Environmental Standards in the Everglades

In Section 5.4.3, we used diatom species composition data to infer historical soil TP concentrations providing a reference of the Everglades soil TP. The current example is about how the ecosystem, represented by various indicators, responded to the increased phosphorus levels in water and soil. Much of the phosphorus-limited Everglades wetland has been lost to agriculture and urban development since the 1950s. Section 1.4.3 summarizes the legal and ecological backgrounds of Everglades research. In this example, we examine the effort of setting the water quality standard for TP summarized in Richardson et al. [2007].

Richardson et al. [2007] used the ecological threshold of TP as the basis for setting the water quality standard for TP in the Everglades. In the Everglades study, many researchers outlined the biological basis of an ecological threshold, measured in terms of changes of indicators of ecosystem attributes along the gradient of interest. In the Everglades study, the gradient is the TP concentration gradient. Biological indicators characterize attributes that represent different aspects of the ecosystem. We have seen the use of EPT taxa richness and richness weighted average tolerance in the EUSE example in this book (e.g., Section 1.4.2) to describe the macroinvertebrate community in streams. In a wetland, we want to use indicators representing ecological functions at different trophic levels to satisfy the legal requirement of setting a standard to protect the balance "in natural populations of aquatic flora or fauna." Accordingly, 12 biological indicators were used in Richardson et al. [2007] to represent algae, macroinvertebrate, and macrophyte communities. These indicators also represent a combination of how fast the indicators would respond to changes in TP concentrations. Indicators with fast response times mostly represent the algae communities, including diatom relative abundance, diatom density, diatom bio-volume, and blue-green algae bio-volume. Indicators with intermediate response times are largely derived from macroinvertebrate and macrophyte communities, including stem densities of an important macrophyte species (*Utricularia* spp., particularly *Utricularia purpurea*), macroinvertebrates biomass, abundance, numbers of Oligochaeta and microcrustacea species, and relative abundances of sensitive species, predators, and gastropoda species; indicators with slow response time are represented by macroinvertebrate community indicators (taxa richness, Bray–Curtis dissimilarity [BCD], and percent calcareous mat cover). For each indicator, a Bayesian change point model was used to estimate the TP threshold [Qian et al., 2003b] (see Section 7.2). The estimated thresholds (Table 6.1) for the 12 indicators are presented here along with the estimated standard error (derived as one fourth of the width of the respective 95% credible intervals).

Richardson et al. [2007] commented that the 12 ecological metrics in Table 6.1 adequately represent the Everglades wetland ecosystem. The ecosystem-level threshold should be a "weighted, integrated threshold." The 12 metrics were selected at each trophic level with at least 100 sampling points with relatively narrow credible intervals (Figure 6.2). The overall mean change point of 15.6 μg/L TP is compared to the change point of the *Utricularia* spp. stem count (15.6 μg/L, and 95% credible interval of 15.0–15.9). Richardson et al. [2007] argued that *Utricularia* spp. is ecologically important in the Everglades wetland by providing a key physical matrix component of the Everglades periphyton mat community; it is, therefore, likely a keystone (and highly

TABLE 6.1: The Everglades TP thresholds of various ecological indicators reported by Richardson et al. [2007].

metric community	change point (μg/L)	width of 95% CI
mat cover	19.2	1.6
BCd (macroinvertebrates)	13.0	6.4
macroinvertebrates		
% tolerant species	13.0	9.6
% sensitive species	12.4	16.2
% predators	8.2	0.8
% microcrustacea	19.9	4.2
% oligochaeta	18.3	1.2
macrophytes (stem counts)		
Utricularia spp.	15.6	0.9
Utricularia purpurea	14.8	2.1
algae		
% diatom on macrophyte stem	14.5	10.2
% diatom on plexiglas	23.5	26.3
% diatom on floating mats	15.3	10.3

sensitive phosphorus indicator) species for the Everglades. Accordingly, Richardson et al. [2007] recommended that the TP threshold for the Everglades should be below 15 μg/L, but above 12 μg/L. This recommendation is largely based on the ecological importance of *Utricularia*, a genus of carnivorous floating aquatic plant commonly known as bladderworts.

Because the legal requirement of setting a TP standard to protect "the natural balance of flora and fauna of the Everglade" is scientifically vague, a threshold based on one species is always less convincing, even though the value is close to the average of the change points of all metrics examined. Each metric represents a specific aspect of the ecosystem (individual species or species groups). These species-specific indicators by themselves cannot describe the natural balance at the ecosystem level. Suppose that there are a total of n indicators to represent the Everglades wetland ecosystem and we have estimates of thresholds of these indicators ($\phi_j, j = 1, \cdots, n$). Although each individual threshold cannot adequately represent the natural imbalance, the distribution of all thresholds should provide a quantitative summary of how TP concentration levels would affect the ecosystem as a whole. Because the 12 metrics were carefully selected to represent the Everglades wetland ecosystems, ecosystem-level threshold distribution can be estimated from these individual-level thresholds. Instead of using the average of the estimated change points of the 12 metrics, we integrate these estimates using a hierarchical model to properly represent the estimation uncertainty we have about these estimates.

The data we have are the estimated change point $\hat{\phi}_j$ and its standard

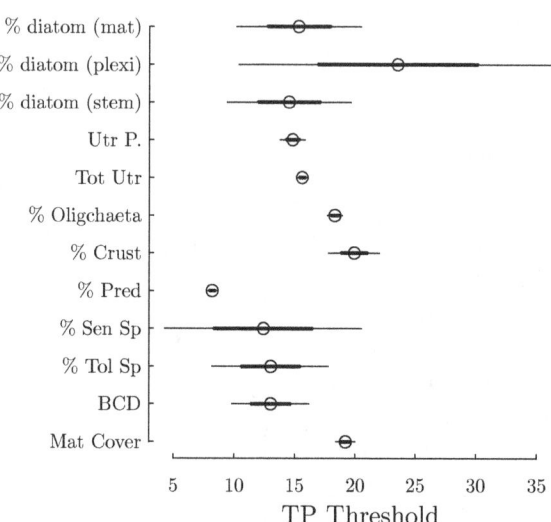

FIGURE 6.2: TP thresholds (in μg/L) for 12 metrics were estimated separately using the change point model. Open circles are the estimated means, and the thick and thin lines are mean $\pm$ 1 and 2 standard errors, respectively.

deviation $\hat{\sigma}_j$. These two numbers provide an indicator-level model:

$$\hat{\phi}_j \sim N(\theta_j, \hat{\sigma}_j^2). \tag{6.4}$$

Information in the data is summarized in the estimated mean and standard deviation $\hat{\phi}_j$ and $\hat{\sigma}_j$. When we have no additional information to determine the relative magnitude of the threshold for different metrics, we can assume that θ_j's can be modeled as follows

$$\theta_j \sim N(\mu, \tau^2), \tag{6.5}$$

that is, assuming a common prior distribution for θ_j. This common prior distribution reflects (1) our understanding that θ_js are likely to be different for different metrics, and (2) our lack of understanding on how θ_js are different from each other. The variance parameter τ^2 is the between metric variance. Using equation (6.5), we expanded the meaning of τ^2 to be the variance among all possible metric means (not just the 12 metrics represented in the data). This model links all metrics together through the common prior distribution $N(\mu, \tau^2)$. As we have no prior knowledge of μ and τ^2, we will use Stan default weakly informative priors. Instead of directly sampling θ_j as random variables, we use the relationship between a normal random variable with mean μ and standard deviation τ and the standard normal random variable $z \sim N(0, 1)$:

$$\theta_j = \mu + \tau \times z_j.$$

This is because θ_j's are often strongly correlated in a hierarchical model. By defining θ_j as a transformed variable, we improve the Stan model's performance by avoiding directly sampling from them:

```
### Stan Model ###
everg_stan <- "
data {
  int<lower=0> J;
  real phi[J];
  real<lower=0> sigma[J];
}
parameters {
  real mu;
  real<lower=0> tau;
  real z[J];
}
transformed parameters {
  real theta[J];
  for (j in 1:J)
    theta[j] = mu + tau * z[j];
}
model {
  z ~ normal(0, 1);
  phi ~ normal(theta, sigma);
}
"
### End ###
```

The model estimated θ_j's are shrunk toward the hyper-mean μ (Figure 6.3), a feature of the hierarchical model. The level of shrinkage is a function of (1) the distance and (2) the ratio of uncertainty between the individual estimated threshold and the overall mean.

The question with regard to setting the TP standard is now whether we use the posterior distribution of μ or the hyper-distribution itself (i.e., $N(\mu, \tau^2)$) as the ecosystem-level threshold distribution. If we use the posterior distribution of μ, we imply that the average of individual thresholds should be used to measure the ecosystem "integrity." As a result, we may use a lower percentile (e.g., 2.5%) of the posterior distribution as a point estimate to reflect the estimation uncertainty (similar to using the lower bound of a 95% confidence interval). If we use the hyper-distribution, which is the distribution of individual thresholds, we assume that the balance of natural flora and fauna is determined by all aspects of the ecosystem. If we use the 2.5 percentile of the hyper-distribution as the threshold for setting the TP environmental standard, we imply that we consider the impact of 2.5% of metrics that represent the "system" is legally acceptable. The difference between the two options is large (Figure 6.4). The 2.5 percentiles of the posterior distribution of μ and

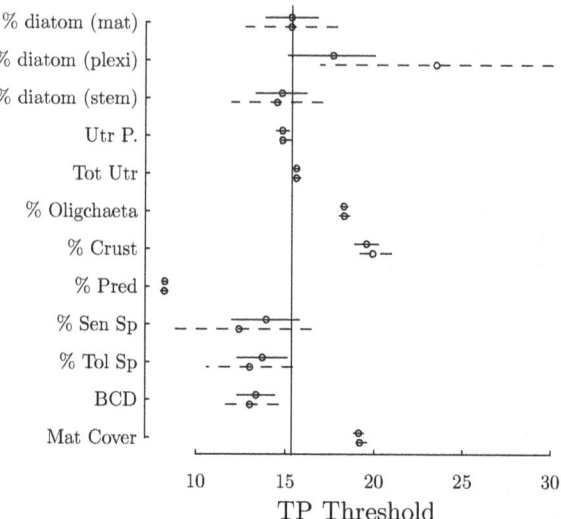

FIGURE 6.3: Hierarchical model estimated TP thresholds (in μg/L) for the 12 metrics (solid lines) are compared to the same estimated separately using a change point model (dashed lines). Open circles are the estimated means, and the thick and thin lines are the 50% and 95% credible intervals, respectively.

the hyper-distribution $N(\mu, \tau^2)$ are 12.67 (in agreement with the recommendation of Richardson et al. [2007] that the standard should be larger than 12 μg/L) and 6.24 μg/L, respectively (Table 6.2).

In this example, we analyzed the reported TP thresholds of a representative sample of ecological indicators and used the hierarchical model to aggregate them into a quantity representing ecosystem-level response to phosphorus enrichment in the Everglades. The hierarchical modeling approach is the natural means for integrating indicator-level thresholds into the ecosystem-level threshold. It is natural because the model properly weighs the individual thresholds based on their respective estimation uncertainty. The model's structure reflects what we know and what we do not know. The Everglades

TABLE 6.2: A comparison of the mean, standard deviation, and selected quantiles of the posterior distribution of μ and the posterior hyper-distribution $(N(\mu, \tau^2))$.

	mean	sd	2.5%	25%	50%	75%	97.5%
$\mu\|y$	15.35	1.31	12.67	14.56	15.42	16.18	17.76
$N(\mu, \tau^2)$	15.32	4.45	6.24	12.55	15.32	18.12	24.47

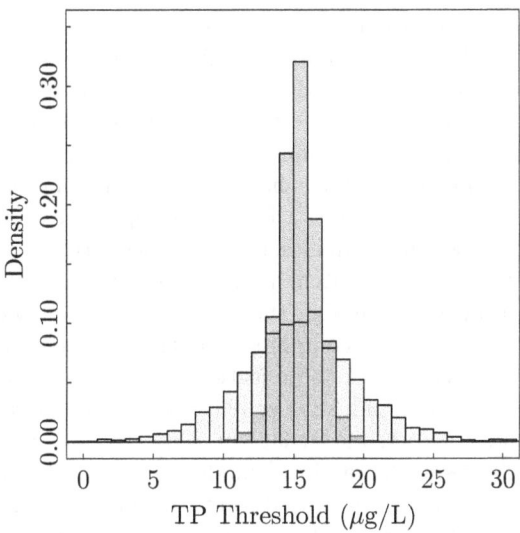

FIGURE 6.4: Histograms comparing the posterior distribution of μ (dark-shaded bars) and the posterior hyper-distribution ($N(\mu, \tau^2)$, light-shaded bars).

wetland ecosystem is affected by nutrient enrichment in many different ways. We know that some aspects of the ecosystem would respond rapidly and some slowly. By selecting ecological indicators that are likely to be affected by eutrophication and by sorting these indicators based on their response time, we ensure that the individually estimated TP thresholds are ecologically relevant. Before data collection, we do not know the range of tolerance of the selected ecological indicators nor their relative magnitude. The result is the hierarchical model structure in equations (6.4) and (6.5).

The hierarchical model, however, presents a choice: whether the ecosystem-level threshold distribution is represented by the posterior distribution of the hyper-mean (the mean of thresholds of all individual indicators) or the posterior hyper-distribution (the distribution of mean thresholds of all indicators). The choice is not a statistical one, rather, an ecological question.

6.4.2 Example 2: Environmental Standard Compliance Assessment

The Everglades TP threshold example is focused on ecological understanding of how the wetland ecosystem responds to the increased nutrient input. The outcome has a policy and management implication in how to set an environmental standard based on our understanding of the ecosystem. Once an environmental standard is set, the next step in environmental management is how to develop appropriate methods for assessing the compliance of the standard. Currently in the U.S., various statistical hypothesis testing approaches are used. Hypothesis-testing based methods are often controversial because of the difficulty in interpreting the statistical significance concept, a concept based on long-run frequency that must also be used to evaluate results from a single realization. Numerous studies have shown that using statistical hypothesis testing is inefficient because of the small sample sizes typically employed for environmental assessment. In classical statistics terms, a small sample size leads to a test with low statistical power (the probability of rejecting the null hypothesis, typically assuming the water is in compliance, when the alternative, the water is not in compliance, is true). Often when a low-power test rejects the null hypothesis, the rejection is frequently due to sampling or other types of error. Qian and Miltner [2018] illustrate these problems using two examples and recommended that the hypothesis testing framework be replaced by the Bayesian hierarchical modeling approach for estimating the posterior distribution of the mean pollutant concentration of a water of interest. They argued that the estimation approach can more effectively leverage information (data) from assessments of similar waters. In this example, we fully explore this recommendation as an extension of the Neuse River water quality assessment example in Chapter 4.

The hypothesis testing based assessment rules, when presented with the Magnitude-Duration-Frequency components (see Section 1.4.4), are often confusing and difficult to interpret. For example, the TP criterion for the Central Florida Bay is expressed as: "the annual geometric mean TP concentration shall not surpass 0.019 mg/L more than once in a three-year period" [FDEP, 2011]. That is, the criterion has a magnitude of 0.019, a duration of 1 year, and a frequency of 1/3. After a careful read of the criterion development document, however, we learned that the criterion is developed to ensure that the long-term (geometric) mean TP concentration is around 0.014 mg/L, a value established as the "healthy existing condition" of the water. In order to derive a rule with a frequency component, Florida Department of Environmental Protection (FDEP) argued that the 80th percentile of the annual geometric mean distribution should be used as the magnitude of TP criterion. This is a level of protection similar to the commonly used engineering practice of adding a safety factor. The frequency of one in three years is based in the binomial test with null hypothesis $H_0 : p \leq 0.2$. (FDEP calculated the 0.8 quantile to be 0.019 using a data set representing the "reference condition.") The null hypothesis can be rejected with a significance level of $\alpha = 0.1$ when more than one exceedance is observed in three trials, where p is the exceedance probability. (If the true exceedance probability is 0.2, the probability of observing 0 or one exceedance in three trials (years) is 0.896). Such a rule attempts to "evaluate a statistical feature that requires the law of large numbers using a sample size of three" [Guttorp, 2006].

The FDEP's TP criterion is common among various compliance assessment approaches based on hypothesis testing. Statistical issues related to these rules can largely be attributed to use of a low sample size to evaluate a statistical feature guaranteed by the law of large numbers. We can, however, avoid these problems by representing the compliance assessment problem as an estimation problem. For example, we can estimate the annual mean and summarize the estimation uncertainty using either the classical frequentist's confidence interval or the Bayesian's posterior distribution. To determine whether a water body is in compliance, we can compare the relevant quantile of the posterior distribution (e.g., 0.8) to the criterion (e.g., 0.019). If the 0.8 quantile is below the criterion, we conclude that the water is in compliance with the standard. This approach of using a confidence interval is in line with the concept of severe testing (Section 8.4). When we approach the problem as an estimation problem, we can effectively reduce the estimation uncertainty by partially pooling data from similar waters.

In the example of setting the Everglades TP standard, we aggregated thresholds of individual ecological indicators to derive the hyper-distribution. The hyper-distribution is seen as the prior distribution of the indicator-level threshold (equation (6.5)). The hierarchical model estimated indicator-level thresholds were shrunk toward the overall mean (Figure 6.3). The shrinkage effect makes the hierarchical estimated threshold less variable. Based on a review of statistical literature on shrinkage estimator, Qian et al. [2015b] suggested that the accuracy of environmental standard compliance assessments can be greatly improved when all available data are used under a Bayesian hierarchical modeling framework.

In a typical environmental standard compliance study, we rely on small sample sizes because of the one-water-at-a-time approach currently used in all states in the U.S. When combining data from similar waters, we can effectively reduce estimation uncertainty by using a shrinkage estimator. Furthermore, the estimated hyper-distribution (e.g., equation (6.5)) can be used as the prior distribution of the mean for a water body that is not included in the current data. Using the sequential updating method we discussed in the Neuse River example (Section 4.4), state agencies can update the hyper-distribution over time for individual water bodies. The sequentially updated hyper-distribution effectively serves as a vessel of information updated each time when new data are available.

The example used in Qian et al. [2015b] was based on data from a U.S. Geological Survey (USGS) study under the National Water Quality Assessment program. The study collected water quality data from wadable rivers in the Great Lakes watersheds. We grouped the rivers by level 3 eco-region (as defined by Omernik [1987]) to develop the hyper-distribution specific for each eco-region and used a river (name unknown) in the far west part of New York State as an example for compliance assessment. The New York river is in eco-region 83 (11th on the list of eco-regions in the data). The watershed land use and land cover pattern of this river (mostly natural land cover) is quite different from other rivers in this region (mostly in Ohio) with strong agriculture influence in their watershed.

The example has two parts. In the first part, we use the multilevel model to derive the relevant hyper-parameters. In the Great Lakes region, nutrient concentrations are affected by seasons: high in spring and early summer (the wet season) and low in summer and fall (the dry season). In addition to regional differences (er), we also use season (sn) and year (yr) as grouping variables. As a result, the multilevel model represents a Bayesian ANOVA:

$$\log(TP) = \beta_0 + \beta_{sn,i} + \beta_{yr,j} + \beta_{er/rv,k} + \epsilon$$

where er/rv represents the nested effects of rivers within an ecoregion.

```
### R Code ###
TP.lmer <- lmer(log(TP)~1+(1|Season)+(1|Year)+
                    (1|Ecoregion)+(1|STAIDer),
               data=GLdata, subset=State!="NEW YORK")
```

For the river in New York, we want to estimate the log TP concentration distribution

$$\begin{aligned} \log(TP) &\sim N(\mu, \sigma_1^2) \\ \mu &\sim N(\mu_0, \sigma_2^2). \end{aligned}$$

The multilevel model result provides prior information for μ_0 and σ_2^2. The prior for μ_0 is set to be normal with the relevant eco-region mean and standard deviation extracted from the fitted multilevel model.

```
### R Code ###
  m <- TP.lmer
  b0 <- fixef(m)[1]+ranef(m)$Ecoregion[11,1]
  seb0 <- sqrt(se.fixef(m)[1]^2+se.ranef(m)$Ecoregion[11,1]^2)
```

The multilevel model provides point estimates of σ_1^2 and σ_2^2. Using the conjugate inverse-gamma prior, the multilevel model provided only the ratio of the two prior parameters (i.e., $\beta/(\alpha-1)$). To quantify the prior of the two variances, Qian et al. [2015b] chose $\alpha = n_0/2$, where n_0 is the sample size of the data in the eco-region where the New York river is located:

```
### R Code ###
  sigma2.sq <- VarCorr(m)$STAIDer[1,1]+VarCorr(m)$Year[1,1] +
    VarCorr(m)$Season[1,1]
  n0 <- 30
  alpha2 <- n0/2
  beta2 <- (alpha2-1)*sigma2.sq
  sigma1.sq <- attr(VarCorr(m), "sc")^2
  alpha1 <- n0/2
  beta1 <- (alpha1-1)*sigma1.sq
### End ###
```

Several TP observations in the New York data were below the method reporting limit (MRL) of 0.01 mg/L. The likelihood function of these "censored" values were evaluated by the cumulative density function.

```
### Stan Model ###
sequp_ch6 <- "
          data{
             int<lower=0> NOBS;
             int<lower=0> ncens;
             real y[NOBS];
             real ycens;
             real alpha1;
             real beta1;
             real alpha2;
             real beta2;
             real mub0;
             real<lower=0> sigmab0;
          }
          parameters{
             real mu;
             real mu0;
             real<lower=0> sigma1sq;
             real<lower=0> sigma2sq;
          }
          transformed parameters{
             real<lower=0> sigma1;
             real<lower=0> sigma2;
             sigma1 = sqrt(sigma1sq);
             sigma2 = sqrt(sigma2sq);
          }
          model{
             sigma1sq ~ inv_gamma(alpha1,beta1);
             sigma2sq ~ inv_gamma(alpha2,beta2);
             mu0 ~ normal(mub0, sigmab0);
             mu ~ normal(mu0, sigma2);
             target += normal_lpdf(y | mu, sigma1);
             target += ncens*normal_lcdf(ycens | mu, sigma1);
          }
          "
### End ###
```

The second part of the example is to use the hierarchical modeling framework to conduct the standard compliance assessment. For the river in New York, we have data from three years (1996 to 1998). The annual assessment would be based on annual data. The U.S. EPA recommended TP nutrient criterion for the eco-region is 0.02413 mg/L [U.S. EPA, 2000]. Using the binomial testing method, we transform the numeric TP concentration values to binary 0 (below the criterion) or 1 (above the criterion) to test whether the probability of observing a success (1) is less than or equal to 0.1. For the three years for which we have data, the resulting p-values were 0.053, 0.013, and 0.028 for 1996, 1997, and 1998, respectively. These results are ambiguous. Using the hierarchical model, we can update the annual mean distribution either using data from all three years or fit the model for each year separately. We will present all the results in the same figure for easy comparison (Figure 6.5). The 33 rivers in the same eco-region were mostly located in Ohio with substantial agricultural activities in their watershed. Consequently, the estimated hyper-distribution mean is higher than nearly all measured concentration values from the New York river. The estimated posterior distribution based on all three years of data is dominated by the river-specific data because of the large sample size. When estimated by year, the influence of the prior distribution is more pronounced, mostly because of the small sample size (e.g., $n = 3$ in 1998). Using the posterior distribution of μ, we can estimate the probability that annual mean TP concentration exceeded the nutrient criterion (they are 0.4185, 0.489, and 0.6925 for years 1996, 1997, and 1998, respectively). All three probabilities are larger than 0.1 (or 0.2, as required by FDEP when setting the surface TP standard for Central Florida Bay), the acceptable exceedance probability [Qian and Miltner, 2018].

The Everglades TP threshold example illustrates the process of aggregating information at individual indicator levels to derive the ecosystem-level TP threshold relevant for the stated objective. This example shows that the aggregated information, likewise, is relevant to individual level inference. For environmental standard compliance assessment, the goal is to estimate the mean concentration of a pollutant based on limited data collected over the assessment period. The traditional statistical estimator of population mean (sample average) is selected because it is unbiased and the least variable among all unbiased estimators. However, the emphasis on the unbiasedness of an estimator often makes us sacrifice overall accuracy. Efron [1975] concluded that some purposefully induced biases in an estimator can often "drastically improve estimation properties." Various shrinkage estimators (including the Bayesian estimator) are such biased estimators. In a Bayesian estimator, the improved estimation properties can only be achieved when we have proper and informative priors. The connection between the James-Stein estimator and Bayesian hierarchical model [Gelman, 2005] suggests that the hyper-distribution of means of exchangeable rivers, in this example, is a proper choice of prior for estimating the means of individual rivers. The hyper-distribution summarizes the distribution of TP means among similar rivers. As long as the rivers used for estimating the hyper-distribution are a representative sample of all similar rivers, we can apply the hyper-distribution as the prior for a future river from the same "population." Mathematically, we define "similar" to mean that the feature we are estimating (i.e., mean TP concentrations) is exchangeable [Lindley and Novick, 1981]. As such, a practical means of defining a proper informative prior would be the distribution of the parameter of interest among exchangeable units.

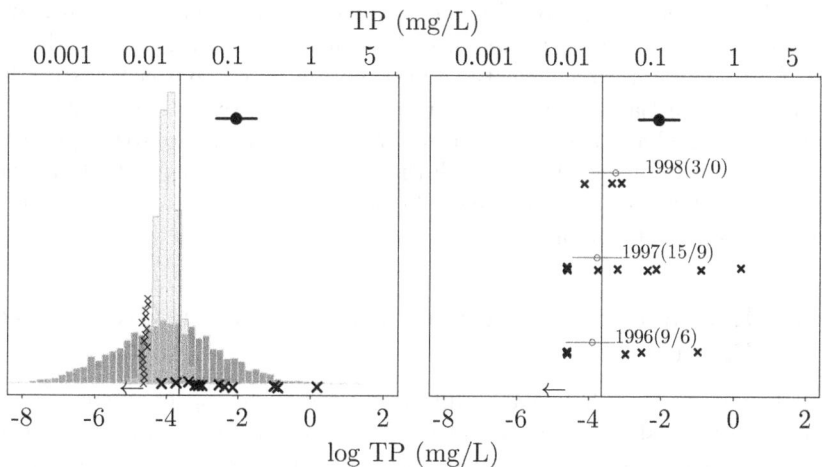

FIGURE 6.5: Posterior (based on all three years data) predictive distributions of site mean (μ, light-shaded histogram) and individual TP values ($\log(TP)$, dark-shaded histogram) in left panel are compared to the prior mean distribution (the dark horizontal line shows the 95% credible interval and the dark filled circle is the mean) derived from similar streams in the same ecoregion in Ohio. The three gray horizontal lines in the right panel show the estimated 95% credible intervals of the posterior predictive distributions of site mean using data from the three years separately (with estimated means shown in open circles and individual data points shown in bold crosses), with sample sizes shown in the parentheses (total/number of censored values). The vertical line is the EPA recommended TP criterion. The bolded crosses at the bottom of the left panel are the observed TP values and the vertically stacked crosses are TP values below MRL (shown at the MRL with slight jitter to avoid complete overlap).

For the current practice of environmental standard compliance assessment, we can improve the accuracy of the assessment by properly grouping rivers and other waters into sub-populations, within which waters (rivers, lakes, wetlands, etc.) to be assessed can be regarded as exchangeable. Using existing data we can derive the hyper-distribution such that future compliance assessment can be conducted using a Bayesian estimator to improve assessment reliability.

Much of the confusion in environmental standard compliance assessment stems from the difference between an ideal standard and a realizable standard [Barnett and O'Hagan, 1997]. An environmental standard, as we discussed, is measured against the mean concentration. In compliance assessment, the underlying mean concentration can only be estimated from data. The uncertainty associated with sampling and estimation complicates the compliance assessment process. Based on the recurring frequency interpretation, Qian [2015] showed that the purpose of the frequency component was to provide a degree of confidence in the compliance assessment process. As long as the degree of confidence is defined clearly, an estimation-based approach is straightforward. Using a Bayesian hierarchical modeling approach can reduce the estimation uncertainty. The Bayesian hierarchical modeling approach provides an informative prior distribution such that even when we have only data from individual waters, we can still take advantage of the shrinkage estimator to improve assessment reliability.

6.4.3   Example 3: Multilevel Modeling with Group-Level Predictors

The concept of exchangeable units is defined with respect to specific parameters of interest. In the Everglades TP threshold example, we assume that the TP thresholds for various ecological indicators are exchangeable. In the environmental standard compliance assessment example, we assume that the annual mean TP concentrations from wadable streams in the same eco-region in Lake Erie watersheds are exchangeable. In both cases, we can interpret the concept of exchangeable units based on whether we have information to determine the relative magnitudes of the parameters of interest among the units. If we do not have such information (and we know that these parameters share certain commonalities), these parameters are exchangeable because the joint likelihood function of these parameters is not affected by the order of these units. Also, because we have no knowledge about their relative magnitude, the rational prior distributions for these parameters should be the same.

In the EUSE example of Qian et al. [2010], the response variable of interest is the measured stream ecological indicator (richness weighted macroinvertebrate tolerance, or RichTOL). If RichTOL is the only variable available, the mean tolerance level for each sampled stream would be exchangeable. In this study, researchers are interested in how watershed urbanization affects stream ecosystems. As a result, each measured RichTOL is accompanied by a co-variate – percent urban land cover in the watershed upstream of the sampling site. The co-variate represents the information we have that makes the watershed mean RichTOL non-exchangeable. When we use a linear model to describe the relationship between RichTOL and percent urban land, we aggregate the watershed-level data (represented by the RichTOL – percent urban land pair) into a regional-level summary. Based on data from 30 watersheds in a region, the linear regression model describes how changes in percent urban land cover would lead to changes in RichTOL using two coefficients, the intercept and the slope. The intercept represents the average RichTOL for watersheds without urban land and the slope represents the rate of change in RichTOL per unit increase in percent urban land. Without additional information to distinguish one region from another, we would treat the intercepts and slopes from different regions as exchangeable. The exchangeable assumption is untenable when we have region-level variables to describe the natural and cultural differences that may also affect stream ecosystems. Because these region-level variables are relatively constant within a region, they are often ignored when a region-specific model is developed. Initially the EUSE data were analyzed region-by-region [Brown et al., 2009, Cuffney et al., 2009]. When data from all nine regions were available, researchers focused on the explanation of the regional differences in how stream ecosystems responded to urbanization. This process was detailed in Qian [2016, Chapter 10] using the classical multilevel modeling. The multilevel modeling is equivalent to the Bayesian hierarchical model with non-informative priors for the hyperparameters. That is,

$$\begin{aligned} y_{ij} &\sim N(\beta_{0j} + \beta_{1j}x_{ij}, \sigma_1^2) \\ \begin{pmatrix} \beta_{0j} \\ \beta_{1j} \end{pmatrix} &\sim N\left[\begin{pmatrix} \mu_{\beta_0} \\ \mu_{\beta_1} \end{pmatrix}, \Sigma \right]. \end{aligned} \tag{6.6}$$

This model is the statistical representation of how information in the data should be properly organized. We took macroinvertebrate samples to represent stream biological conditions, which vary among watersheds in the same region because of variation in watershed urban land covers. The model coefficients (β_{0j}, β_{1j}) are summaries of how stream ecological conditions change as watershed urbanization changes at a regional scale. The region-specific model aggregates watershed-level data to regional models. The regional-level model coefficients (β_{0j}, β_{1j}) in this model are assumed to be exchangeable. They share the same joint prior specified by the cross-region means $(\mu_{\beta_0}, \mu_{\beta_1})$ and the variance-covariance matrix Σ. The priors for $\mu_{\beta_0}, \mu_{\beta_1}$ can be the typical reasonable weakly informative prior for independent coefficients, such as $N(0,5)$. When more information about these regression coefficients is known, we can modify the prior. See the hockey-stick model example in Section 7.2 for an example.

The inverse Wishart distribution is often recommended to be the prior for Σ, largely because it is the conjugate prior for a multivariate normal distribution. Conjugacy, however, does not guarantee a smooth MCMC process. Barnard et al. [2000] proposed a more convenient specification of the covariance matrix that is applicable to modeling regression coefficients in a Bayesian hierarchical modeling setting. The prior covariance matrix is decomposed into a vector of scales (standard deviations) and a correlation matrix. Specifically,

$$\Sigma = \text{diag\_matrix}(\tau) \times \Omega \times \text{diag\_matrix}(\tau) \tag{6.7}$$

where Ω is a correlation matrix and τ is the vector of coefficient scale (standard deviation of β_{0j} and β_{1j}). Mathematically, the link between τ, Ω and Σ decomposition of the covariance matrix can be derived directly from a known Σ as follows:

$$\tau_k = \sqrt{\Sigma_{k,k}} \text{ and } \Omega_{ij} = \Sigma_{ij}/(\tau_i \tau_j).$$

As such, we can specify weakly informative priors for τ and Ω to model the covariance matrix. The Stan User's Manual recommends a half-Cauchy distribution as the prior for τ (e.g., $\tau_k \sim \text{Cauchy}(0, 2.5)$). For the correlation matrix, we can propose a uniform prior on the joint distribution of individual correlation coefficients. With the positive definite constraint of a correlation matrix, the marginal priors for individual correlations are more concentrated around 0. In other words, such a uniform joint prior favors values close to 0 over values close to ± 1. As the dimension of the correlation matrix increases, the marginal priors of correlation coefficients tighten up around 0 [Barnard et al., 2000]. The Stan User's Manual recommends the LKJ prior with shape $\eta > 1$ as the prior for the correlation matrix (e.g., $\Omega \sim \text{LKJCorr}(\eta = 2)$). The LKJ prior in Stan is based on the efficient computation algorithm for generating random correlation matrices by Lewandowski et al. [2009]. The joint LKJ prior is uniform (-1,1) when $\eta = 1$.

Specifically in Stan, we declare Ω as a correlation matrix and τ as a vector. The covariance matrix is reconstructed using the function `quad_form_diag`. The prior in equation (6.6) and the scale-correlation decomposition (equation (6.7)) can be implemented in Stan using the following code snip:

```
### Partial Stan Code ###
...
parameters{
  vector[K] beta[Nreg];
  corr_matrix[K] Omega;
  row_vector[K] mu_b;
  vector[K] tau;
...
}
model{
  tau ~ cauchy(0,2.5);
  Omega ~ lkj_corr(2);
  beta ~ multi_normal(mu_b, quad_form_diag((Omega, tau));
  ...
### End ###
```

Note that we declared the regression coefficient as an array of vectors (`vector[K] beta[Nreg]`) to take advantage of the vectorized multivariate normal specification.

To optimize computation, we can parameterize the correlation matrix Ω directly in terms of its Cholesky factors $\boldsymbol{L}$ (i.e., $\boldsymbol{LL}' = \Omega$) using Stan's Cholesky LKJ correlation distribution. Just like we can draw a random sample from a normal variable with mean μ and standard deviation σ (i.e.,

$y_i \sim N(\mu, \sigma^2))$ through drawing random samples from the standard normal distribution $(z_i \sim N(0,1))$, that is, $y_i = \mu + \sigma \cdot z_i$, we can draw random samples from a multivariate normal vector $\boldsymbol{y} \sim MVN(\boldsymbol{\mu}, \Sigma)$ using random samples of $\boldsymbol{z} \sim N(0,1)$, that is $\boldsymbol{y} = \boldsymbol{\mu} + \boldsymbol{z} \times \sqrt{\Sigma}$). The Cholesky decomposition of the correlation matrix $\Omega = LL'$ is a lower triangle matrix that satisfies the definition of the square root of the correlation matrix. The covariance matrix is then $\Sigma = (\text{diag\_matrix}(\tau) \cdot L)(L \cdot \text{diag\_matrix}(\tau))^T$. As a result, we can specify the "square root" of the covariance matrix as `diag_-pre_multiply(tau,L_Omega)`. The specialized products function `diag_pre_-multiply` takes a row vector (i.e., `tau`) and a matrix (`L_Omega`) as input and returns the product (i.e., $(\text{diag\_matrix}(\tau) \cdot L)$). Stan comes with the Cholesky LKJ correlation distribution `lkj_corr_cholesky(k)`. When we declare a correlation matrix L as `parameters{cholescky_factor_corr[k] L;}`, we mean that $LL' \sim LKJcorr(\eta = k)$, and we can use the Cholesky factorization of the correlation matrix Ω by changing the above code as follows:

```
#### Partial Stan Code ####
parameters {
  matrix[K,Nreg] z;
  cholesky_factor_corr[K] L_Omega;
  row_vector[K] mu_b;
  vector<lower=0>[K] tau;
}
transformed parameters {
  matrix[Nreg,K] beta;
  beta = rep_matrix(mu_b, Nreg) +
            (diag_pre_multiply(tau,L_Omega)*z)';
}
model {
  //prior
  to_vector(z) ~ std_normal();
  L_Omega ~ lkj_corr_cholesky(2);
  // likelihood
...
}
"
```

End

Although the maximum likelihood (ML) implementation (e.g., the R function `lmer` from package `lme4`) of the simple multilevel model is satisfactory for most applications, implementation under Stan is still necessary for more complicated settings, especially for nonlinear regression problems where an efficient self-starter function is not available. The Bayesian implementation of a hierarchical model has two advantages – more accurate estimation of uncertainty parameters (standard deviations and correlations) and the ability to incorporate prior information to resolve non-identifiable issues (e.g., the mixture of two normal distributions example in Chapter 2). However, the Bayesian implementation in Stan requires writing specific code and the running time is usually much longer than the MLE implementation. As such, we often use MLE implementation such as `lmer` and **glmer** in R to explore the appropriate model form and use Stan to execute the most appropriate model. In this section, we use data from Qian [2016, Section 10.4] and Tang et al. [2019] to illustrate the Stan implementation of multilevel models.

The EUSE example in Qian [2016] started with the simple multilevel linear regression model as in equation (6.6). In this model the response is the richness weighted average taxon tolerance (*RichTOL*) and the predictor is percent urban land cover.

The Stan code using the scale-correlation matrix decomposition is shown below:

```
### Stan Code ###
euse_stan1 <- "
data {
  int<lower=0> N;
  int<lower=0> Nreg;
  int<lower=1> K;
  int<lower=1,upper=Nreg> region[N];
  matrix[N,K] x;
  vector[N] y;
}
parameters {
  vector[K] beta[Nreg];
  corr_matrix[K] Omega;
  row_vector[K] mu_b;
  vector<lower=0>[K] tau;
  real<lower=0,upper=10> sigma_y;
}
transformed parameters {
  vector[N] mu_y;
  for (i in 1:N)
    mu_y[i] = x[i] * beta[region[i]];
}
model {
  tau ~ cauchy(0,2.5);
  Omega ~ lkj_corr(2);
  beta ~ multi_normal(mu_b, quad_form_diag(Omega, tau));
  y ~ normal(mu_y, sigma_y);
}
"
### End ###
```

To use the Cholesky LKJ correlation distribution, we modify the above code as follows.

```
#### Partial Stan Code ####
parameters {
  matrix[K,Nreg] z;
  cholesky_factor_corr[K] L_Omega;
  row_vector[K] mu_b;
  vector<lower=0,upper=pi()/2>[K] tau_unif;
}
transformed parameters {
  matrix[Nreg,K] beta;
  vector<lower=0>[K] tau;
  for (k in 1:K) tau[k]=2.5*tan(tau_unif[k]);
  beta = rep_matrix(mu_b, Nreg) +
              (diag_pre_multiply(tau,L_Omega)*z)';
}
model {
  to_vector(z) ~ std_normal();
  L_Omega ~ lkj_corr_cholesky(2);
  y ~ normal(rows_dot_product(beta[region], x), sigma_y);
}
"
### End ###
```

The simple multilevel model resulted in similar estimates from the MLE estimates – regression coefficients (intercept and slope) vary by region. In the next step, regional-level predictors were used to explain the region-to-region variation. The obvious explanations of the variation may be the regional differences in weather/climate. Stream macroinvertebrates are known to prefer cooler and wetter conditions. Therefore, regional annual mean temperature and annual mean precipitation may be important factors explaining why stream ecosystems responded to changes in watershed urbanization differently from region to region. The next explanation for variations in watersheds may be due to different human impacts on streams (other than urbanization) in different parts of the country. Agriculture development also results in increased nutrient and sediment loading to streams. As a result, the impact of urban development in areas without agriculture (i.e., developed from natural land cover) would be more severe than the impact of urbanization in previously agricultural land. The next step was to explore whether various regional-level predictors can be used to explain the differences in regression coefficients (β_0's and β_1's in equation (6.6)). The exploration led to the use of annual mean temperature and antecedent agricultural land cover as two regional-level predictors. The antecedent agriculture land cover is usually unavailable. In the EUSE study, this variable was estimated based on the average current agriculture land cover in watersheds with less than 10% urban land cover. As a result, antecedent agricultural land cover is treated as categorical, either high or low. Knowing the regional differences in annual mean temperature and antecedent agricultural land cover makes the regression coefficients non-exchangeable. Instead, we further summarize the regional differences in model coefficients using another linear model:

$$\begin{pmatrix} \beta_{0j} \\ \beta_{1j} \end{pmatrix} \sim N \left(\begin{pmatrix} a_0 + a_1 Temp_j + a_2 Ag + a_3 Ag_j \times Temp_j \\ b_0 + b_1 Temp_j + b_2 Ag + b_3 Ag_j \times Temp_j \end{pmatrix}, \Sigma \right). \quad (6.8)$$

With this change, the model coefficients are now a_0, a_1, a_2, a_3 and b_0, b_1, b_2, b_3. The regional-level intercept (β_0's) and slope (β_1's) can be coded as transformed parameters in Stan:

```
### Partial Stan Code ###
parameters {
  matrix[K,Nreg] z;
  cholesky_factor_corr[K] L_Omega;
  vector<lower=0,upper=pi()/2>[K] tau_unif;
  matrix[J,K] gamma;
  real<lower=0,upper=10> sigma_y;
}
transformed parameters {
  matrix[Nreg,K] beta;
  vector<lower=0>[K] tau;

  for (k in 1:K)
    tau[k] = 2.5*tan(tau_unif[k]);
    beta = gr*gamma + (diag_pre_multiply(tau,L_Omega)*z)';
}
model {
  to_vector(z) ~ std_normal();
  L_Omega ~ lkj_corr_cholesky(2);
  to_vector(gamma) ~ normal(0,5);
  y ~ normal(rows_dot_product(beta[region], x), sigma_y);
}
"
### End ###
```

Alternatively, we can reexpress the model as:

$$\begin{aligned} \beta_{0j} &= a_0 + a_1 Temp_j + a_2 Ag + a_3 Ag_j \times Temp_j + \epsilon_{1j} \\ \beta_{1j} &= b_0 + b_1 Temp_j + b_2 Ag + b_3 Ag_j \times Temp_j + \epsilon_{2j} \end{aligned}$$

and model the residuals (ϵ_{1j} and ϵ_{2j}) as exchangeable among regions:

$$\begin{pmatrix} \epsilon_{1j} \\ \epsilon_{2j} \end{pmatrix} \sim N \left(\begin{pmatrix} 0 \\ 0 \end{pmatrix}, \Sigma \right)$$

In equation (6.8) we did not consider the interaction between $Temp_j$ and Ag_j because the interaction was shown to be unnecessary in Qian [2016].

The two regional-level variables are examples of non-nested groups: regions are either high or low in antecedent agricultural land cover. Because there are only nine regions (three with high antecedent agricultural land cover), we expect model fitting issues (e.g., slow convergence) as the model included eight group-level coefficients and two variances. As in Qian [2016], we coded `Ag` as numeric (binary 0 or 1). That is, the estimated intercepts (a_0 and b_0) and slopes (a_1 and b_1) are for regions with low antecedent agricultural land cover. This is the default treatment in many statistical software packages. The convergence issue can be avoided by dropping the interaction terms and increasing the option `adapt_delta` from the default of 0.8 to 0.9. The model runs slowly. This may be an example where small regional sample size (we have three regions with high antecedent agricultural land cover) makes the resulting model less reliable.

The model is graphically summarized by plotting the estimated regional intercepts (β_{0j} in equation (6.8) and `be0` in the Stan code) slopes (β_{1j} and `be1`) against the regional annual average temperature (Figure 6.6). In comparison to the same figure in Qian [2010, Figure 10.10], the standard deviations of the Bayesian estimated region-level regression coefficients (especially the intercepts) are higher than the standard deviation from the respective MLE estimates. The standard deviations of the MLE estimated region-level intercepts were nearly 0. The estimated region-level intercepts form two nearly perfect lines. (The `lmer` algorithm for this model did not achieve convergence.) The level of uncertainty in Figure 6.6 are more reasonable.

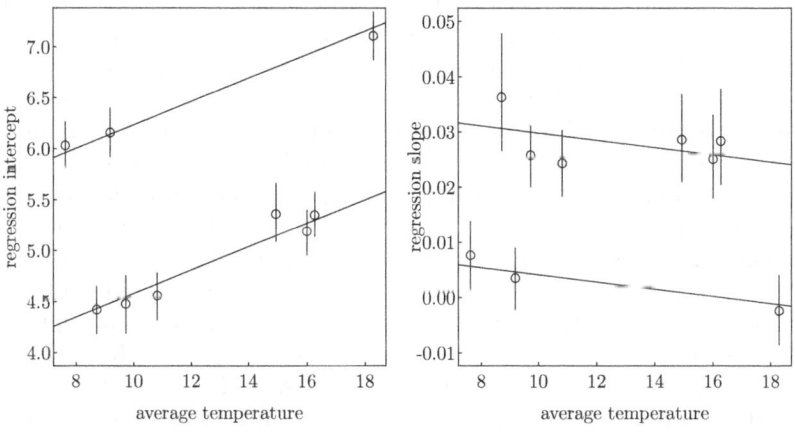

FIGURE 6.6: Regression coefficients from the nine regions as functions of regional annual mean temperature and antecedent agriculture land cover.

The outcome of this model showed that the three regions with high antecedent agricultural land cover all have higher intercepts and lower slopes than the other six regions with low antecedent agricultural land cover. In these models, intercepts represent the average tolerance without urban development, and slopes are the rate of increase in average tolerance per unit increase in watershed urban land cover. For regions with high antecedent agricultural land cover, agricultural activities in the watershed had already lowered water quality (and altered the stream macroinvertebrate community to a higher tolerant community) before urban development (hence a high intercept). In these watersheds, converting agricultural land cover to urban land does not represent as dramatic a change as cutting down forests for housing development (hence a smaller slope). The reduced stream ecosystem response to watershed urbanization in regions with high antecedent agricultural land cover reinforced our recognition that impact of various human activities may not be easily separated. In a subsequent study focused on the impact of climate change on stream ecosystems in the southeastern U.S., we used watershed percent natural land cover as a more general representation of human activities [Qian et al., 2021a].

Tang et al. [2019] present another example of how multilevel modeling improved our understanding of the roles of variables operating over different spatial scales. The underlying statistical model presented by Tang et al. [2019] is nearly identical to the EUSE example, except that this is an example of nested groups. This study further illustrates the common theme in many ecological studies where the roles of predictor variables operating over different spatial and temporal scales should be analyzed according to the proper hierarchical structure of the data. Tang et al. [2019] explored the role of soil iron level on phosphorus sedimentation and phosphorus bio-availability in lakes and reservoirs. They hypothesized that (1) nutrient concentration changes in response to changes in precipitation may differ between natural lakes and reservoirs because of their differences in the strength of summer stratification and in hydraulics, and (2) bio-availability of phosphorus in lakes and reservoirs may be affected by regional-level soil iron content. They collected summer monitoring data from 77 lakes and 112 reservoirs distributed throughout eastern China, ranging from tropical southern China to temperate northern and northeastern China. Natural lakes in China are typically shallow (lakes included in the study have an average depth less than six meters), while reservoirs are mostly deeper typically with strong thermal stratification. Shallow lakes tend to have weak thermal stratification, which may be mixed during heavy precipitation events, thereby, increase the release of particulate phosphorus from the sediment. Strong thermal stratification typically present in deep reservoirs prevents diffusion of phosphorus from hypolimnion. Furthermore, reservoirs can discharge water through outlets at depths reaching the phosphorus-enriched hypolimnion. As a result, Tang et al. [2019] hypothesized that the phosphorus concentration-precipitation relationship in natural lakes and in reservoirs are likely different. In addition, iron oxides derived from catchment soil directly influence phosphorus sedimentation (hence changing the TP-precipitation relationship) and bio-availability (changing the Chla-TP relationship). A natural north-to-south gradient in soil iron content in east China creates an ideal case study. Tang et al. [2019] divided the study area into seven regions along large river basins. As these rivers (and almost all rivers in China) flow generally from west to east, these seven regions represent slices (from west to east) of the north-to-south soil iron gradient. Reservoirs were represented in all seven regions and lakes were represented in five of the seven regions. Observations from lakes/reservoirs within the same region are considered replicates (i.e., no lake/reservoir-specific models). That is, data from the 189 lakes and reservoirs are grouped into seven groups: natural lakes were represented in five of the seven groups and reservoirs were represented in seven. Within each group, we further divide the data into categories of lake versus reservoir. We can use the same multilevel model as in the EUSE example, except that the lake-reservoir categories are specified at the lake (or observational) level. Specifically, the nesting is expressed as

$$\begin{aligned} \beta_{0ij} &= a_0 + a_1 Fe_j + R_i(\delta_{a0} + \delta_{a1} Fe_j) + \epsilon_{1j} \\ \beta_{1ij} &= b_0 + b_1 Fe_j + R_i(\delta_{b0} + \delta_{b1} Fe_j) + \epsilon_{2j} \end{aligned}$$

where Fe_j is the region-level average soil iron content and R_i is a binary variable indicating whether the ith observation is from a lake ($R_i = 0$) or a reservoir ($R_i = 1$). The model error terms (ϵ_{1j} and ϵ_{2j}) are exchangeable among regions:

$$\begin{pmatrix} \epsilon_{1j} \\ \epsilon_{2j} \end{pmatrix} \sim N \left(\begin{pmatrix} 0 \\ 0 \end{pmatrix}, \Sigma \right).$$

As before, we use a relatively non-informative LKJ-prior to model the covariance matrix Σ (through Cholesky decomposition):

Partial Stan Code

```
...
parameters {
  matrix[2,Nreg] z;
  cholesky_factor_corr[2] L_Omega;
  vector<lower=0,upper=pi()/2>[2] tau_unif;
  real a[4];
  real b[4];
  real<lower=0,upper=10> sigma_y;
}
transformed parameters {
  vector[N] mu_y;

  ...

  matrix[Nreg,2] beta;
  vector<lower=0>[2] tau;

  for (k in 1:2)
```

```
      tau[k] = 2.5*tan(tau_unif[k]);
    beta = (diag_pre_multiply(tau,L_Omega)*z)';
...
    for (i in 1:N)
      mu_y[i] = (beta[region[i],1]+be0[region[i]]+
                 typ[i]*be0Ag[region[i]]) +
                 (beta[region[i],2]+be1[region[i]]+
                 typ[i]*be1Ag[region[i]])*x[i];
}
model {
  to_vector(z) ~ std_normal();
  L_Omega ~ lkj_corr_cholesky(2);
  y ~ normal(mu_y, sigma_y);
}
"
```

End

Tang et al. [2019] implemented a similar model in R without modeling lake type as nested under regions, similar to equations (6.6) and (6.8). They assumed the effects of lake type and regional soil iron content on regression intercepts and slopes are additive (lake- and reservoir-specific intercept/slopes share the same slope on region-level soil iron content) for the TP-precipitation model, while allowing an interaction effect on both the intercept and slope between region-level soil iron content and lake type for the Chla-TP model. As a comparison, we fit our model (with interaction and accounting for the nested data structure) to the Chla-TP data (Figure 6.7). The estimated region-level model for the intercept and slope are somewhat different from the ones presented in Tang et al. [2019], although the main conclusions are the same.

Gelman and Hill [2007] recommended a workflow for modeling data with multilevel structures. The workflow starts with fitting classical regressions using the lm() and glm() functions in R to understand the basic relationship in the data. Once a proper model form is selected, we increase the complexity of the model by allowing intercepts and slopes to vary by using R functions lmer() or glmer(). We can start with using non-nested groupings when appropriate. Once a final model is determined, we fit fully Bayesian multilevel models using Stan to obtain simulations representing inferential uncertainty about all the parameters in a model. The MCMC samples can be used to summarize uncertainty about coefficients, predictions, and other quantities of interest. We follow this workflow in this section and in Section 6.4.4. Although the multilevel models in Section 6.4.4 were used in the project, only the fully Bayesian models were presented in the cited references for uncertainty inference. The models in the EUSE example in this section had convergence issues when using lmer(), largely because of the small number of groups and strongly correlated regression coefficients. Many convergence issues are related to difficulties in inverting the correlation matrix (e.g., in a linear regression problem, $(\boldsymbol{X}\boldsymbol{X}^T)^{-1}$. An appropriately selected prior can often be seen as adding

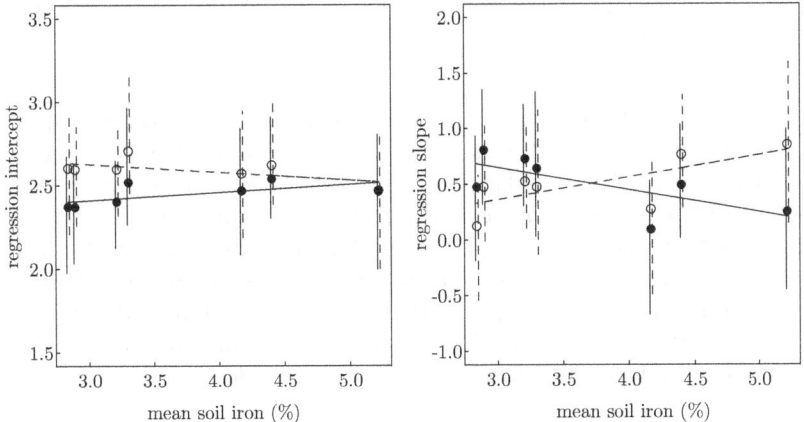

FIGURE 6.7: Regression coefficients for lakes and reservoirs from seven regions in eastern China are shown as functions of average regional annual soil iron content and lake type (lake – solid lines or reservoir – dashed lines).

additional data points to the regression design matrix, which might make the inversion possible. As a result, the full Bayesian model with weakly informative priors should be used when fitting a multilevel model for which fitting with `lmer()` returns a convergence warning. In some cases, the convergence problem is because of the strongly correlated model coefficients as in the example in Section 6.4.4.1. As such, centering the predictor can be an effective strategy. Centering the predictor can also improve the Stan model's performance. The nested-group example of Tang et al. [2019] further illustrates the benefit of this workflow. The `lmer()`-based analysis provided an exploratory tool that led to the appropriate model structure. In this example, the conceptual understanding of the varying slopes enhances our understanding in the role of regional environmental differences in how lakes and reservoirs respond to increased nutrient input. In addition, the study highlighted the different patterns of responses between natural lakes and reservoirs.

6.4.4 Example 4: Multilevel Modeling for Evaluating Fisheries Sampling Methods

Fishery-independent sampling methods are widely used to obtain data for estimating fish abundance. Because fisheries sampling methods are always imperfect, fishery independent estimates, often recorded as catch-per-unit-effort (CPUE), are taken as proportional to true abundance. This assumption implies that a fraction of the population captured (catchability) is constant with increasing abundance. Unfortunately, this proportionality assumption is rarely met. To describe the concept of catchability, Harley et al. [2001] used a power function to quantify the change in catchability for a sampling method:

$$U_i = q N_i^\beta e^{\epsilon_i}$$

where U_i is CPUE and N_i is the unknown abundance in time or space (i), q is the catchability coefficient, and e^{ϵ_i} is a multiplicative error term. The proportion of fish in a population at a given location or time that a sampling method (or gear) can capture is the method's catchability (U_i/N_i). Under proportionality (i.e., $\beta = 1$), the proportion is q. It is a constant with respect to N_i. If $\beta < 1$, the proportion decreases as the abundance increases (hyperstable). If $\beta > 1$, the proportion increases as the abundance increases (hyperdepletion). The catchability equation can be linearized to meet normal regression assumptions by taking the log of both sides:

$$\log(U_i) = \log(q) + \beta \log(N_i) + \epsilon_i \tag{6.9}$$

where ϵ_i represents normally distributed estimation error.

While equation (6.9) is a general approach for characterizing a sampling method or gear, different species of fish may have different susceptibility to a type of gear and a type of gear may perform differently when environmental conditions change. As such, a sampling method's catchability may vary by species and locations. How to combine data collected from a large space over a long time is of interest. In this section we use two examples from studies of Lake Erie walleye to show how regional differences in Lake Erie affect how we interpret standard monitoring data, which may have important implications in regional fisheries management.

6.4.4.1   Regional Differences in Gill-net Catchability

Lake Erie walleye is an internationally important species in the Laurentian Great Lakes region. These fish support valuable commercial and recreational fisheries. As a result, management jurisdictions (the states of Michigan, Ohio, Pennsylvania, and New York in the U.S., and the Canadian province of Ontario) invest a lot of resources in monitoring the population and fisheries. The Ohio Department of Natural Resources - Division of Wildlife (ODNR-DOW) conducts one of the fishery independent surveys, which consists of 53 gill-net sets across the Ohio waters of Lake Erie during the fall. Information from this survey is used in statistical catch-at-age (SCAA) models to annually estimate total abundance, assess the impact of harvest related mortality, and set sustainable levels of total allowable catch (TAC).

The ODNR-DOW gill-net survey is standardized, meaning the survey time (fall) and sample locations (53) are fixed. The survey is conducted the same way each year, and ideally the strict sampling protocols lead to a proportional relationship between the survey catch-per-unit-effort (CPUE) and population abundance (N). As with all fisheries sampling methods, gillnetting is imperfect, in that it has an unknown probability of false negative. For some sampling methods, the false negative probability is nearly impossible to quantify. Furthermore, we know that the false negative probability varies by species and by local environmental conditions. In fisheries literature, the imperfection is commonly represented by the catchability. Although not explicitly stated, the standardized sampling protocol is intended to ensure a relatively constant catchability, such that the resulting CPUE can be directly compared and used to infer fish population trend.

The proportionality assumption (i.e., constant catchability/efficiency) is not likely met across the ODNR-DOW gill-net survey, due to regional differences in environmental conditions and fish distributions across the survey. For example, in general, the lake environment in Lake Erie changes from west to east and onshore to offshore with respect to depth, turbidity, temperature, and trophic state. During the fall (survey time) fish are actively migrating from eastern foraging habitats back toward western spawning habitats. However, within the fall survey window, the fish population's distribution may vary from year to year, depending on year-specific environmental conditions causing the nucleus of the population to encounter the survey in different regions. If the survey catchability changes from west to east, a similar abundance of fish could produce different CPUE indices, which could, in turn, affect the harvest management process.

To explore the impact of varying catchability and fish migratory patterns, DuFour et al. [2019] collected paired gill-net and hydroacoustic data at 52 locations from Lake Erie during 2012 and 2013 in the western portion of the survey area. The gill-net data included a count of walleye captured during overnight sets, representing CPUE data (catch/set). The hydroacoustic data included counts of walleye-sized targets in the acoustically sampled water volume (i.e., density) which were then expanded to abundance in a fixed area encompassing all gill-net samples. These data approximated the true walleye abundance at each sample location. Each sample was collected from one of three regions, whose characteristics potentially influenced catchability from west to east, as the lake transitions from shallow, warm, and turbid to deeper, cooler, and more clear water conditions.

Based on all of the information above, DuFour et al. [2019] fit a hierarchical model, sharing information among region-level parameters (equation (6.10)).

$$
\begin{aligned}
\log(U_{ij}) &= \log(q_j) + \beta_j \log(N_{ij}) + \epsilon_{ij} \\
\begin{pmatrix} \log(q_j) \\ \beta_j \end{pmatrix} &\sim MVN \left[\begin{pmatrix} \mu_q \\ \mu_\beta \end{pmatrix}, \Sigma \right]
\end{aligned} \tag{6.10}
$$

In R, equation (6.10) can be fit using the function `lmer`:

```
### R Code ###
GNq.lmer <- lmer(y~x+(1+x|region))
```

In the R code, y and x are log transformed gill-net walleye catch and hydroacoustic estimated walleye density in the vicinity of the gill net, respectively.

Because there were a few 0 acoustic detections in the data, we added the minimum acoustic estimated nonzero density (137) to all values to make the log transformation possible. The regression intercept represents the log of CPUE when the density is 1, far away from the observed data. As a result, the estimation uncertainty in the estimated intercept is large. In this case, the `lmer` model did not converge.

```
### R Output ###
> summary(GNq.lmer)
Linear mixed model fit by REML ['lmerMod']
Formula: y ~ x + (1 + x | region)
   Data: data

REML criterion at convergence: 117.4

Scaled residuals:
     Min       1Q   Median       3Q      Max
-2.48990 -0.55789  0.06998  0.61852  1.97376

Random effects:
 Groups    Name        Variance Std.Dev. Corr
 region    (Intercept) 6.3988   2.5296
           hydroN      0.1026   0.3204   -1.00
 Residual              0.4806   0.6933
Number of obs: 52, groups:  region, 3

Fixed effects:
            Estimate Std. Error t value
(Intercept)   1.6268     1.7194   0.946
x             0.4092     0.2191   1.867

Correlation of Fixed Effects:
     (Intr)
x    -0.995
optimizer (nloptwrap) convergence code: 0 (OK)
Model failed to converge with max|grad| = 0.00348979
   (tol = 0.002, component 1)
### End ###
```

The strong correlation between the intercept and slope is often the reason for computational difficulties. In a regression problem, centering the predictor does not change the model; rather, positions the intercept to the mean of the predictor variable data reducing correlation between the intercept and the slope to 0. In a multilevel/hierarchical model, centering the predictor will reduce the correlation, but usually not to 0. Centering the predictor in this problem avoided the non-convergence issue.

```
> summary(GNq.lmerC)
Linear mixed model fit by REML ['lmerMod']
Formula: y ~ x.cen + (1 + x.cen | region)

REML criterion at convergence: 117.4

Scaled residuals:
      Min        1Q    Median        3Q       Max
-2.48863  -0.55819   0.06962   0.61857   1.97537

Random effects:
 Groups    Name        Variance Std.Dev. Corr
 region    (Intercept) 0.05762  0.2400
           x.cen       0.10373  0.3221   -0.40
 Residual              0.48042  0.6931
Number of obs: 52, groups:  region, 3

Fixed effects:
            Estimate Std. Error t value
(Intercept)   4.7241     0.1775  26.621
x.cen         0.4089     0.2200   1.859

Correlation of Fixed Effects:
      (Intr)
x.cen -0.297
### End ###
```

The estimated region-specific model coefficients are

```
### R Output ###
> coef(GNq.lmerC)
$region
   (Intercept)      x.cen
1     4.569587 0.7089376
2     4.931516 0.3321168
3     4.671112 0.1855892
```

Because the predictor is centered at the overall mean, the regional specific $\log(q)$ in equation (6.10) is the difference between the reported intercept and the product of the reported slope and the mean (7.5681):

```
### R Output ###
> coef(GNq.lmerC)[[1]][,1]-mean(hydroN)*coef(GNq.lmerC)[[1]][,2]
[1] -0.7957549  2.4180080  3.2665461
```

When pooling data from the three regions into a single regression, the estimated log-log linear regression model intercept and slope are 0.1155 and 0.6058, respectively, masking the region-specific variability.

DuFour et al. [2019] conducted a series of simulations to illustrate how ignoring the regional differences may lead to a substantial underestimation of walleye population. This example emphasizes the importance of properly combining data from different sources based on our knowledge. When using the hierarchical modeling approach, we can properly organize the model to represent what we know and what we don't know.

Here, we used the maximum likelihood estimator (MLE) implemented in the R function `lmer`. In many simple problems, the speed of classical MLEs makes them ideal for model exploration. The same hierarchical model can be implemented using Stan. As we discussed in Section 6.4.3, once a model form is decided, we implement the model in Stan:

```
GNq_cor_cent <- "
data {
  int<lower=0> N;              // num individuals
  int<lower=1> L1;             // num ind predictors (level 1)
  int<lower=1> J;              // num groups
  int<lower=1> L2;
                    // num group level predictors (level 2)
  int<lower=1,upper=J> jj[N];// group for individual
  matrix[N,L1] x;             // individual predictors (level 1)
  vector[N] y;                // outcomes
  matrix[J,L2] u;             // group level predictors (level 2)
  }

parameters {
  matrix[J,L1] z_B;
  corr_matrix[L1] Omega;      // prior correlation
  vector<lower=0>[L1] tau;    // prior scale
  matrix[L2,L1] mu_B;         // group coefs
  real<lower=0> sigma;        // prediction error scale

  }

transformed parameters {
  matrix[J,L1] B;
  vector[N] log_mu;
  vector[J] log_q;
  vector[J] beta;

  B = u * mu_B + (z_B * quad_form_diag(Omega, tau));

  log_mu = rows_dot_product(B[jj] , x);

  log_q = B[,1];   // rename intercept parameter
  beta = B[,2];    // rename slope parameter
```

```
    }

model {
    to_vector(z_B) ~ std_normal();
    tau ~ cauchy(0, 5);
    Omega ~ lkj_corr(2);
    to_vector(mu_B) ~ normal(0, 10);

    y ~ normal(log_mu, sigma);

    }"
### End ###
```

We used the same method discussed in Section 6.4.3 to decompose the covariance matrix into a vector of standard deviations and a correlation matrix using the quad-form decomposition function in Stan. Again, we define the regression coefficients as transformed parameters in Stan to improve the sampling efficiency by avoiding sampling over Neal's funnel [Neal, 2003]. See discussions of Cholesky decomposition of the correlation matrix implemented in the code on page 253.

The model showed regional differences in model coefficients (Figure 6.8). The seemingly slight differences lead to different characterization of the three regions in terms of catchability (Figure 6.9).

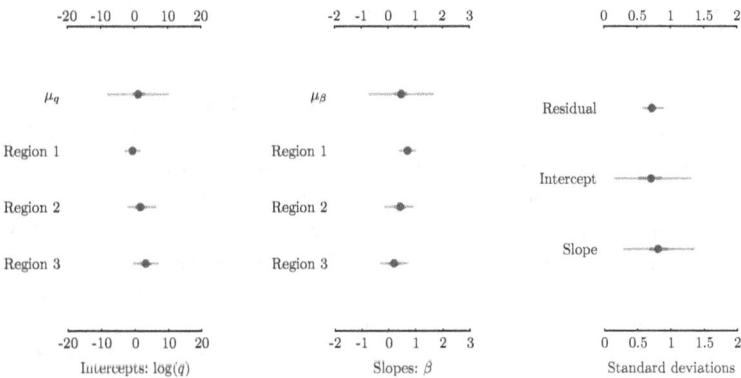

FIGURE 6.8: Estimated catchability model (equation (6.9)) coefficients vary by regions. The left column shows the estimated regional intercepts and the hyper-intercept (μ_q in equation (6.10)), the middle column shows the estimated region slopes and the hyper-slope (μ_β), and the right column shows the estimated residual standard deviation and the among-region standard deviations of the model intercept and slope.

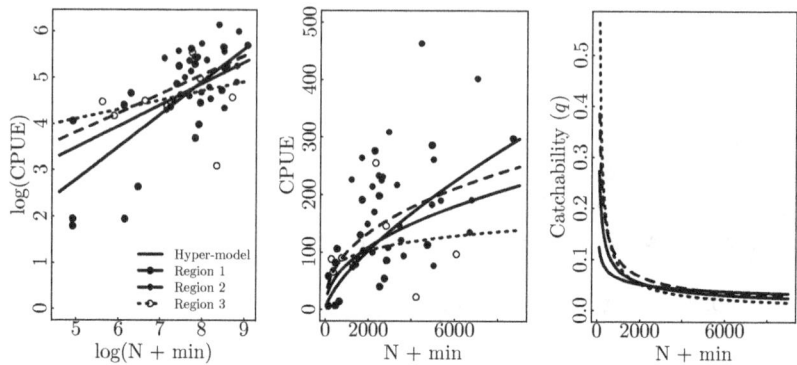

FIGURE 6.9: Walleye catchability characterization varies by region.

During the model evaluation process, we recommend fitting the final model in Stan to generate the most accurate uncertainty and parameter estimates and facilitate post-processing and visualization of results. The final model described here was identified though the iterative model formulation, estimation, and evaluation process which we've summarized in Chapter 8.

6.4.4.2   Species-length relationships

While the catchability example showed the importance of properly combining data based on the underlying hierarchical structure, our next example illustrates how the hierarchical modeling approach also allows us to explore potential causes of regional differences. DuFour et al. [2021] used data from the 2014 ODNR-DOW fishery independent gill-net survey described above. This included counts of fish by species and total length measurements (mm) for each individual fish. Gill-net samples were collected from a fraction of the sample grids within the survey area, while environmental data were collected from all grids during the hydroacoustic portion of the survey.

In Section 2.3.5, we used a logistic regression model to predict whether a gill-net caught fish was a walleye based on its length. DuFour et al. [2021] showed that the logistic regression coefficients varied with changes in environmental conditions, especially water clarity measured as turbidity. Here, using data from the coupled gill-net and hydroacoustic survey grids, we fit a logistic regression and used the grid average turbidity as a group-level predictor [Qian, 2016, Chapter 10]. We can fit this model using `glmer` by including the individual (centered total length) and region level (turbidity) predictors as well as thier interaction.

```
data$Grid <- as.numeric(ordered(data$Grid))
data$Turb <- data_g$turb[data$Grid]
wly.glmer <- glmer(walleye ~ len.c+Turb+Turb:len.c+
```

```
(1+len.c|Grid),
    data=data, family="binomial")
```
End

The estimated coefficients show that both the intercept and slope are positively correlated to turbidity (Figure 6.10). The intercept in this model is the logit of the probability an average sized fish is a walleye and the slope is the rate of increase in the probability that a fish is a walleye when its size increases. That is, as turbidity increases (visibility decreases) the proportion of walleye at a given size increases, and the odds of a fish being a walleye increases more rapidly with the length in more turbid water.

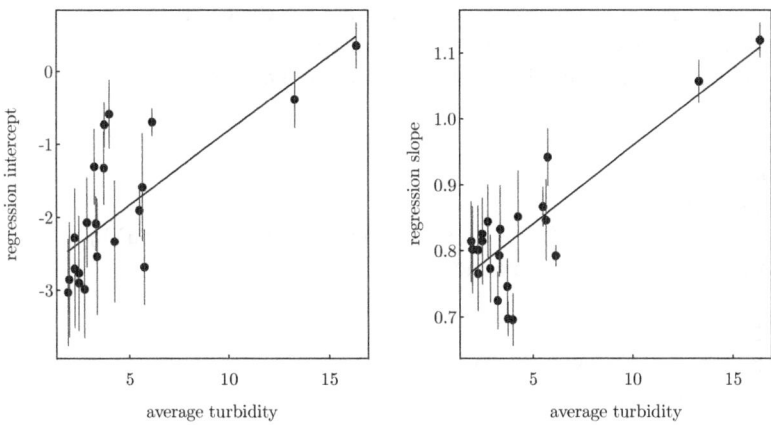

FIGURE 6.10: The walleye apportionment model coefficients are positively related to turbidity of the water.

This model allows correlation among the grid-level α_j and β_j parameters while sharing information through the global intercept ($\delta 1$, $\gamma 1$) and slope ($\delta 2$, $\gamma 2$) parameters from the second level regressions (equation (6.11)).

$$
\begin{aligned}
y_{ij} &\sim Bernoulli(p_{ij}) \\
\text{logit}(p_{ij}) &= \alpha_j + \beta_j len.c_{ij} \\
\alpha_j &= \delta_1 + \delta_2 Turb_j \\
\beta_j &= \gamma_1 + \gamma_2 Turb_j \\
\begin{pmatrix} \alpha_j \\ \beta_j \end{pmatrix} &\sim MVN \left[\begin{pmatrix} \delta_1 + \delta_2 Turb_j \\ \gamma_1 + \gamma_2 Turb_j \end{pmatrix}, \Sigma \right]
\end{aligned}
\tag{6.11}
$$

Following the hierarchical structure described above, we fit the logistic regression model in Stan:

```
### Stan Model ###
walleye_id <- "
data {
    int<lower=0> N;              // num individuals
    int<lower=1> L1;             // num ind predictors (level 1)
    int<lower=1> J;              // num groups
    int<lower=1> L2;             // num group predictors (level 2)
    int<lower=1,upper=J> jj[N]; // group for individual
    matrix[N,L1] x;             // individual predictors (level 1)
    int<lower=0, upper=1> y[N]; // outcomes
    matrix[J,L2] u;             // group predictors (level 2)
}
parameters {
    matrix[J,L1] z_B;           // centered parameters
    corr_matrix[L1] Omega;      // prior correlation
    vector<lower=0>[L1] tau;    // prior scale
    matrix[L1,L2] mu_B;         // group coeffs
}
transformed parameters {
    matrix[J, L1] B;
    vector[N] theta;
    B = u * mu_B + (z_B * quad_form_diag(Omega, tau));
    theta = rows_dot_product(B[jj] , x);
}
model {
    to_vector(z_B) ~ std_normal();
    tau ~ cauchy(0, 2);
    Omega ~ lkj_corr(2);
    to_vector(mu_B) ~ normal(0, 5);

    y ~ bernoulli_logit(theta);
}"
### End ###
```

This model differed from the gill-net catchability model in three specific ways: (1) the data are binary and read in as integers; (2) rather than including dummy variables in the group-level predictors (u) we included the grid-specific turbidity estimates; and (3) the likelihood statement (y~Bernoulli_logit(theta)) which provides a logit link for the logistic regression and includes a single model parameter, theta. This model demonstrated the turbidity relationships vary across the survey area with the strongest influence generally in Region 1 and weaker influence moving east to Regions 2 and 3. The change in species-size relationships becomes evident when plotting the grid-specific logistic curves by region, and shading the curves by their turbidity values (Figures 6.11 and 6.12).

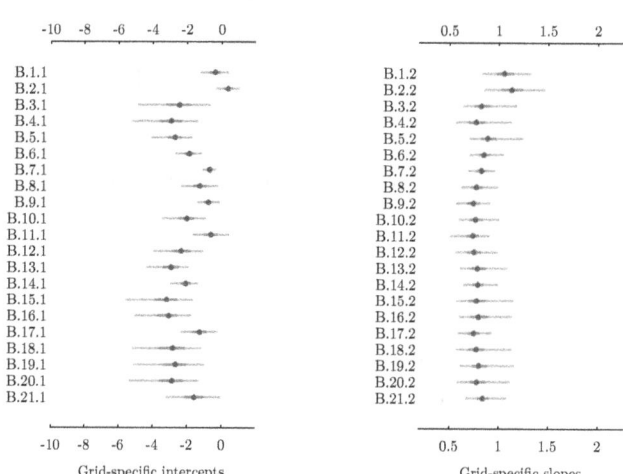

FIGURE 6.11: Species-length model coefficients (α_j and β_j) vary by grid with turbidity.

In effect, the logistic curves shifted right and flattened as turbidity decreased within the survey area, moving west to east and onshore to offshore. One explanation for this pattern was the associated change in species composition. In the west, high-turbidity waters were dominated by smaller sized walleye, where the probability of being a walleye increased rapidly at small sizes. Further east and offshore, small walleye were replaced by similarly sized white bass and the proportion of other larger bodied fishes increased, where the probability of being a walleye increased more gradually at larger sizes.

6.4.5 Censored Data and Imperfect Detection

A common problem in environmental data analysis is the data censoring issue. The most common censoring is a measured concentration value below the method detection limit (MDL, also known as the method reporting limit). When a value is detected as below its MDL, we know that the actual concentration value is below MDL and otherwise uncertain. Historically, a censored value was often replaced by a fixed number (e.g., 0, 0.5MDL, or MDL) before analysis. Gleit [1985] introduced several methods for properly analyzing data with censored values to environmental scientists. These methods rely on various iterative procedures to "estimate" the censored values. They are only

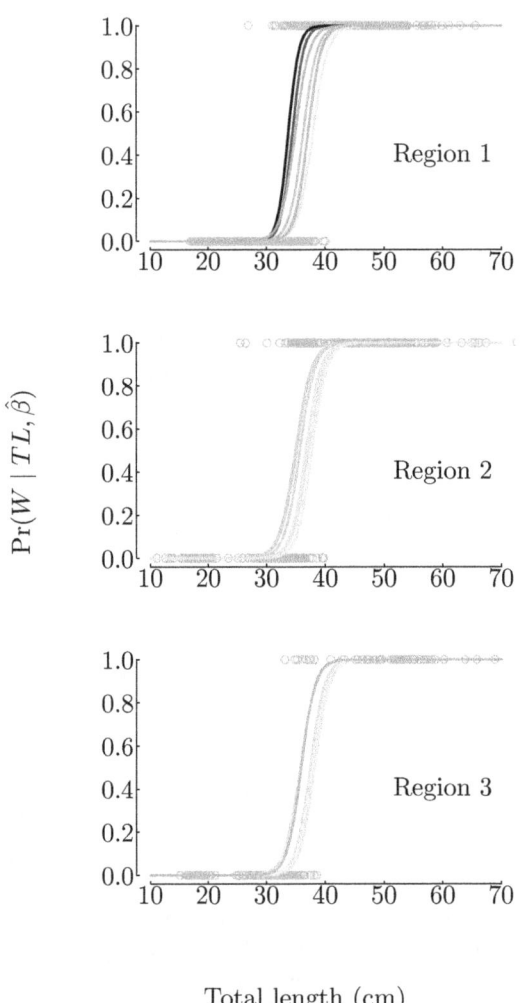

Total length (cm)

FIGURE 6.12: Probability of a fish being a walleye changes with size, and varies by grid with turbidity (Darker lines indicate higher turbidity). Grid specific estimates are grouped into three west to east regions highlighting a shift in species-length relationship across the survey area.

viable when the number of censored values is relatively low, compared to the sample size. In classical statistics, a censored response variable value can be used in a maximum likelihood estimator as a data point with a likelihood specified by the cumulative density function (CDF) [Little and Rubin, 2019], instead of the probability density function (PDF) of an uncensored value. The apparent problem of a likelihood function of a mixture of CDF's and PDF's is computational. With MCMC, computation is no longer a challenge (as we saw earlier in this chapter in the Stan code on page 247). We use data from Qian et al. [2004b] and Wu et al. [2011] as examples of censored response variable data. Both examples are related to environmental management, specifically, for ensuring drinking water safety.

6.4.5.1 Example 5: Drinking Water Safety Review in the US

In the U.S., public drinking water safety is regulated by the Safe Drinking Water Act (SDWA), enacted in 1974 and amended in 1986 and 1996. The law requires many actions to protect drinking water and its sources – rivers, lakes, reservoirs, springs, and ground water wells. It authorizes the United States Environmental Protection Agency (EPA) to set national health-based standards for drinking water to protect against both naturally occurring and man-made contaminants that may be found in drinking water. These health-based standards are mostly in the form of maximum contaminant levels (MCLs) for particular contaminants in drinking water. These standards also include requirements for water systems to test for contaminants in the water to make sure standards are achieved. EPA, states, and water systems then work together to make sure that these standards are met. Specifically, the 1996 amendment requires that EPA review "no less often than every six years," each national primary drinking water regulation. The primary goal of the Six-Year Review (SYR) process is to identify national primary drinking water regulations for possible regulatory revision. Part of the six-year review process is to evaluate contaminant occurrence, specifically to estimate the number of public water systems in which contaminants occur at levels between the existing MCL and a new potential MCL, or other threshold value. These threshold levels are based on health effects or analytic methods information. In addition, the review will also evaluate the number of people potentially exposed to these levels of interest. This occurrence and exposure information indicate how changing an MCL or required treatment technique may affect health risks of water consumers and impact compliance costs for public water systems. For example, if EPA were to lower an MCL for a particular contaminant, the occurrence analysis can estimate the additional number of water systems that will have to incur costs to treat or otherwise reduce the level of the contaminant in drinking water. Determining the number of people currently exposed to these levels of contaminant occurrence can help determine if a meaningful opportunity exists for health risk reduction by modifying a drinking water regulation. This is an example of how statistical aggregation of system-level information supports national-level management decision-making processes.

Data for SYR were obtained from voluntary submission of historical drinking water system monitoring data for a specified period of time in response to EPA's "Information Collection Request (ICR)." During the first SYR, data from 16 states were used as a representative sample of the potential of pollution from manufacturing and agriculture in each state. Drinking water systems were divided into 10 categories based on two source water types (groundwater versus surface water) and five population-served sizes (<500, 501–3300, 3301–10000, 10001–50000, and >50001). The model uses system-level observations to estimate system means, which are then aggregated into category means using a hierarchical model:

$$
\begin{aligned}
y_{ijk} &\sim N(\theta_{jk}, \sigma_y^2) \\
\theta_{jk} &\sim N(\gamma_k, \sigma_{1k}^2) \\
\gamma_k &\sim N(\mu, \sigma_2^2)
\end{aligned}
\tag{6.12}
$$

where the subscript ijk represents the ith observation from system j in category k. The distribution of θ_{jk} (i.e., $N(\gamma_k, \sigma_{1k}^2)$) is the distribution of system means in category k, which is the basis for evaluating the cost and benefit of revising an MCL. When an MCL is revised, the system mean distribution is used to estimate the expected number of affected drinking water systems in each of the 10 source water type-population-served categories. These categories can also provide estimates of population affected by the change.

Implementing this model in Stan is straightforward when using the incremental log density (target +=) to specify the log-likelihood function, separately for censored and non-censored observations:

```
### Stan Code ###
occ_stan1 <- "
data {
  int<lower=0> N;
  int<lower=0> Ncens;
  int<lower=0> Ngrp;
  int<lower=0> Nsys;
  int<lower=1,upper=Nsys> sid[N];
  int<lower=1,upper=Nsys> sidcens[Ncens];
  int<lower=1,upper=Ngrp> sys_grp[Nsys];
  vector[N] y;
  vector[Ncens] ycens;
}
parameters {
  vector[Nsys] theta;
  vector[Ngrp] gamma;
  real mu;
  real<lower=0,upper=10> sigma_1[Ngrp];
  real<lower=0,upper=10> sigma_2;
  real<lower=0,upper=10> sigma_y;
}
model {
  mu ~ normal(0, 10);
  gamma ~ normal(mu, sigma_2);
  for (j in 1:Nsys)
```

```
   theta[j] ~ normal(gamma[sys_grp[j]], sigma_1[sys_grp[j]]);
 for (i in 1:N)
   target += normal_lpdf(y[i] | theta[sid[i]], sigma_y);
 for (i in 1:Ncens)
   target += normal_lcdf(ycens[i] | theta[sidcens[i]],
                                     sigma_y);
}
"
```

End

In our GitHub repository, we use the relationship between a normal distribution ($N(\mu, \sigma^2)$) and the standard normal distribution to reparameterize the system and strata means as derived parameters as we first did in the Gulf of Mexico example (Section 4.2.2, in the code on page 105) to speed up the sampling process. Data from the second and third SYRs are available from EPA's web page. We downloaded the atrazine data from the third SYR for this example. The Bayesian hierarchical model was used only in the first SYR. During the second and third SYR, EPA used a simplified analysis by directly calculating averages for all systems after replacing censored values by 0, 0.5MDL, and MDL to represent the range of system means exceeding selected thresholds (the replacement method). The first SYR was based on data from a 16-state cross-section. EPA deemed that as less representative of the county, thereby a modeling approach was necessary. With the second and third SYRs, the ICR data set came from 45 and 46 of the 50 states, and EPA considered the data to be reasonably complete and nationally representative as the basis of the contaminant occurrence estimates. As a result, a multilevel/hierarchical modeling approach was considered as not essential. This argument is largely due to the widespread confusion on the difference between fixed effects and random effects. Gelman and Hill [2007, Section 11.4] outlined why the hierarchical modeling approach is always preferred. For the drinking water assessment data, the difference between the Bayesian hierarchical model and the maximum likelihood estimator (system means) lies in the treatment of the between-system variance. When estimating system means using MLE, we estimate the system means conditional on the among-system variance (in this problem, σ_{1k}^2 and σ_2^2) being infinity, whereas the Bayesian hierarchical model estimated system means are conditional on σ_{1k}^2 and σ_2^2 estimated from the data. Because the among-system variances cannot be infinity, the hierarchical model estimated variances are more realistic and the shrinkage effect on the estimated system means improves the overall estimation accuracy, we recommend that the hierarchical model always be used in analyzing SYR data, as did Gelman and Hill [2007], who recommended to "always use multilevel modeling." Furthermore, drinking water quality data have large proportions of censored values and the replacement method for the censored data problem is always questionable.

Using the atrazine data, we estimate the fraction of systems with mean atrazine concentrations exceeding the current maximum contaminant level

(MCL) of 3 μg/L in each of the 10 source water-size strata (Table 6.3). In addition to EPA's MCL, the U.S. Centers for Disease Control and Prevention (CDC) sets an acute exposure limit of 1 μg/L, the World Health organization's (WHO) guideline for atrazine in drinking water is 2 μg/L, and Switzerland's (CHE) drinking water is 0.1 μg/L. The replacement method yielded a wide range and the mid-level estimates are uniformly above the respective BHM estimates (Table 6.3).

TABLE 6.3: The estimated fraction of systems with atrazine concentration means exceeding selected drinking water safety thresholds (set by EPA, WHO, CDC, and CHE) in each of the 10 source water-size strata (1-10) using the Bayesian hierarchical model (BHM) and the EPA's replacement method with upper bounds, mid-levels, and lower bounds calculated by replacing censored values with the respective MDLs, 0.5MDLs, and 0, respectively.

threshold	1	2	3	4	5	6	7	8	9	10
					EPA upper bounds					
EPA	8.5×10^{-5}	0	0.000711	0	0	0	0.002155	0	0	0
WHO	8.5×10^{-5}	0.00022	0.000711	0	0	0	0.00431	0.002041	0.00177	0
CDC	0.001111	0.002639	0.001422	0.001427	0	0.023256	0.051724	0.05102	0.035398	0.015528
CHE	0.962817	0.961302	0.931721	0.938659	0.932203	0.925581	0.982759	0.963265	0.957522	0.92236
					EPA mid-levels					
EPA	0	0	0	0	0	0	0	0	0	0
WHO	0	0.00022	0	0	0	0	0.002155	0.002041	0.00177	0
CDC	8.5×10^{-5}	0.00044	0.001422	0	0	0.009302	0.032328	0.016327	0.010619	0
CHE	0.34285	0.299252	0.303698	0.338088	0.542373	0.427907	0.515086	0.493878	0.481416	0.546584
					BHM					
EPA	0	3×10^{-6}	3×10^{-6}	1×10^{-6}	4×10^{-6}	3×10^{-6}	1.7×10^{-5}	5×10^{-6}	0	0
WHO	10^{-6}	10^{-5}	10^{-5}	3×10^{-6}	2.5×10^{-5}	1.2×10^{-5}	9.8×10^{-5}	0.000105	3.2×10^{-5}	3×10^{-6}
CDC	1.7×10^{-5}	7.8×10^{-5}	0.000129	3.4×10^{-5}	0.000585	0.000843	0.004342	0.004681	0.001967	6.4×10^{-5}
CHE	0.002959	0.009946	0.02835	0.027839	0.052468	0.041106	0.152442	0.156068	0.11428	0.106508
					EPA lower bounds					
EPA	0	0	0	0	0	0	0	0	0	0
WHO	0	0.00022	0	0	0	0	0.002155	0.002041	0.00177	0
CDC	0	0.00044	0	0	0	0.009302	0.025862	0.014286	0.010619	0
CHE	0.003248	0.010774	0.030583	0.031384	0.067797	0.037209	0.142241	0.155102	0.129204	0.121118

6.4.5.2   Example 6: Water Quality Survey of China's Drinking Water Sources

Wu et al. [2011] used the first national water quality survey of drinking water source water to explore the proper stratification of drinking water sources. The drinking water sources were stratified with the goal of making source water systems within a stratum more or less exchangeable. Using the Bayesian hierarchical model, Wu et al. [2011] explored three approaches and evaluated them based on the among-strata variance of the stratum means, similar to the criterion of a classification and regression tree model [Qian, 2016, Chapter 6]. The Chinese drinking water survey was exploratory because each source water within an administrative jurisdiction was represented by only one water sample. As a result, we cannot derive mean pollutant concentrations for individual source waters. The natural stratification was the administrative jurisdictions, a result of the top-down management and regulatory system. For this example, because each source water within a city was represented by only one observation, the model we used for the Six Year Review is directly applicable, that is, by replacing the source water type-size stratum with provinces and water systems with cities. Because of the small number of source waters in some cities (about 150 of the 350 cities with data had one source water), the variance σ_{1k}^2 in equation (6.12) cannot be calculated directly. As a result, we assume a common within-system/source water variance. Using the fluoride concentration data as an example, we show how the hierarchical modeling results can be used for identifying subsequent monitoring priorities, and more importantly, how we can leverage the analysis for improving future studies within a regulatory jurisdiction by deriving meaningful prior distributions. In the SYR example, the estimated system means are not directly relevant to EPA's review process. As a result, when running the Stan model, system means are not recorded. For the Chinese drinking water example, the estimated city means are directly relevant to understanding the among-city differences in source water quality. The among-city variation is an important consideration when setting drinking water treatment policies, in this case, whether fluoridation of drinking water should be considered.

Fluoride can help reduce dental caries. As a result, some U.S. cities started adding fluoride to community drinking water in the 1940s. In the 1960s, the U.S. government recommended fluoridation of drinking water to prevent tooth decay. Currently, the U.S. Public Health Service has recommended a concentration of 0.7 mg/L in drinking water. Long-term exposure to high levels of fluoride, however, can cause a condition called skeletal fluorosis, the buildup of fluoride in the bones. This can eventually result in joint stiffness and pain, and can also lead to weak bones or fractures in older adults. As a result, government agencies and health organizations established legal or recommended limits for fluoride in drinking water. For example, EPA set a legally enforceable MCL at 4 mg/L and a secondary (recommended) MCL at 2 mg/L to help protect children (under the age of 9) from dental fluorosis (fluoride build-up in developing teeth, preventing tooth enamel from forming normally); the World Health Organization has a fluoride guideline of 1.5 mg/L in drinking water [U.S. EPA, 2016a].

Fluoridation of drinking water can be a controversial topic in China. Wei and Wei [2002] reported that the southern city of Guangzhou started fluoridation in 1964. In the 1970s and 1980s, epidemiology studies indicated an increase in dental fluorosis in children born after the start of fluoridation, but no decrease in dental caries. Fluoridation was promptly stopped after 20 years. Experts argued that drinking water is only one of many sources of fluoride intake. Other sources include air pollution caused by widespread use of coal burning stoves for cooking and the popularity of brick tea [Wei and Wei, 2002]. As a result, fluoridation may lead to overdose of fluoride. The current drinking water fluoride MCL is 1 mg/L in China [Wu et al., 2011]. Information about source water fluoride concentration is, therefore, relevant to drinking water treatment.

We compare the estimated posterior distributions of city means for two provinces: Inner Mongolia and Sichuan (Figure 6.13). In Figure 6.13, the two probability density plots (top row) compare the estimated posterior distributions of fluoride concentrations of individual cities (θ_{jk} in equation (6.12)) in the two provinces to the posterior distribution of the provincial mean (γ_k in equation (6.12)). The two cumulative density function plots (bottom row) compare the posterior distributions of θ_{jk} and the posterior distribution of city means (i.e., $N(\gamma_k, \sigma_1^2)$). While the posterior distribution of a specific θ_{jk} is directly relevant to the city in question, the distribution of the city means is relevant to the development of provincial-level management policies. For example, cities in Sichuan Province have very similar fluoride concentration distributions (Figure 6.13, left column). Consequently, a uniform drinking water treatment standard with regard to fluoride for all cities in the province is reasonable. All source waters in Sichuan have very low fluoride concentrations, far below the U.S. recommended 0.7 mg/L for preventing dental caries. Cities in Inner Mongolia, on the other hand, have a wide range of city-level concentration distributions (Figure 6.13, right column). The recommended concentration of 0.7 mg/L is close to the 0.6 quantile and the Chinese MCL of 1 mg/L is near the 0.8 quantile of the posterior distribution of city means (bottom right panel of Figure 6.13), suggesting that the mean concentrations of about 40% and 20% of the source waters in Inner Mongolia exceed 0.7 and 1 mg/L, respectively. Based on these data and this analysis, a uniform policy with respect to fluoride treatment in Inner Mongolia may not be advisable.

At a national level, the estimated provincial means (γ_k) show a general north-to-south decreasing trend [Wu et al., 2011].

6.4.5.3   Example 7: Developing a Drinking Water Regulatory Standard in the U.S.

The last example in Qian [2016, Chapter 10] discussed the initial process of exploring whether the U.S. should regulate the harmful microorganism *Cryptosporidium* in drinking water. *Cryptosporidium* is a parasitic coccidian protozoan found in the intestinal tract of many vertebrates. When ingested, it causes the diarrheal disease cryptosporidiosis. The disease and the parasite are commonly known as "Crypto." There are many species of Crypto that infect animals, some of which also infect humans. The parasite, protected by its outer shell, is tolerant to chlorine disinfection during drinking water treatment and can survive in the environment for a long time. Crypto is present in almost all aquatic environments. They live in the gut of infected humans or animals. An infected person or animal sheds Crypto parasites in their feces. As a result, nearly all surface water that is used for drinking water supply can be occasionally contaminated. Crypto is the leading cause of waterborne disease in the U.S. [Painter et al., 2015, 2016]. The most effective treatment a drinking water treatment plant can deploy is to irradiate the finished water with UV light [Morita et al., 2002], which "inactivates" Crypto (rendering them unable to reproduce once ingested). As installing and operating a UV treatment

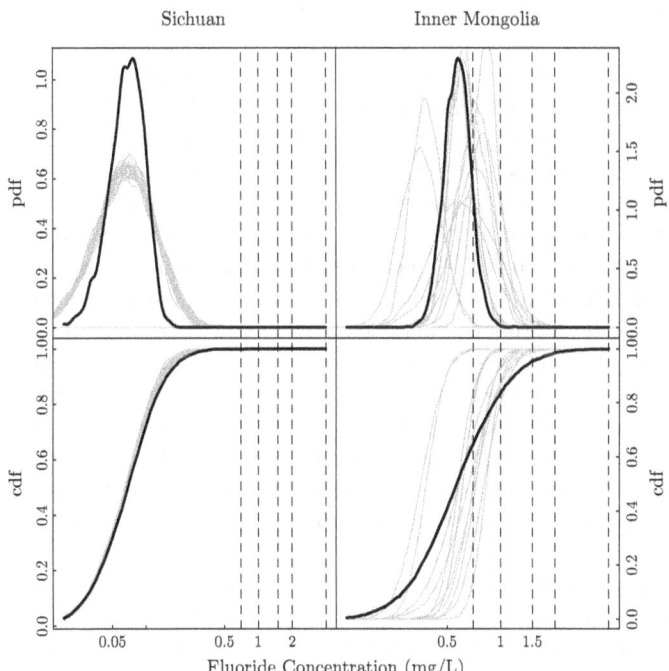

FIGURE 6.13: Posterior distributions of city-level mean (θ_{jk} in equation (6.12)) fluoride distributions (gray lines) from two provinces (Sichuan, left column, and Inner Mongolia, right column) are displayed in probability density functions (PDF, upper row) and cumulative density functions (CDF, bottom row). The black lines in the PDF plots are the estimated PDF of the posterior distribution of the mean of city-level means (γ_k), and the black lines in the CDF plots are the posterior distribution of city-level mean distribution ($N(\gamma_k, \sigma_2^2)$). The dashed lines are the various criteria (0.7, 1, 1.5, 2, and 4 mg/L) discussed in the main text.

facility is costly, the study was aimed at (1) understanding the prevalence of Crypto in U.S. drinking water and (2) identifying indicators of high likelihood of Crypto contamination. The EPA, through its Data Collection and Tracking System (DCTS), collected data for Crypto, *E. coli*, and turbidity in source waters of U.S. public drinking water systems. The goal of the study was to estimate the magnitude of Crypto contamination in the U.S. [U.S. EPA, 2016b]. The intended final product is a distribution of system mean concentrations. In Qian [2016], the observed Crypto count is modeled using a multilevel Poisson regression model. When checking the model results, Qian [2016] showed that the Poisson regression model cannot account for the large proportion of zeros in the data. Using this data set, we estimate the distribution of system mean concentrations of Crypto by using a model that captures the data-generating process.

The data EPA obtained consist of the observed number of Crypto oocysts in a water sample with a known volume. Unlike the previous two drinking water quality assessment examples, the observation has no detection limit. However, the method used for detecting Crypto in a water sample is imperfect. If a Crypto oocyst is in the water sample, the detection method will be able to detect its presence on average about 44% of the time based on "spiked" tests conducted by many EPA certified labs. In other words, the detection method has an average false negative probability of 0.56. Furthermore, unlike measuring concentrations of chemicals such as atrazine and fluoride, where we can assume that concentrations in the sample analyzed and in the water body are more or less the same, Crypto oocysts are discrete particles: even they are present in the source water, we may not capture one in the water sample. As a result, when we observe a zero, it is a result of both the imperfect detection and the random process of capturing an oocyst in the sample. These two processes combined are the cause of the overwhelming number of 0s in the data.

The model used in Qian [2016] assumes the observed number of oocysts is a Poisson random variable, using the average recovery rate of $r = 0.44$ and the sample volume to parameterize the Poisson distribution parameter:

$$
\begin{aligned}
y_{ij} &\sim Pois(\lambda_{ij}) \\
\lambda_{ij} &= rc_j v_{ij}
\end{aligned}
\tag{6.13}
$$

where the subscript ij represents the ith water sample from system j, c_j is the true concentration in the water from the jth system, and v_{ij} is the volume of the water sample analyzed. On average, the number of oocysts in the sample is $\lambda = cv$. The multilevel Poisson model used in Qian [2016] imposes a common prior on system means c_j:

$$
\log(c_j) \sim N(\mu_c, \sigma_c^2).
$$

The posterior hyper-distribution $N(\mu_c, \sigma_c^2)$ is the estimated national distribution of system means. In Qian [2016], the estimated mean system means $(\bar{c}_j)$ were used to estimate a cumulative distribution of system means to compare to the cumulative distribution of the posterior hyper-distribution. The comparison and a simulation showed that the model is adequate in estimating the upper quantiles of the distribution, but it cannot account for the large proportion of zeros in the data.

The model failed to account for the two-step data-generating process: (1) taking a water sample and (2) analyzing the sample in the lab. Although we can reasonably assume a constant Crypto concentration in the source water, the small volume of water sample is taken at random and the actual number of oocysts included in the sample is, therefore, random. When a water sample is analyzed in the lab, the number of oocysts captured in the sample is fixed (but unknown). As a result, the observed oocysts is a binomial random variate with an unknown actual number of oocysts in the sample (N_{ij}). This unknown number itself can be modeled as a Poisson random variable.

$$\begin{aligned}
y_{ij} &\sim Binom(p = r, N_{ij}) \\
N_{ij} &\sim Pois(c_j v_{ij}) \\
\log(c_j) &\sim N(\mu_c, \sigma_c^2)
\end{aligned} \tag{6.14}$$

We did not divide drinking water systems into the usual source water type and population served categories as in the model discussed in Section 6.4.5.1, although the city means ($\log(c_j)$) in equation (6.14) can be further divided into the same categories as in equation (6.12) on page 274. The emphasis in the rest of this example is computational.

Equation (6.14) is a latent variable model, similar to the models we used in Section 5.3.1, where we recommended specifying the joint likelihood function of the latent variable (N_{ij}) and the variable of interest (c_j) and then deriving the marginal likelihood of the variable of interest by marginalizing out the latent variable. The joint likelihood is

$$\pi(y_{ij}, N_{ij} \mid c_j, v_{ij}) = \pi(y_{ij} \mid p, N_{ij})\pi(N_{ij} \mid c_j, v_{ij}) \tag{6.15}$$

where $\pi(y_{ij} \mid p, N_{ij})$ is the binomial probability function and $\pi(N_{ij} \mid c_j, v_{ij})$ is the Poisson probability function. The likelihood function is then

$$\pi(y_{ij} \mid c_j, v_{ij}) = \sum_{N_{ij}=y_{ij}}^{\infty} \pi(y_{ij} \mid p, N_{ij})\pi(N_{ij} \mid c_j, v_{ij}) \tag{6.16}$$

and the log-likelihood is now

$$\log\left(\pi(y_{ij} \mid c_j, v_{ij})\right) = \log\left(\sum_{N_{ij}=y_{ij}}^{\infty} e^{\log(\pi(y_{ij} \mid p, N_{ij})) + \log(\pi(N_{ij} \mid c_j, v_{ij}))}\right).$$

To make the model more general, we consider the recovery rate as a random variable. As part of the DCTS, EPA required certified commercial labs to include at least one "spiked" sample for each 20 field samples. A spiked sample is a sample with a known number of oocysts. The number of oocysts recovered from these spiked samples was used to calculate an average recovery rate. The recovery rates in these spiked samples vary widely. For simplicity, we assume that the recovery rate is a random variable that can be approximated by a beta distribution:

$$r \sim beta(\alpha, \beta). \tag{6.17}$$

We consider equation (6.17) as the prior distribution of r and the parameters ($\hat{\alpha} = 15.5$ and $\hat{\beta} = 19.7$) were estimated using data from spiked samples. This model is a mixture of binomial and Poisson distributions. Henceforth, we refer to it as the Poisson mixture model. The model is similar to the N-mixture model [Kéry et al., 2005], popular in conservation biology/ecology studies for estimating population sizes without using mark-recapture data.

In theory, the upper bound of N_{ij} is infinity. However, the number of oocysts in a typical 10-liter water sample cannot be too many. In the data we used, although the range of the observed oocysts is from 0 to 121, 13,088 of the 13,102 observations are less than 10 and only 2 observations are larger than 35. We can set a reasonable upper bound for N_{ij} and program the log-likelihood function using the Stan function log_sum_exp:

```
### Partial Stan Code ###
transformed parameters {
  real lambda[Nobs];
  for (i in 1:Nobs)
    lambda[i] = exp(lconc[pwsid[i]]) * vol[i];
}
model{
  int k;
  r ~ beta(alpha, beta);
  lconc ~ normal(mu, sigma);
  for (i in 1:Nobs){
    vector[Nmax-y[i]+1] temp;
    for (j in y[i]:Nmax){
      k = j-y[i]+1;
      temp[k] = binomial_lpmf(y[i] | j, r) +
                poisson_lpmf(j | lambda[i]);
    }
    target += log_sum_exp(temp);
  }
}
### End ###
```

Because the value of Nmax directly affects the computation, we can use a small value (e.g., 200) initially and use a few larger values once the model is ready. But, for this example, the large sample size and the large number of drinking water systems (884) made the model run very slow even for a relatively small value of Nmax. Running the model using 10000 MCMC iterations with eight parallel chains took more than 10 days to finish on a reasonably fast personal computer. To explore the effect of the upper bound value on model results, we took a subset of systems with more than 20 and less than 25 observations from the data. The model with an upper bound of 75 took about one hour and the model with an upper bound of 150 took more than 90 minutes to complete 10000 MCMC iterations with eight parallel chains. In our subset of the data, there were 24 systems. The estimated system means are very similar (Figure 6.14). The estimated hyper-parameters are also very similar (Table 6.4). This comparison indicates that a reasonable upper bound can be found, but we do not have theoretical guidance on how to properly determine the right value.

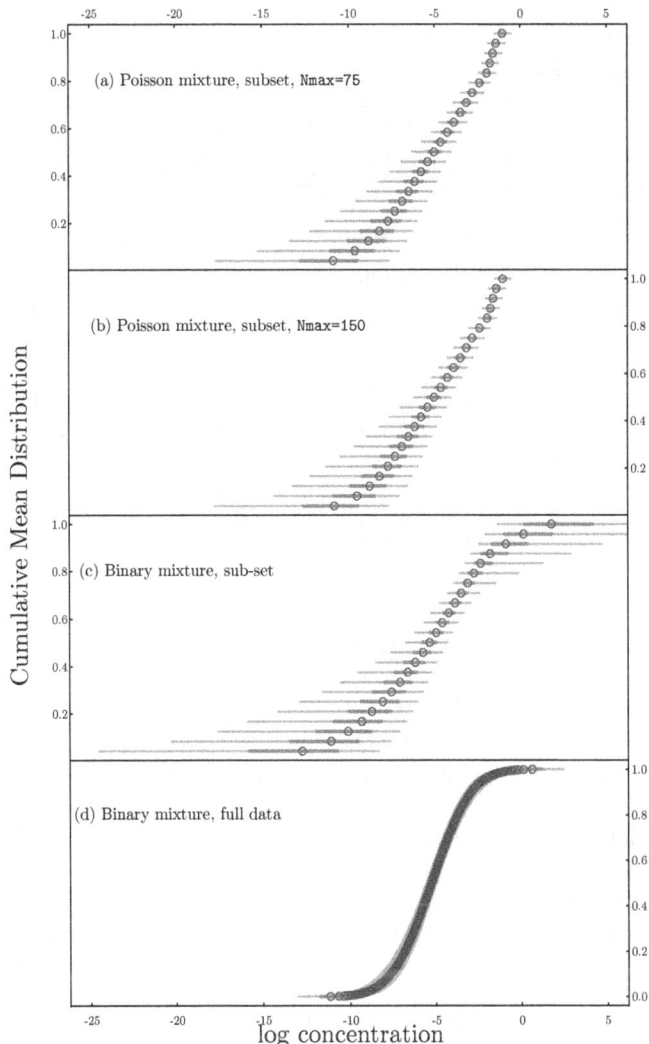

FIGURE 6.14: Estimated log system mean of Crypto concentrations from Poisson mixture model with `Nmax` set to 75 (a) or 150 (b), respectively. The two lower panels show the same estimates from the binary model with the subset of 24 systems (c) and with the full data (d).

The Crypto count data in this example are mostly zeros (93.2% of the observations). The 6.8% non-zero observations are mostly less than 5. Of the

TABLE 6.4: A comparison of the estimated posterior distribution (mean, standard deviation, and selected percentiles) of hyper-parameters (μ_c, σ_c, and r in equation (6.14)) from three Poisson mixture model runs (using data from a subset of 24 systems and setting `Nmax` set to 75 or 150, and full data set), as well as the two binary mixture model runs, using the subset and full data.

Parameter	Nmax/Model	mean	sd	2.5%	25%	50%	75%	97.5%
σ_c	75	3.171	0.902	1.905	2.527	2.999	3.634	5.422
σ_c	150	3.18	0.896	1.902	2.562	3.012	3.634	5.322
σ_c	full data	1.966	0.104	1.772	1.894	1.963	2.033	2.181
σ_c	Bin, subset	4.263	1.623	2.006	3.061	3.914	5.124	8.332
σ_c	Bin, full data	1.85	0.138	1.608	1.752	1.839	1.941	2.145
μ_c	75	-5.132	0.876	-7.178	-5.64	-5.046	-4.528	-3.648
μ_c	150	-5.152	0.899	-7.138	-5.660	-5.053	-4.534	-3.636
μ_c	full data	-5.263	0.223	-5.694	-5.415	-5.272	-5.109	-4.807
μ_c	Bin, subset	-5.383	1.169	-7.982	-5.971	-5.275	-4.651	-3.342
μ_c	Bin, full data	-5.297	0.156	-5.609	-5.4	-5.297	-5.194	-5.000
r	75	0.441	0.082	0.286	0.385	0.439	0.496	0.607
r	150	0.44	0.083	0.276	0.383	0.439	0.497	0.604
r	full data	0.441	0.080	0.285	0.387	0.439	0.494	0.602
r	Bin, subset	0.425	0.063	0.314	0.379	0.422	0.468	0.552
r	Bin, full data	0.454	0.046	0.373	0.421	0.451	0.485	0.551

884 systems included in the data, only 284 of them reported at least one positive detection. For every sample with a positive detection in one of these 284 systems, there were, on average, 7 samples with zero detection. In a way, differences in Crypto concentrations between two systems are largely reflected in the fraction of positive samples. Therefore, reformulating the model using a binomial distribution can be advantageous, especially with respect to computation.

If we consider the lab result of a sample as binary positive (1, or Crypto is detected) or negative (0, Crypto is not detected), the data for each system are a series of 0s and 1s. We can model the outcome as a Bernoulli random variable. The probability of observing a positive result is the product of recovery rate and the probability that at least one oocyst was present in the sample:

$$
\begin{aligned}
y_{ij} &\sim bern(\theta_{ij}) \\
\theta_{ij} &= r \times p0_{ij}
\end{aligned}
\tag{6.18}
$$

where θ is the probability of observing a positive result, $p0_{ij}$ is the probability that at least one oocyst was captured in the ith water sample in system j, and y_{ij} is the observed result (0 or 1).

In doing so, we are confusing two probabilities involved in the process. One is the recovery probability r, a conditional probability of detecting an oocyst when it is present, estimated from the spiked studies. This probability is the probability of success in the binomial model used in equation (6.14).

The other probability is the probability of detecting at least one oocyst, or the probability of a positive result (p_p). Using the binomial distribution formula, the probability of detecting at least one oocyst should be $p_p = 1 - (1 - r)^N$, where N is the unknown number of oocysts in the water sample. The two probabilities are the same only when $N = 1$. We should, therefore, use this approximation only when we are reasonably convinced that the number of oocysts in a typical sample is small.

Now considering the number of oocysts in a water sample as a Poisson random variable, the expected number of oocyst is $\lambda_{ij} = c_j v_{ij}$, and the probability that at least 1 oocyst is in the water sample is

$$p0_{ij} = 1 - e^{-\lambda_{ij}}. \tag{6.19}$$

As in the Poisson mixture model, we assume that the recovery rate is a random variable that can be approximated by a beta distribution (equation (6.17)). The model in equations (6.18), (6.19), and (6.17) is a mixture of two binomial processes (binomial mixture model) and it is a simplified version of the model we discussed in Chapter 5 (Section 5.3.1, equation (5.18) on page 176, with $f_p = 0$). As in the Poisson model (equation (6.14)), we use the data augmentation (or latent variable) approach to derive the log-likelihood function.

- For each observation y_{ij}, we use z_{ij} to indicate whether at least one oocyst was included ($z_{ij} = 1$) or not ($z_{ij} = 0$) in the water sample.

- The joint distribution of y_{ij} and z_{ij} is then derived using the conditional probability formula:

$$p(y_{ij}, z_{ij} \mid r, p0_{ij}) = p(y_{ij} \mid z_{ij}, r)p(z_{ij} \mid p0_{ij})$$

where

$$p(y_{ij} \mid z_{ij}, r) = \begin{cases} r & \text{if } z_{ij} = 1 \\ 0 & \text{if } z_{ij} = 0 \end{cases}$$

and

$$p(z_{ij} \mid p0_{ij}) = \begin{cases} 1 - e^{-\lambda_{ij}} & \text{if } z_{ij} = 1 \\ e^{-\lambda_{ij}} & \text{if } z_{ij} = 0 \end{cases}.$$

- By marginalizing out the latent variable Z, the resulting marginal probability function integrates both $z_{ij} = 1$ and $z_{ij} = 0$. Because z_{ij} is binary, the joint probability can be easily marginalized to derive the probability of y_{ij}:

$$p(y_{ij} \mid r, p0_{ij}) = p(y_{ij}, z_{ij} = 0 \mid r, p0_{ij}) + p(y_{ij}, z_{ij} = 1 \mid r, p0_{ij}).$$

Specifically:

$$
\begin{aligned}
p(y_{ij} \mid r, p0_{ij}) &= p(y_{ij} \mid z_{ij} = 0, r)p(z_{ij} = 0 \mid p0_{ij}) + \\
&\quad\; p(y_{ij} \mid z_{ij} = 1, r)p(z_{ij} = 1 \mid p0_{ij}) \\
&= \begin{cases} 0 \times e^{-\lambda_{ij}} + r \times (1 - e^{-\lambda_{ij}}) & \text{if } y_{ij} = 1 \\ 1 \times e^{-\lambda_{ij}} + (1 - r) \times (1 - e^{-\lambda_{ij}}) & \text{if } y_{ij} = 0 \end{cases}.
\end{aligned}
$$

- Recall that $\lambda_{ij} = c_j v_{ij}$, the log-likelihood for observation ij is:

$$
\begin{aligned}
LL_{ij} &= y_{ij} \log(p(y_{ij} = 1 \mid r, p0_{ij})) + (1 - y_{ij}) \log(p(y_{ij} = 0 \mid r, p0_{ij})) \\
&= y_{ij} \log \left[r(1 - e^{-c_j v_{ij}}) \right] + \\
&\quad (1 - y_{ij}) \log \left[e^{-c_j v_{ij}} + (1 - r)(1 - e^{-c_j v_{ij}}) \right] \\
&= y_{ij} \left[\log(r) + \log(1 - e^{-c_j v_{ij}}) \right] + \\
&\quad (1 - y_{ij}) \log \left[e^{-c_j v_{ij}} + (1 - r)(1 - e^{-c_j v_{ij}}) \right] \\
&= y_{ij} \left[\log(r) + \log(1 - e^{-c_j v_{ij}}) \right] + \\
&\quad (1 - y_{ij}) \log \left[e^{-c_j v_{ij}} + e^{\log(1-r) + \log(1 - e^{-c_j v_{ij}})} \right].
\end{aligned}
$$

The Stan model for this likelihood is then

```
#### Partial Stan Code ####
transformed parameters{
  vector[Npwsid] conc;
  real lambda[Nobs];
  for (i in 1:Nobs)
    lambda[i] = exp(lconc[pwsid[i]]) * vol[i];
  conc = exp(lconc);
}
model{
  real temp1;
  real temp2[2];
  r ~ beta(alpha, beta);
  for (i in 1:Nobs){
    temp1 = log1m_exp(-conc[pwsid[i]]*vol[i]) + log(r);
    temp2[1] = -conc[pwsid[i]]*vol[i];
    temp2[2] = log1m_exp(-conc[pwsid[i]]*vol[i])+log(1-r);
    target += y[i]*temp1 + (1-y[i])*log_sum_exp(temp2);
  }
}
### End ###
```

Running this model using the full data set with 10000 iterations and 8 parallel chains took about 1.5 hours. In both the Poisson mixture model and the binomial mixture model, we assumed that system means c_j are exchangeable (equation (6.14)). The shrinkage effect induced by the hierarchical structure moves individual system means toward the overall mean.

As a comparison to the Poisson model, we apply the binary mixture model to the same subset of data from the 24 systems with 20 to 25 observations. The estimated model parameters (system means, Figure 6.14; hyper-parameters and recovery rate, Table 6.4) from the binary model are more variable than the respective estimates from the Poisson model. The estimated variances are larger for systems with all 0 observations and systems with nearly all positive observations because the variance of the binary model estimated probability of observing a positive observation ($p0$ in equation (6.18)) increases when the estimated value is approaching 0 or 1. In the Poisson mixture model, the variance of the estimated system means decreases when the system mean increases. Because the amount of shrinkage is inversely related to the among-system variance (σ_c^2), the estimated among-system standard deviation (σ_c) based on data from all 884 systems is substantially smaller than the same estimated from the subset from the selected 24 systems. As a result, the estimated system means from the full data are well concentrated.

The Stan code can be further simplified if the sampling volume is standardized (i.e., the same volume for all samples). Instead of looping through observations, each system can report the number of positive samples (Y_{1j}) and the number of negative samples (Y_{2j}). The likelihood function becomes:

$$LL_j = Y_{1j}\left[\log(r) + \log(1 - e^{-c_j v_j})\right] + \\ Y_{2j}\log\left[e^{-c_j v_j} + e^{\log(1-r)+\log(1-e^{-c_j v_j})}\right].$$

In this example, we did not fully explore the hierarchical structure of the data in our model. Rather, we focused on the computational details to illustrate the advantage of Bayesian statistics in developing models according to the underlying data-generating processes. The binomial mixture model in equations (6.18) and (6.19) can be applied in analyzing many types of fisheries monitoring data, especially to estimate the population of rare species. For example, long-term monitoring data such as the ones discussed in Section 6.4.4 occasionally capture rare endangered species (e.g., sturgeon) and rare early-stage invasive species. Catch data for these rare species are often not used for understanding the population trend. In addition to gill-net monitoring, regional and local fisheries management agencies also maintain a routine trawl survey of fish populations. Although such monitoring efforts are largely designed for monitoring important commercial or recreational fisheries (e.g., walleye in Lake Erie), these long-term monitoring data can be readily used in a similar way as we discussed in this example.

6.5   When Data from Nonexchangeable Units Are Mixed

Simpson's paradox is a well-known and yet repeatedly encountered statistical phenomenon. When the paradoxical outcome fortunately appears, we are forced to understand and explain the phenomenon. But the effect of Simpson's paradox was unfortunately less obvious in many published works, especially in studies where only one level of aggregations was presented. With the increased availability of "large data" (data collected across multiple regions over multiple years), empirical analyses of data across multiple levels of spatial and temporal aggregation become feasible. However, combining and analyzing data from multiple sources (hence, likely collected for different purposes) should proceed with a clear understanding of the implications of Simpson's paradox. While we emphasize the statistical concept of exchangeable units, Simpson's paradox is often a result of improper representation of the underlying cause-effect relationship. We close this chapter with such an example.

In explaining the concept of exchangeability, Qian et al. [2019] used hypothetical data representing the Chla-TP relationship from four lakes (Figure 6.1), where the Chla-TP correlations within each of the three lakes are positive, while the correlation of the lake means of Chla and TP is negative. In this hypothetical example, observations from the same lake are exchangeable (assuming that data we have were random samples), whereas the lake means of Chla and TP are exchangeable among lakes, but not exchangeable with individual lake observations. Because the Chla-TP relationship can be influenced by other factors (e.g., Section 6.4.3), the Chla-TP relationship based on data within a lake is likely lake-specific. When these factors are unknown, we can assume that coefficients of the lake-specific Chla-TP models are exchangeable: these coefficients vary by lake, but we cannot determine their relative magnitude without knowing these other factors. A lake-specific Chla-TP model is not exchangeable with the same relationship based on lake means. While the Chla-TP relationship based on lake means can be meaningful (e.g., explaining the gradient of another factor across multiple lakes), it cannot be used to quantify the Chla-TP relationship in a given lake.

Yuan and Pollard [2017] used data from the National Lake Assessment (NLA), a cross-lake data set including randomly selected lakes in all 48 contiguous states of the United States [Pollard et al., 2018], to develop a dose-response model to describe the relationship between microcystin (MC) concentration and total nitrogen (TN) concentration. The resulting model was used to propose a national nitrogen criterion for controlling harmful algal blooms. Because nutrient criteria are part of lake eutrophication management practices for enforcing the U.S. Clean Water Act, they are applied to evaluate whether individual lakes are impaired. Consequently, a model based on a national database (i.e., NLA) is likely a misrepresentation of the lake-specific MC-TN relationship. A national nutrient criterion is, therefore, almost always irrelevant to lake-specific eutrophication management, a point illustrated by Liang et al. [2020] using data from 93 lakes and reservoirs in China with long-term monitoring data. They demonstrated that coefficients of the log-log linear models of Chla-TP and Chla-TN estimated using combined data from lakes within an eco-region are nearly always different from the same model coefficients estimated using lake-specific data. Figure 4 of Liang et al. [2020] showed a situation similar to Figure 6.1 – the Chla-TP relationship has a negative slope when estimated using combined data and the slopes estimated using lake-specific data are all positive. Liang et al. [2020] used the term "ecological fallacy" to represent a more general faulty inference due to the confusion of correlations at different levels of aggregation. Simpson's paradox is often viewed as a special case of ecological fallacy. Because the word "ecological" in this term means "aggregate" or "group," we prefer "Simpson's paradox" to avoid the potential confusion to the now more common meaning of the word "ecology."

6.5.1 Example 8: Are Small Wetlands More Effective in Nutrient Retention?

There are numerous discussions on the causes of and the means to avoiding Simpson's paradox. We discussed two main lines of arguments. Lindley and Novick [1981] emphasized the concept of exchangeable units, suggesting that the fallacy lies in applying results of a model to subjects that are not exchangeable with the data used for model development. Pearl et al. [2016] stressed the importance of properly outlining the causal structure of the problem, particularly, identifying hidden causes. We use the paper by Cheng and Basu [2017] to illustrate the importance of these two lines of arguments. Cheng and Basu [2017] analyzed a large cross-sectional data set to study nutrient retention capacities of lakes, reservoirs, and wetlands. We use the wetland data to show how causal analysis and identifying exchangeable units can avoid the misleading conclusion of the paper.

Cheng and Basu [2017] compiled a data set of 600 lentic water bodies (lakes, reservoirs, and wetlands) around the globe from several dozen studies, including the North American Treatment Database (NATD) v2.0 for constructed wetlands. In NATD, most wetlands were represented by a small number of records which were often the temporal (e.g., annual) and spatial (e.g., segments) averages of each of the key relevant factors examined in their study (i.e., flow, hydraulic residence time, and nutrient loading). Using the data, they calculated, for each water, the nutrient retention as a ratio of the amount nutrient retained in the water over the input loading:

$$R = \frac{M_{in} - M_{out}}{M_{in}}$$

where M_{in} is the input mass loading and M_{out} is the output loading. In addition, they estimated two parameters that are part of water quality models commonly used to simulate the fate and transport of contaminants. Specifically for model phosphorus retention in wetlands, they are the effective removal rate constant k and the hydraulic residence time τ. In a typical simplified water quality model based on the first-order reaction mechanism, these two parameters are used to estimate nutrient retention:

- Assuming the water is well mixed, use the continuously stirred tank reactor (CSTR) model

$$k = \frac{R}{1-R}\left(\frac{1}{\tau}\right).$$

- Assuming the water flows from inlet to outlet without longitudinal diffusion and dispersion, use the plug-flow reactor (PFR) model

$$k = \log(1-R)\left(\frac{1}{\tau}\right).$$

Once k and τ were estimated separately for each wetland, lake, and reservoir, Cheng and Basu [2017] fit a regression model using τ as the predictor variable and k as the response variable:

$$\log(k_j) = \beta_0 + \beta_1 \log(\tau_j) + \epsilon_j \tag{6.20}$$

where j represents individual waters. They showed that the estimated slope β_1 is negative, suggesting that the shorter the hydraulic residence time (τ) is, the larger the phosphorus effective removal rate constant (k) is. Because a wetland's τ is positively correlated with its surface area, Cheng and Basu [2017] concluded that small wetlands are more effective in removing phosphorus over the landscape than large wetlands on a per unit area basis (k).

We illustrate the issues with this analysis in two steps.

First, we examine the meaning of model coefficients using the exchangeable concept. The model in equation (6.20) is inevitably a model for individual waters. As a result, fitting the model using combined data from lakes, reservoirs, and wetlands is susceptible to Simpson's paradox. We fit the model in equation (6.20) using combined data from lakes, reservoirs, and wetlands, and compare the resulting model coefficients to the coefficients from the same model fit to data from lakes, reservoirs, and wetlands separately. The slope estimated using the combined data is much lower than the slopes estimated using data from the three types of water separately (Figure 6.15).

We can further fit the model to data from individual wetlands. Using six wetlands in the database (with more than 10 observations), we estimate the wetland-specific slopes using a hierarchical model assuming the wetland-specific regression coefficients are exchangeable. The six wetlands range in mean size (by volume) from 5.24 to 47,585.27 m^3. Using the concept of exchangeable units, we recognize that observations from the wetland with an

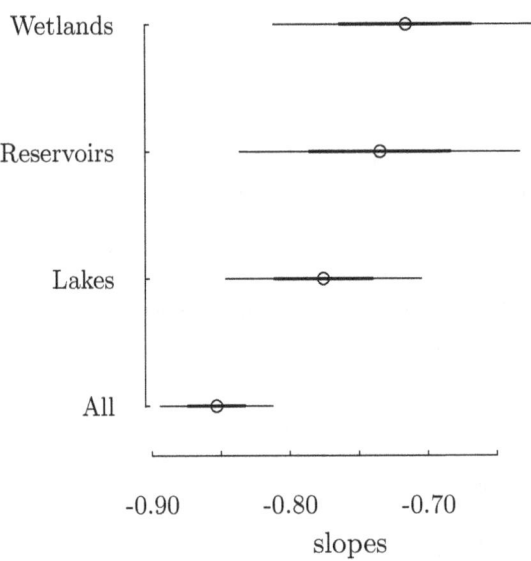

FIGURE 6.15: The slope in equation (6.20) (β_1) were estimated using data derived based on the PFR model. The slope estimated using the combined data and the slopes separately estimated using data from lakes, reservoirs, and wetlands are not comparable. The open circles represent the estimated means, and the thick and thin lines represent the mean plus/minus 1 and 2 times estimation standard errors, respectively.

average volume of 5.24 m³ cannot be exchangeable with observations from the wetland with an average volume of 47,585.27 m³. Consequently, we cannot directly combine data from these wetlands. However, by assuming individual wetlands are exchangeable with respect to the regression model coefficients, we can partially pool data from multiple wetlands using a hierarchical model. The slopes for the smallest and the largest wetlands are not different from 0 (larger than the slope estimated using the combined wetland data), while the slopes of the four intermediate sized wetlands are either highly uncertain (wetland 514) or well below the slope estimated using the combined wetland data (Figure 6.16). By now, we recognize that the variation in estimated slopes is a manifestation of Simpson's paradox. The average model coefficients for all wetlands (labeled "Mean slope") are parameterized by the hyper-distribution model (i.e., $\beta_j \sim N(\mu_\beta, \sigma_\beta^2)$). The hyper-distribution mean (μ_β) is most likely different from the estimated slope using combined wetland data. The hyper-distribution mean has a clear physical meaning (the mean of the wetland-specific coefficients), whereas the slope estimated using combined data does not.

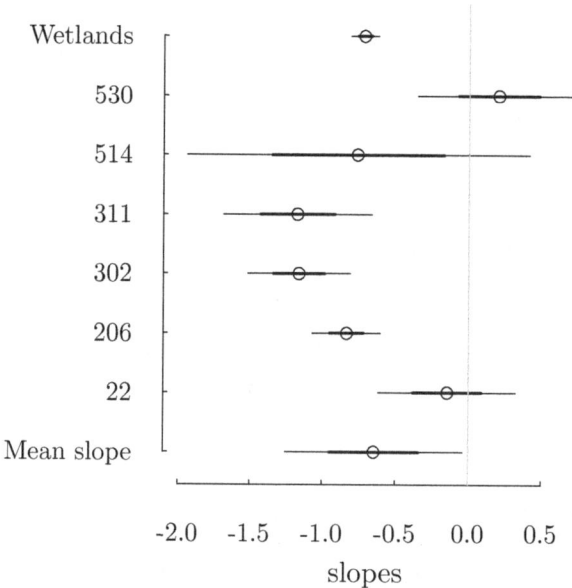

FIGURE 6.16: Slopes in equation (6.20) (β_1) were estimated using PFR data from six constructed wetlands in the North American Database using a multilevel model. The "fixed" effect slope ("Mean slope") represents the mean of wetland-specific slopes (labeled by NADB wetland identification numbers). The slope estimated using combined wetland data is labeled with "Wetlands." The open circles represent the estimated means, and the thick and thin lines represent the mean plus/minus 1 and 2 times estimation standard errors, respectively.

Second, we can explain the differences in estimated slopes at different levels of aggregation using causal inference, as in Tang et al. [2019]. In this case, we don't have additional variables for such analysis. However, we can examine equation (6.20) from a causal analysis angle. The two parameters in question (k and τ) represent two different aspects of a wetland and they are most likely independent of each other [Carleton and Montas, 2007, Hejzlar et al., 2007, Vollenweider, 1975]. In this case, the link between the two parameters is established by the percent removal (R in the CSTR or PFR models). The parameter k reflects the intrinsic characteristics of a wetland, while τ is a parameter determined by external input of water relative to the size of the wetland. The percent removal is a function of both k and τ (approximating the amount of time the nutrient mass stays in the system). In other words, the causal diagram for wetland phosphorus removal should be represented as $k \rightarrow R \leftarrow \tau$, which means that k and τ together determine R, but k and τ are independent of each other. A spurious correlation between k and τ arises when R is set to vary within a narrow range. In computer science literature, k and τ are known to be direction-separated (d-separated) by R. If two variables are d-separated, the apparent correlation between them is most likely spurious. We can use a simulation to demonstrate the effect of this d-separation. We randomly generate values of k and τ to calculate R using the CSTR model plus random noise ($R_i = k_i\tau_i/(1 + k_i\tau_i) + \epsilon_i$). In this case, the parameters k_i and τ_i were independently drawn from log-normal distributions with log means ($\mu_k = -2.726$ and $\mu_\tau = 1.914$) and log standard deviations ($\sigma_k = 1.371$ and $\sigma_\tau = 1.269$) calculated from the log values for k and τ for TP from the data used by Cheng and Basu [2017]. We then use a scatter plot of the randomly drawn k and τ to show the spurious correlation by highlighting the data points with k and τ values resulted in R values between 32% and 65% (Figure 6.17). Cheng and Basu [2017] indicated that wetlands with a percent removal (R) between 32% and 65% are of "no significant differences between systems and across constituents." The (spurious) negative correlation between k and τ shown by the highlighted data points in Figure 6.17 is remarkably similar to the pattern reported in Cheng and Basu [2017] in their data analysis, which suggests that the conclusion that small wetlands are more effective in phosphorus retention on a per unit area basis is a result of the spurious correlation induced by the d-separated relationship between k and τ.

6.6 Summary

In this chapter, we discussed what we considered as the key advantages of the Bayesian hierarchical approach – the exchangeable assumption and the use of the hierarchical modeling approach to properly aggregate data across multiple spatial and temporal scales. In setting up the hierarchical structure of the data, we clearly present what we know and what we do not know. The conscious steps of establishing a hierarchical model based on our objective knowledge and subjective ignorance lead to models that are conceptually appealing and epistemologically advantageous. From a properly constructed hierarchical model, not only we can clearly explain the assumptions of the

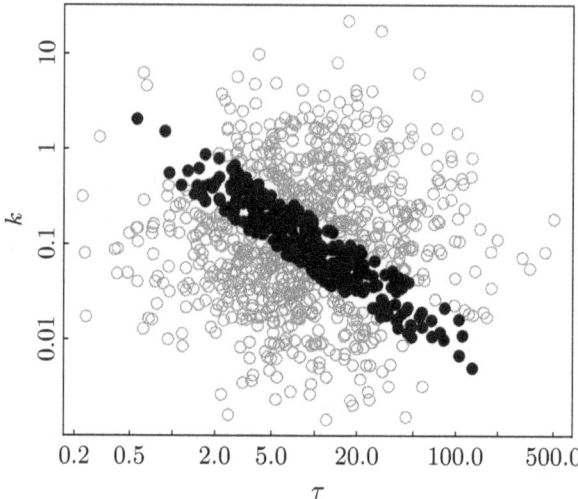

FIGURE 6.17: Random samples of k are independent of random samples of τ, both generated based on data reported by Cheng and Basu [2017] (grey circles). Pairs of k and τ resulting in TP retention (R) between 32% and 65% are highlighted (black dots) and appear to be strongly correlated.

model, but also carry out further exploration based on model results. The process of analyzing the EUSE data (Section 6.4.3) is an example of why the hierarchical model is appealing for analyzing large data (data from multiple sources). We started our initial analysis using simple linear regression and other classical statistics tools. The regression models as presented by Brown et al. [2009] and Cuffney et al. [2009] were unsatisfactory. In reviewing these regression models while studying the multilevel models from Gelman and Hill [2007], we recognized the value of modeling the data using a hierarchical modeling approach. The initial multilevel model without group-level predictors [Qian, 2016, equation 10.14] was an indication that the nine regions are very different and the shrinkage effect of the multilevel model is negligible, a sign that EUSE was a well-designed study. However, our geographer and ecologist colleagues quickly recognized what distinguished the three regions with high antecedent agriculture land cover from the other six regions. As a result, we systematically explored group-level predictors. The modeling process captured in Qian [2010, Chapter 10] is an accurate representation of our learning experience. Additional applications of the multilevel modeling approach similar to the EUSE example [Tang et al., 2019, Rizo et al., 2019, e.g.,] led us to the broad implications of the exchangeable assumption with regard to Simpson's paradox [Qian et al., 2019, Liang et al., 2020]. The Everglades example (Section 6.4.1) prompted us contemplate the practical meaning of the hyper-distribution in a hierarchical model. The hyper-distribution (equation (6.5)) does not apply to any individual ecological metric. Mathematically, it serves as a vehicle to link all metrics in the data. But, when interpreting equation (6.5), we recognized the practical meaning of the distribution – distribution of the means of all metrics. The interpretation of the hyper-distribution as the cross-metric distribution of means of exchangeable metrics prompted us to extrapolate the meaning of the hyper-distribution as the prior distribution for a metric that is not included in the current data. This interpretation resulted in the sequential updating idea, where the hyper-parameter is updated repeatedly when new data are available. A likely future application is to update the ambient water quality standard compliance assessment process (Section 6.4.2). A hierarchical model can be developed using existing data from a state and the hyper-distribution from this state-wide model can be used as the prior when evaluating the compliance of individual waters, as explained by Qian and Miltner [2018] that an estimation-oriented approach can effectively use data from similar waters to effectively reduce estimation uncertainty. The same approach can be used in the national drinking water quality compliance assessment (the Six Year Review). Instead of compiling data from all drinking water systems every six years, the current assessment estimated hyper-distributions can be used as prior distributions. Subsequent analysis can then be based on random samples of systems in each of the ten strata. Such a sampling-based assessment approach is perhaps more cost-effective to allow more frequent assessment and the trajectory of the posterior distributions can be used to understand the country's drinking water quality trend.

Chapter 7

Bayesian Applications

We introduce two areas of application of the Bayesian statistics: the Bayesian networks (BNs) model and the Bayesian change point model. We group these two topics because they represent unique challenges in Bayesian statistics. The BN is mainly a model for categorical variables, using the discretized Bayes' theorem as the computation tool. Each variable has several states modeled by the multinomial distribution, with parameters representing the probabilities of the states occurring. The probabilistic dependencies among variables of a BN model are presented as a directed acyclic graph (DAG) made up of nodes (variables) and directed arcs (arrows) connecting among variables. A child node represents a variable whose state distribution is dependent on at least one other variable (parent node). The model formulation process is the process of establishing the DAG of a BN model. Model parameters are the conditional probabilities of a node's states conditional on the states of its parent node(s). These conditional probabilities are often tabulated. As such, parameters of a BN model are the conditional probability tables (CPTs) of all nodes. Because of the scarcity of data in most BN applications, we are unlikely to estimate these CPTs entirely from data. As a result, the CPTs of a BN model are often populated based on information sources other than raw data. From a Bayesian statistics perspective, these estimated CPTs represent prior information that can be updated once new data become available. However, data scarcity often prevents us from updating these CPTs. As a result, most BN applications focus only on the process of model formulation and prior elicitation. Model evaluation is rarely possible, while model sensitivity analysis is rarely done. We provide a review of the BN literature with an emphasis on model structure identification.

Meanwhile, the challenge in a change point model is mainly computational because of the discontinuity of the model or the first derivative of the model. We discuss computational options to overcome this hurdle, and their implementation in Stan including alternative model forms to circumvent the computational difficulties caused by the discontinuity.

7.1   Bayesian Networks

A Bayesian Network (BN) is a graphical representation of the probabilistic dependencies among the variables in a model. BNs were first introduced in the early 1980s by Pearl [1982] and Spiegelhalter and Knill-Jones [1984]. Their adoption in the environmental field started in the late 1990s [Reckhow, 1999, Varis, 1997] and have since increased. BNs now represent an important environmental modeling platform, as they are used more as a meta-modeling tool [Barton et al., 2008] that can successfully integrate inter-disciplinary knowledge and a diverse set of information types (e.g. expert elicitation, multiple linear regression model predictions, observational/experimental data, and mass balances) [Johnson et al., 2010]. Moreover, BNs can easily account for uncertainties both with regards to model parametrization and the strengths of certain pathways. Thus BNs allow for the transparent evaluation of uncertainties in a manner that can be easily communicated with stakeholders. These features are some of the main reasons behind the increased interest in adopting BN in environmental and resource management applications [Bromley et al., 2005, Barton et al., 2008, Pollino and Henderson, 2010, Fienen et al., 2013, Death et al., 2015, Chee et al., 2016, Moe et al., 2016, Couture et al., 2018, Giné-Garriga et al., 2018, Uusitalo et al., 2018]. Additionally, their legible graphical interface that is user-friendly for non-technical users and their ability to incorporate decision variables and associated utility values have allowed them to be adopted as decision support tools [Fienen et al., 2013, Molina et al., 2013, Gonzalez-Redin et al., 2016, Rachid et al., 2021].

BNs have both a qualitative aspect and a quantitative aspect. The qualitative aspect is the underlying model structure, which is comprised of a directed acyclic graph (DAG) made up of nodes and directed arcs representing our understanding on the causality of the process we are trying to model. The DAG nodes represent the important concepts (variables) in the system of interest, while the arrows represent the probabilistic relations between those concepts. As such, the DAG represents the structural assumptions of the domain under study. The DAG structure ultimately is represented by the joint probability distribution over the set of statistical variables in the model. The variables or nodes of the model take certain values or states. These nodes are often discrete and as such the values are Boolean, ordered, or integral ranges [Das and Ghosh, 2020]. The probabilities of the conditional probability tables (CPTs) represent the strength of the relationships between the nodes in the DAG, conditional on the states of each of those nodes. As such, the quantitative aspect of the BN involves populating the marginal and conditional probabilities of the BN model [Woodberry et al., 2005]. One of the advantages of BNs is their ability to reduce the dimensionality of the joint probability distribution space of the implied model, which is often intractable and hard to assess. This is possible through the application of the chain rule (equation (7.1)) [Korb and Nicholson, 2010, Nielsen and Jensen, 2009, Pearl, 2000],

$$P(X_1, \ldots, X_n) = \prod_{i=1}^{n} P(X_i | pa(X_i)) \tag{7.1}$$

where X_i's are the variables, and $pa(X_i)$ are variables represented by the parent nodes of node X_i.

The BN allows for the decomposition of the complicated system of joint distributions into a set of simpler conditional probabilities that describe the distribution for each separate child node (a node with arrows pointing into it) given values of variables represented by its parent nodes (nodes from where the arrows originate). Child nodes are then themselves modeled as parent nodes of subsequent child nodes. Ultimately, a BN is a model that quantifies the probabilities of each node to be in a particular state given the likelihood of the states of all other nodes in the model [Kashuba, 2010]. In BNs, any node is conditionally independent of its non-descendants given its parents [Acid et al., 2004]. Moreover, the BN's probabilistic structure allows it to represent uncertainties explicitly and to propagate them through the network [Stritih et al., 2020].

While we are seeing an increase in the popularity of BNs in the environmental field, their adoption still faces major limitations, including the availability of data, the need to discretize continuous variables, difficulties associated with model representation, challenges of implementing quantitative validation and sensitivity analysis, and complications associated with the representation of space and time [Sperotto et al., 2017].

7.1.1 Model Structure and Conditional Probability Tables

A BN is made of nodes that take certain values or states and arrows connecting nodes. The arrows represent probability dependencies among the nodes. BNs allow for the seamless forward and backward propagation of information, especially when the data are discrete. Most BN applications opt for discretizing nodes into states, where each node is defined over a set of k non-overlapping states that are commonly referred to as intervals. As such, the probability to be in any given state is governed by a multinomial distribution (7.2) with probability vector θ given a number of trials n. Note that the length of the vector θ will be equal to the number of states defined minus 1.

$$f(x_1, \cdots, x_n) = \begin{cases} \frac{n!}{x_1! \cdots x_k!} \theta_1^{x_1} \times \cdots \times \theta_k^{x_k}, & \text{where } \sum_{i=1}^{k} x_i = n \\ 0 & \text{otherwise} \end{cases} \tag{7.2}$$

The prior on the vector of probabilities is distributed as a Dirichlet distribution (equation (7.3)). Just as the multinomial is a multivariate generalization of the binomial, the Dirichlet is a multivariate generalization of the beta distribution. Given the conjugacy between the multinomial and the Dirichlet distribution, the posterior distribution of the vector of probabilities for a given node is also a Dirichlet distribution (equation (7.4)):

$$\text{Dir}(\theta|\alpha) = \frac{1}{B(\alpha)} \prod_{i=1}^{K} \theta_i^{\alpha_i - 1} \tag{7.3}$$

where $B(\alpha)$ is the multivariate beta function, given by $\frac{\prod_{i=1}^{K}(\alpha)}{\left(\sum_{i=1}^{K} \alpha_i\right)}$ and $\alpha_i = (\alpha_1, \cdots, \alpha_K)$. They describe the possible values of the vector θ, with $\sum_{i=1}^{K} \theta_i = 1$ and $\theta_i \geq 0$ for $i \in \{1, \cdots, K\}$.

Based on that, the expected value of the θ_i is $\frac{\alpha_i}{\sum_{i=1}^{K} \alpha_i}$ and its variance is

$$\frac{\frac{\alpha_i}{\sum_{i=1}^{K} \alpha_i} \times \left(1 - \frac{\alpha_i}{\sum_{i=1}^{K} \alpha_i}\right)}{\left(\sum_{i=1}^{K} \alpha_i + 1\right)}$$

$$(P(\theta|D) \propto P(D|\theta)P(\theta) \propto \prod_{i=1}^{K} \theta_i^{N_i + \alpha_i - 1} = Dir(\theta|\alpha_1 + N_1, \ldots, \alpha_k + N_k,)$$
$$(7.4)$$

where N_1 through N_k are the respective observations in each of the k intervals defined for the given node.

The prior vector α can be viewed as representing the number of observations in each category that we have already seen before the evidence is introduced to the BN model. This conjugacy allows new evidence to be easily incorporated and propagated in the model as soon as it is made available. This is possible because of the analytically tractable compound distribution that permits for the easy application of Bayes' theorem to update beliefs in response to any new addition of data without having to resort to computationally intensive processes like MCMC. Interestingly, most environmental and ecological BN applications develop only a prior model and make inference through evidence propagation without actually updating the model parameters themselves. As such, most BN applications are not truly Bayesian (Kashuba 2010).

7.1.1.1   Building a BN Model

The construction of a BN model is a time-consuming endeavor [Madsen et al., 2003]. So far, the method of developing the model structure of a BN has largely depended on previously accumulated subject-matter information. Previous knowledge is often extracted through expert elicitation, sometimes supplemented by literature synthesis. This information leads to a conceptual diagram consisting of boxes and arrows, which becomes an initial BN structure with variables and dependencies among the variables [Bromley et al., 2005, Marcot et al., 2006, McNay et al., 2006, Pollino et al., 2007]. Yet with the uniqueness of data in some situations and the indefiniteness of experts and the literature in certain instances, there has been a push toward learning the model structure from the data.

Expert Elicitation

Most BN models in the environmental field are built through knowledge elicitation from subject matter experts. These experts can provide an integrated view of the relationships and uncertainties of the subject area that will be modeled based on their assimilated knowledge that they have accrued over their entire careers. Thus many think that opting for expert elicitation is more appropriate as it goes beyond simple data summary [Kashuba, 2010]. Subject matter expert elicitation has proven to be effective in constructing causal links that dictate the resulting CPTs.

Expert elicitation of the model structure has also been very helpful to overcome data limitations, particularly in poorly monitored systems. This feature has made BNs a preferred modeling technique in data-poor situations, where significant expert knowledge (and uncertainty estimates) can be elicited and used to guide model development, provide transparent predictions at meaningful endpoints, as well as identify gaps and the relative sensitivities of decisions to parameter uncertainties.

The main difficulty with expert elicitation is the need to ensure that the adopted elicitation method is capable of adequately capturing the expert's conceptual understanding of the problem at hand. This elicitation is often done by conducting several open-ended expert interviews, where probing questions for different parts of the model are posed. The ultimate goal is to make sure that these sessions generate a directed causal narrative of the process/system under study [Nadkarni and Shenoy, 2004]. During the expert elicitation process, it is important to ensure that the same concepts are not repeated, that the causal pathways are clearly understood, and that the ultimate model structure is not over-parameterized in order to avoid overfitting [Kashuba, 2010]. If the CPTs of the elicited model will themselves be elicited from the experts, one has to keep in mind that people cannot think in terms of more than a few conditioning factors [Morgan et al., 1990]. As such, the model elicitation process should stipulate the maximum number of parents a child node may have [Kashuba, 2010]. Throughout the elicitation process, one has to ensure that the ultimate structure should remain a directed, acyclic graph with no feedback loops. Following structure elicitation, it is recommended that the validity of the model structure is checked and its structure further refined by conducting additional elicitations with a new set of subject area experts.

Qian and Miltner [2015] developed a BN to predict the streams' abilities to meet their designated uses for aquatic life as a function of nutrient concentrations, background land use, habitat quality index, and other relevant physio-chemical factors. Inference was focused on two macroinvertebrate metrics, namely the Invertebrate Community Index (ICI) and the EPT taxa richness (EPT is the number of Ephemeroptera (mayfly), Plecoptera (stonefly), and Trichopera (caddisfly) taxa in a collected sample). Their model structure was based on eliciting the structure from experts and integrating previously developed models into one BN. This process resulted in including theoretically important and/or management-relevant predictors even when their relationships were found to be statistically insignificant. Their proposed model structure is shown in Figure 7.1. We will use this example throughout this chapter to discuss different aspects of BN models. We note that Qian and Miltner [2015] developed a continuous variable BN (cBN) and that much of our discussion with this example is based on assuming that the model was fit with discretized variables.

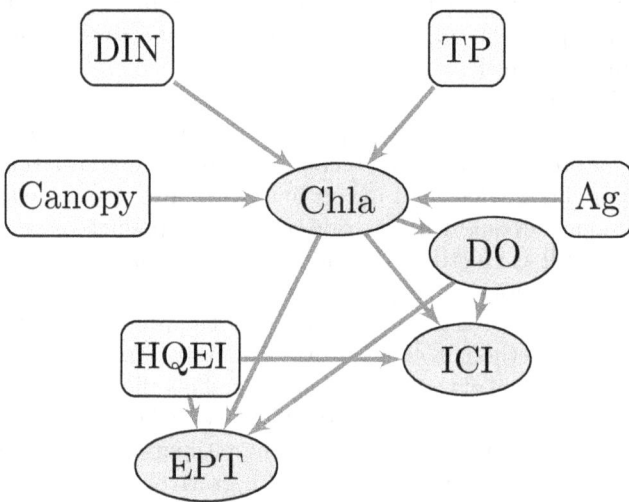

FIGURE 7.1: BN model proposed by Qian and Miltner [2015] to predict stream aquatic ecosystem indicators as a function of nutrient concentrations, tree canopy, agricultural landcover and habitat quality index.

Structure Learning

While using expert elicitation to build the model structure is adequate in many instances and may often be the only option when lacking observational data, this process is often hindered by the absence of a widely accepted interpretation of the process at hand. Moreover, expert elicitation is a difficult and time-consuming activity given that experts may have incomplete knowledge of the domain, may be uncomfortable in specifying and combining probabilities, and may be unsure about the causal direction of influences between variables [Woodberry et al., 2005]. Experts may tend to generate elaborate models with a large number of variables, a high degree of interconnections between variables, and include feedback loops that violate the acyclic nature of BN models

[Alameddine et al., 2011]. Additionally, experts often do not agree on a common model structure. For example, many new environmental problems are contentious subjects on which experts may not agree on a single structure. As such, letting the data speak and guide us with regards to which model structure it supports is useful. Interest in adopting model structure learning in the environmental field has recently peaked, given the worldwide increased interest in data mining and the increase in data availability.

Structure learning based on data assumes 1) the existence of a "true" network in the real world that describes the process at hand; 2) the data are actually sampled from that "true" network; 3) the data were collected with no bias; 4) the data are large enough to cover the network adequately; and 5) there are no hidden variables in the system [Alameddine et al., 2011, Pearl, 2000, Korb and Nicholson, 2010, Nielsen and Jensen, 2009]. Even under these assumptions, structure learning may only be able to generate a set of Markov equivalent model structures that share the same set of variables and are equally supported by the joint probability distribution of the available data [Alameddine et al., 2011, Korb and Nicholson, 2010, Kjaerulff and Madsen, 2008].

For BNs, it is possible to "learn" the structure of the network from a set of data using one of several algorithms that have been developed [see Korb and Nicholson, 2010, Nielsen and Jensen, 2009, for an in-depth discussion of some of these algorithms]. Structure learning is thus based on identifying a DAG structure from a set of (conditional) dependence and independence relations that are derived from the data using a set of classical statistical tests [Madsen et al., 2003]. In the Bayes net program Hugin[1], several structure learning algorithms are available: the PC (named after its authors, Peter and Clark) algorithm, the NPC (Necessary Path Conditions) algorithms, the Greedy search-and-score algorithm, the Chow-Liu tree algorithm, the Rebane-Pearl polytree algorithm, and the Tree Augmented Naive Bayes algorithm [Hugin Expert, 2021].

Structure learning algorithms prune the space of all possible structures given the available data since the number of possible BNs that describe a given set of variables grows faster than exponential with the number of variables [Robinson, 1977]. Two of the most commonly used algorithms are the constraint-based PC and the NPC algorithms. The PC algorithm was proposed by Spirtes et al. [1993] for structural equation models and was subsequently applied for BNs. Both the PC and NPC algorithms try to assess the likelihood of the data given the model, or $\Pr(\text{Data} \mid M)$. This is computed by determining the probability of the observed data set using a given model M. For the PC algorithm, it begins with a fully connected network; in other words, all nodes (variables) are directly connected to all other nodes. The connections in the network are sequentially thinned by first removing edges with zero-order conditional independence relationships then thinning those

---

[1]http://www.hugin.com

with first-order conditional independence relationships, and so on [Acid et al., 2004]. Connections are evaluated using the statistical significance of partial correlation coefficients. Taking a simplistic example with three nodes A, B, and C, where A and B are "parents" (predictors) of C. The PC algorithm starts with all three nodes initially connected. If it finds that the partial correlation between A and C, given B, is not significantly different from zero, then the connection between A and C is removed. This assessment of "conditional independence" is the basis for learning the structure. Given that most BN models are made of discrete nodes, the PC algorithm uses the χ^2 test to test for the statistical significance of the partial correlations. The χ^2 tests are conducted assuming a fixed confidence level such as 0.99 or 0.95 [Acid et al., 2004]. Using the same example as above, one will have to look at the χ^2 test to see if the expected frequency in the cell (or bin) of the conditional probability table (CPT) for node C conditional on nodes A and B is the same as the expected frequency for node C conditional on node B only. If that is the case, then the link between A and C is removed. In effect, these tests (partial correlation and χ^2) indicate whether A provides useful information on C, given B. This process is continued until a reduced DAG skeleton is generated with no directed arrows. Table 7.1 [Alameddine et al., 2011, from] summarizes the main steps of the PN algorithm. Once the BN model structure has been adequately thinned, its links need to be converted into directed arrows so that the model can be considered as a directed DAG. This process is made possible by four prioritized principles [Nielsen and Jensen, 2009]. The first principle requires creating a number of local v-structures (or colliders) that are also known as converging structures (i.e., $A \rightarrow B \leftarrow C$). V-structures are possible when A and C are found to be conditionally (or marginally) independent given any set of nodes that excludes B. These v-structures allow for the incorporation of the "explaining away" concept that allows for intercausal inference in BN [Kjaerulff and Madsen, 2008]. After introducing as many v-structures as possible given the model skeleton, the second and the third principle are applied with the aim of preventing adding a directed arc that would lead to the creation of another v-structure or to the creation of local directed cycles. When the principles 1 to 3 are exhausted and if there still remain any undirected links, the fourth principle assigns random directions to all the remaining undirected links. Due to this arbitrary nature of the fourth principle, a structure learning procedure can result in multiple parallel equivalent solutions [Alameddine et al., 2011]. The correctness and faithfulness of the PC algorithm has been proven under the assumption of infinite data sets [Madsen et al., 2003]. Yet in realistic applications, the data sets used for the learning are finite; thus the faithfulness of the generated structure to the theoretical one is not guaranteed. With limited data, it is often found that too many conditional independence relations are generated by the PC algorithm [Madsen et al., 2003].

Applying the PC algorithm on the data used by Qian and Miltner [2015], generated a model structure that is significantly different from that elicited by

Qian and Miltner [2015] (Figure 7.2). Many of the links generated by the PC algorithm have no scientific meaning, with many of the directed links pointing from the cause toward the effect (e.g., EPT→QHEI; Chla→DIN). One important point to note and discuss in the PC-generated model is the link EPT→ICI. The Qian and Miltner [2015] BN model did not incorporate that link, as they modeled these two variables independently, because they are the two end points used to evaluate a river's biological conditions according to Ohio's water quality assessment rules. Yet, the high correlation between the two variables supported the addition of that link in the PC-generated model. Knowing that a site has a high EPT would provide valuable information on the state of the ICI as both are similar metrics, and vice versa. As such, one would argue that keeping that link is informative. The absence of many of the directed links from the Qian and Miltner [2015] PC-generated model structure is to a large extent a result of the relatively small sample size of the data used (less than 200 measurements) and the weak linkages among the variables. It should be noted that several linkages in the Qian and Miltner [2015] model were found to be statistically insignificant based on their exploratory data analysis, but they decided to keep them because they had scientific and management implications. Under situations where we have data limitations, relatively weak correlations, the potential for latent variables, and/or a partial view of the complex ecological/environmental processes at hand, the PC algorithm appears to fail to re-create a defendable model structure that can help inference and decision making.

TABLE 7.1: PN structure learning algorithm.

Step 1	Start with a complete undirected graph.
Step 2	Start with $i = 0$.
Step 3	Look for all variables with at least $i + 1$ neighbors and place these nodes in a set which we will call Δ.
Step 4	Look for the neighbors of each variable node that is an element of Δ. Each element in Δ will have a set of neighbors as identified from the undirected graph.
Step 5	Start with the first variable in Δ and see if it is conditionally independent of any of its identified neighbors, given the rest of its neighbors that are to be combined into sets of size i.
Step 6	If conditional independence is proven between that variable and one of its neighbors given the rest of the neighbors, then proceed to remove the arc linking the variable and that neighbor. Proceed until you have analyzed all identified neighbors.
Step 7	Move on to the next variable in Δ and repeat the process identified in Steps 5 and 6 until all the variables in Δ have been cycled through. This will generate an un-directed graph that has less than or an equal number of arcs as compared to the one we started out with.
Step 8	Increment i by one ($i = i + 1$) and repeat Steps 3 through 7.
Step 9	The PC algorithm is terminated once there are no variables with $i + 1$ neighbors.

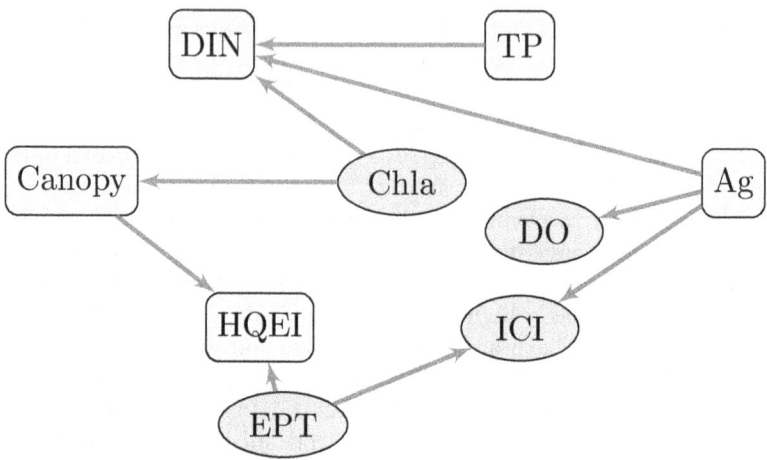

FIGURE 7.2: PC-generated structure for the Ohio stream model.

The NPC algorithm shares the same basic procedure with the PC algorithm; yet it entails an additional criterion called the necessary path condition. That criterion assesses the independence between X and Y given a set $Z(X \perp Y \mid Z = [C, D, E])$ only if the elements in Z appear on a path between X and Y [Nielsen and Jensen, 2009]. This logic makes it possible to introduce ambiguous regions to the model structure. An ambiguous region is caused by a set of inconsistent statements of conditional independence and dependence. In these regions, there exist inter-dependent uncertain links that will require the intervention of the modeler to settle [Kjaerulff and Madsen, 2008]. Software like Hugin allow the user to interact with and resolve these ambiguous regions based on the user's judgment, although the software can resolve them by incorporating the smallest number of ambiguous links, which in turn leads to assigning the largest number of independent nodes [Hugin Expert, 2021]. Integrating ambiguous regions in the NPC algorithm enables it to better address the inconsistencies of conditional independent and dependent relations as compared to the PC algorithm. As a result, the NPC algorithm is particularly useful when structure learning is based on a limited data set or a data set with a high uncertainty level that adversely affects structure determination. These conditions can lead to ambiguity as to whether a link should be present or absent in a particular BN and to determine in which direction the arrow should point. To resolve these ambiguities, the Hugin software provides the user with a graphical screen that displays the ambiguous links, and the user is allowed to interact with this screen to resolve these ambiguous connections based on substantive knowledge.

The generated model structure resulting from applying the NPC algorithm on the Ohio stream data after the data were discretized using an equal frequency method and limiting the states in each node to 3 is shown in Figure 7.3. The generated model structure is similar to that produced by the PC algorithm and is significantly different from that elicited by Qian and Miltner [2015]. The NPC algorithm produced only one vague region. That region was *Canopy − −DO − −Chla*. We resolved this vague region by accepting the link between *Chla* and *DO* and eliminating the other link. Similar to the PC-generated model, many of the links had no scientific meaning and the directed links pointed from the cause to the effect (e.g., EPT→QHEI; Chla→DIN). The link EPT→ICI was once again part of the final model given the high correlation between the two variables.

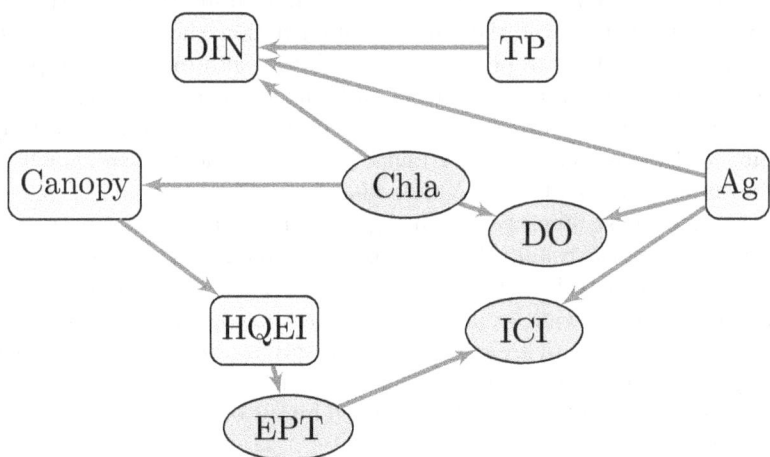

FIGURE 7.3: NPC-generated structure for the Ohio stream model.

Both the PC and NPC algorithms can be effective methods for discovering the underlying structure in multivariate data. Since both algorithms allow the user to input prior substantive knowledge about links (either through their known presence or absence), they will generally yield a plausible model structure in the presence of a scientific expert and an informative data set. However, neither is guaranteed to yield the best model. In terms of performance, the PC algorithm is faster than the NPC, since fewer tests are performed and the algorithm does not account for ambiguous regions, whose resolution requires additional computations. As such, the PC algorithm is able to direct more edges than the NPC algorithm; yet the PC algorithm tends to generate more randomly directed arcs than the NPC [Madsen et al., 2003].

Other BN structure learning algorithms have been developed based on scoring functions and search procedures rather than on testing for conditional independence [Acid et al., 2004]. These algorithms attempt to find the DAG that maximizes a predefined selected score. These methods start with an initial DAG and, at each step, local changes in the form of arc addition, deletion, and/or reversal are tested until a local maximum of the scoring function is reached. The score is usually defined as a measure of fit between the graph and the data. Scores include the use of entropy, the Minimum Description Length (MDL), and Bayesian approaches [Acid et al., 2004].

Few studies in the environmental and ecological fields have opted for the use of structure learning. In their paper, Alameddine et al. [2011] adopted the NPC algorithm and then attempted to resolve the ambiguous arcs with substantive knowledge. Then they consulted the generated Akaike information criterion (AIC) and Bayesian information criterion (BIC) scores, statistics used to evaluate model fit, in an effort to generate a more parsimonious model (fewer arcs). Finally, they examined the mutual information $(I(X; Y))$ to remove additional arcs if their mutual information showed that the arc contributed little to the goal of their model. Mutual information, as reported in Hugin, represents the information shared by nodes X and Y. Thus the mutual information tells us how much knowledge of X reduces our uncertainty concerning Y. Correspondingly, if X and Y are independent, then knowing X tells us nothing about Y, then $I(X; Y) = 0$.

Interestingly, most steps taken during the structure learning process for BN models are not Bayesian. Moreover, once the model is proposed and accepted, it is assumed to be true without any uncertainty associated with its structure. Prior beliefs can be introduced by adding hard constraints (connections) between nodes or by restricting connectivity between model nodes. Unfortunately, in most applications the model structure is never revisited once new data are acquired. Only the CPTs implied by the existing model structure are updated by the new data.

Overall, opting for the implementation of structure learning when developing a BN model should be taken with care, as depending on the DAG and the associated node states in the model, the resulting model size may have data requirements that exceed the ones at hand and as such, the structure learning accuracy can be compromised [Kashuba, 2010]. For example, this situation was one of the main reasons why we ended up with the inferior model structures generated by the PC and NPC algorithm given the limited Ohio stream data (89 complete data points). de Campos and Castellano [2007] found that in many instances both the PC and NPC algorithms couldn't re-create the model structure from which the simulated data were sampled. Additionally, Alameddine et al. [2011] found that both algorithms were sensitive to the binning process adopted as we will discuss later on. In fact, Uusitalo [2007] has questioned the validity of using structure learning in the environmental and ecological field altogether, given the inherent complex environmental interactions, which often lead to large variabilities and uncertainties that preclude the ability to reliably infer the structure of the process based on collected data sets. Pollino et al. [2007] proposed a hybrid system that tries to combine real data with the elicited information when field data are available. They proposed a knowledge engineering-based method for parameterizing and evaluating a BN. Yet, in most cases, structure learning is done through a combination of domain expert knowledge and mining the collected observational data [Madsen et al., 2003].

7.1.1.2 Populating the CPTs

All nodes in a BN are associated with a CPT. The CPT is simply a table that has one probability for every possible combination of parent and child states. CPTs for parent nodes describe the marginal probability distribution of those nodes, as a function of the adopted discretization. For child nodes, the CPTs represent the probabilities that a given state in the child node occurs, conditional on every possible combination of the states defined for its parents. This means that the number of parameters in the CPT for a child node is exponential to the number of its parents. For example, a simple BN model with three nodes $(A \rightarrow C \leftarrow B)$, each with three states $(a_1, a_2, a_3; b_1, b_2, b_3, c_1, c_2, c_3)$, has three CPTs, one for each node. The CPTs for the two parent nodes $(A$ and $B)$ consist of simplexes of three probabilities for the three states (i.e., $\{\Pr(a_1), \Pr(a_2), \Pr(a_3)\}$ and $\{\Pr(b_1), \Pr(b_2), \Pr(b_3)\}$). The CPT for node C consists of nine sets of simplex of conditional probabilities of the three states, one for each unique combination of the two parent node states. That is, $\Pr(c_1 \mid a_i, b_j), \Pr(c_1 \mid a_i, b_j), \Pr(c_1 \mid a_i, b_j)$ for $i = 1, 2, 3$ and $j = 1, 2, 3$. Populating the CPTs of a BN is an arduous task that often drives environmental modelers away from using BNs. CPTs are often constructed based on data and/or domain expert knowledge. Moreover, these two sources of knowledge can be fused together, making use of the properties of the Dirichlet distribution.

Expert Elicitation

Eliciting the probabilities of CPTs from experts is a long and arduous process, particularly as the size of the model increases (both in terms of the number of nodes and the number of states in each node). As such, the size of the model and the resulting number of CPT entries to be elicited should be kept reasonably low in an effort to reduce the elicitation burden [Rohmer, 2020]. There are two types of expert elicitations to populate CPTs, the direct and the indirect elicitation. Direct elicitation employs asking experts questions such as "What is the probability that variable A takes a given state knowing that its parents have taken these values?" The elicitation process can also ask experts to provide frequencies or odds rather than probabilities, as most experts may not feel comfortable giving probabilities. Another option that has been used is the adoption of qualitative elicitation, where experts are asked to provide answers using terms such as "almost certainly," "fifty-fifty chance," or it is "impossible" to describe the probability of a given state in the child node, given that we know the states of the parents (Rohmer 2020). Yet, this type of elicitation requires an additional step of mapping these responses to actual probabilities that are needed for the CPTs. This mapping can be done using fuzzy sets [Zadeh, 1975]. Several BN models have adopted this technique [D'Angelo et al., 2014, Zhang et al., 2016]. Yet, this process involves uncertainties that are introduced by the mapping and that are often left unrecognized and unquantified [Woodberry et al., 2005]. Another direct approach of expert elicitation is based on eliciting probabilities based on pairwise comparisons. Chin et al. [2009] adapted the Analytical Hierarchy Process method developed by Saaty [1990] to elicit the parameters of CPTs from experts. Their method attempted to elicit pairwise comparisons about the relative likelihood of possible events using predefined scores instead of directly asking the experts to provide probability values for each entry in the CPT. Yet, this method results in a significant increase in the number of comparisons as the number of conditional probabilities increases.

Kashuba [2010] adapted the direct fixed value elicitation method proposed by Clemen [1996] to apply to multinomial elicitations, following the Stanford Research Institute Elicitation Protocol [Spetzler and Stael von Holstein, 1975] in an effort to minimize bias and error. Her method included five steps:

1. establishing motivation and rapport,

2. structuring and the definition of uncertain qualities,

3. conditioning through nudging the experts to think about all the evidence,

4. encoding and quantifying the expert judgment, and finally

5. validating and verifying the elicited probabilities.

Indirect methods of expert elicitation also exist but they are less commonly used. These include the Filling-up methods and the use of the Noisy-OR gates [Rohmer, 2020]. Yet, these methods have not been adopted in environmental and ecological applications.

Whatever elicitation process is adopted, care should be taken so as to ensure that no zero probabilities are assigned to any entry within the CPT. Assigning a zero probability is congruent to stating that this event cannot occur with 100% certainty. This strong proclamation leads to an inability to update the CPT with data as a result of the application of Bayes' theorem with a prior set to zero. It is therefore essential that experts are made aware that zero should only be assigned for impossible events and not for highly unlikely outcomes [Kashuba, 2010].

One commonly overlooked step in the elicitation process is the elicitation of prior weights. While these weights do not affect the elicited prior CPTs themselves, they are an integral part of the Bayesian updating of the probabilities within the CPTs. Often the weights should be elicited in terms of units of equivalent data points. Kashuba [2010] tested three different methods of expert prior weight elicitation including (1) direct elicitation, (2) hypothetical sample [Winkler, 2003], and (3) probability range [Cowell, 1999, Nielsen and Jensen, 2009]. She reported that the probability range elicitation method showed the lowest within-method variability and the most consistent prior weights among the model nodes. Additionally, the experts that undertook the three types of elicitation preferred it to the other methods, especially since they thought that being asked to report ranges expressed their uncertainty more intuitively and accurately than reporting equivalent data points for the priors.

CPTs from Data

The CPT of a BN can be learned from a set of previously observed cases assuming that these cases are a random sample from the population we are modeling. In this case, we can assume that the frequencies observed in the collected data approximate the desired vector of probabilities for a given node [Company, 2010]. This approach is considered to be a purely data-driven approach that works most of the time under data rich contexts. This method corresponds to finding the maximum likelihood estimation (MLE) for each entry in the CPT. The MLE aims at maximizing the log-likelihood function of θ given D [Rohmer, 2020].

$$L(\theta|D) = \log(P(D|\theta)) = \sum_{i,j,k} N_{i,j,k} \log(\theta_{i,j,k}),$$

for which the MLE is $\frac{N_{i,j,k}}{N_{i,j}}$, where $N_{i,j}$ is the total number of records found in the data for which the parents $pa(X_i)$ are in a given set of states j and where $N_{i,j,k}$ is the data record available for which the node of interest (X_i) is in state k and its parents $pa(X_i)$ are in the state j. Complications arise when the data are not complete and include missing values. This is often dealt with using Expectation–Maximization (EM) [Dempster et al., 1977] and/or Gibbs sampling [Geman and Geman, 1984]. Both methods assume that the values are missing at random. The Hugin Expert software implements the EM method to estimate the conditional probability tables of discrete chance nodes and the conditional probability densities of continuous chance nodes. Yet, Hugin allows the user to provide prior knowledge about the conditional distributions for the variables in the model. The inclusion of prior knowledge before the CPT learning step ensures that the resulting probabilities will be based on both the prior knowledge and the data. Weight on the prior knowledge is inserted by specifying the previous experience through an equivalent number of data counts. That number is used to weight the prior information against the cases coming in through the collected data files.

7.1.1.3 Discretization and Its Impacts on a BN

Most environmental variables are continuous, taking real values or integer values. They are best described by continuous distribution functions (e.g., normal, lognormal, gamma distributions) or by count distributions (e.g., Poisson, negative binomial). Yet, most BN inference algorithms can only work with categorical data. This makes data discretization a required step when implementing BNs in the environmental/ecological field. In a review of BN applications in the environmental field, Aguilera et al. [2011] reported that

53% of all published BN applications used discrete data to build their models, while 31% resorted to a discretization method to convert their continuous data into discrete classes.

Discretization invariably results in a loss of information and can thus impact model inference and decision-making. Yet, some of its benefits include substantially increasing information propagation in the model, providing an intuitive graphical interface, and improving the parameterizability of complex, multivariate relationships that would have been prohibitive to describe with unknown continuous functions [Kashuba, 2010]. It is important that the full implications of data discretization not be overlooked in environmental studies. The impact that discretization may have on information loss has been highlighted by several studies that recommended a verification process to ensure that the conclusions made are not an artifact of the adopted discretization approach [Alameddine et al., 2011, Ames et al., 2005, Death et al., 2015, Dlamini, 2010, Nojavan A. et al., 2017].

While increasing the number of states defined for a given node will result in a better characterization of the marginal distribution of the data in that node, this needs to be done while accounting for the amount of data available for building the CPTs of the BN model. As such, one has to ensure that the CPT resulting from the discretization process does not lead to sparse entries. The size of the CPT for a node increases multiplicatively as the number of bins increases either in the node itself or in one of its parents (equation (7.5)).

$$\text{CPT}_{\text{size}} = N_{\text{Bins}} \times \prod_{i=1}^{n} N_{\text{parent}_i} \tag{7.5}$$

where N_{Bins} is the number of bins in the actual node, n is the number of parents affecting the node, and N_{parent_i} is the number of states for the ith parent node.

Therefore care must be taken to ensure that the size of the CPTs in a BN model remains significantly less than the amount of data available, while also respecting the dispersion of the data and ensuring that all resulting states are well covered by the available data. Beuzen et al. [2018] discussed how the performance of a BN model can suffer when the number of states increases beyond the available data, with CPTs suffering from the sparse data needed to develop the implied conditional relationships. As such, it can be important to try to keep the number of states as low as possible to account for the need to populate the CPTs from the collected data [Chen and Pollino, 2012, Forio et al., 2015].

As an example of how the size of the model increases as a function of the number of nodes and states, the structure proposed by Qian and Miltner [2015] that has 9 nodes and 11 edges will have a total CPT of 429 entries if all nodes are restricted to three states. Should discretized variables be used for the BN model, the chlorophyll-a node alone would have a CPT with 81 entries. However, sample size is only 109. Clearly, discretization in such a case is not recommended, as there is a high risk of introducing sparse entries if the CPTs are learned from the data. As a result, Qian and Miltner [2015] developed a continuous variable BN (cBN).

The process of discretizing the data, both in terms of defining the number of states and their associated cutoffs, is often based on reported literature, natural thresholds, software defaults, statistical modeling, mathematical methods, or stakeholders' elicitation [Keshtkar et al., 2013, Phan et al., 2016, Sperotto et al., 2017]. Interestingly, Aguilera et al. [2011] reported that around half of all published environmental BN studies didn't discuss their adopted discretization process. Moreover, around one fourth of all studies reported resorting to expert elicitation and less than 10% of the papers used either equal intervals (3%), equal quantiles (3%), or software defaults (2.9%).

Methods of Discretization

Expert elicitation is the most commonly used method adopted for the discretization of continuous data in BN applications. Several studies have opted to use experts to help them discretize their continuous data [Dlamini, 2010]. Woodberry et al. [2005] proposed that experts be elicited for the acceptable ranges for the parameters. They proposed asking experts to provide 95% confidence intervals for capturing the desired parameters. While this appears to be a straightforward method, several questions remain, particularly related to how many experts should be sought, how to normalize the data collected from different experts, and how to formulate the questions posed to the experts [Vilizzi et al., 2013]. Most often, expert elicitations are through focus groups or aggregated by several mathematical and behavioral approaches such as those outlined by Clemen and Winkler [1999]. Yet, it has been shown that no single expert elicitation combination process is best across all circumstances [Clemen and Winkler, 1999]. As such, expert elicitation remains an open area of research.

Probably the best approach to discretize continuous data is to account for natural agreed-upon thresholds and/or significant cutoffs with management implications. These cutoffs can incorporate environmental standards (e.g., dissolved oxygen levels above 4 mg/L; TMDL defined loads), agreed-upon definitions of environmental states (e.g., Carlson's trophic index; stratification status; environmental flows; salinity levels), or modeled environmental thresholds (refer to Section 7.2). Unfortunately, most nodes in a BN lack this correspondence to significant cutoffs.

Kashuba [2010] adopted a three-step process for discretization. She first asked the experts whether there were any thresholds of ecological or environmental significance that can be mapped to a low, medium-low, medium-high, or high state for any of the chosen continuous model variables. For variables that lacked clear thresholds, the data were split into quartiles (i.e., equal frequency in each bin). Lastly, starting from the a priori threshold and quartile bin definitions, the final bin endpoints were refined via expert elicitation that occurred in tandem with the elicitation of the CPTs.

A significant number of BN models opt for software defaults such as the use of equal intervals or equal quantiles [Aguilera et al., 2011]. Both of these methods are implemented by most BN software [Aguilera et al., 2011, Chen and Pollino, 2012]. The equal interval method of discretization is ideal when the data distribution is roughly uniformly distributed over its natural range [Nojavan A. et al., 2017]. While equal intervals can retain the natural distribution of the data (the frequency), they are sensitive and can often be skewed by a few extremes, especially when the node in question represents a process that is known to follow a skewed distribution. This can often result in very few states (sometimes even one) holding most of the data and the remaining ones having to be populated by a sparse set of realizations. This sparseness is compounded if the variable in question is also a child node to several parents. Furthermore, the equal interval discretization is not invariant to nonlinear transformations and thus decisions on variable transformation will impact interval definition and thus final model results.

Meanwhile, the adoption of equal quantiles for discretization guarantees that the marginal data are equally spread between the defined states. This discretization approach is often suitable for data with clearly defined modes [Nojavan A. et al., 2017] as the actual magnitude of each observations is irrelevant, with the exception of allowing for the relative ordering of the observations. Hence, equal frequency (quantile) discretization is unaffected by transformations of the data. Yet, this comes at the risk of eroding and muting the impact of extremes as these are lumped with more mediocre data, which can have major implications on the utility of the model, where predictions of the probabilities of extreme events are often of interest.

In addition to these default methods of discretization, several studies have proposed alternative methods of discretization such as the moment-matching discretization method proposed by Nojavan A. et al. [2017] and the supervised discretization approach recommended by Beuzen et al. [2018]. In the moment-matching discretization method, the moments of the generated discretized distribution for a pre-selected number of states are matched to the moments of the continuous data by applying a set of moment equations. These equations include the mean along with the higher-order central moments. The number of moment equations that need to be solved increases with the number of discrete states defined for that node. While the discrete distribution becomes a more accurate approximation of the continuous distribution as the number of states increases, the number of moment-matching equations that need to be solved increases by a factor of $(2 \times s - 1)$, where s is the number of states predefined for that node. Under this approach, the location of the breaks will be determined using non-convex nonlinear optimization. As such, solutions become intractable as the number of break points (states) exceeds four [Nojavan A. et al., 2017]. Additionally the number of states will most often be limited by the available data and the need to guarantee an adequate number of cases in each of the predefined states.

The supervised discretization approach recommended by Beuzen et al. [2018] attempts to optimize the discretization of the parent nodes of an already discrete child node by minimization entropy. Yet, this approach requires that the child node is itself discrete. If not, then it will need to be discretized by one the above-mentioned methods prior to the implementation of this approach. Two supervised classifiers were tested by Beuzen et al. [2018], namely the Fayyad & Irani (F&I) [Fayyad and Irani, 1993] and Kononenko (KO) [Kononenko, 1995] algorithm. Both classifiers are available in R under the packages RWeka [Hornik et al., 2009], discretization [Kim, 2012] and FSelectorRcpp [Zawadzki and Kosinski, 2021].

Several studies have tried to compare the performance of different discretization methods. However, the studies have found that none of the methods consistently outperformed all others across a set of comparison criteria. As such, these studies have recommended caution when discretization was to be implemented [Beuzen et al., 2018, Nojavan A. et al., 2017]. Moreover, these studies have also shown that most of these discretization methods will end up with states that often lack a physical meaning [Beuzen et al., 2018]. A dynamic discretization method has been proposed by Neil et al. [2007] specifically to perform inference in hybrid BNs that include both continuous and discrete variables.

As expected, the choice of the discretization method has great impact on the model structure generated by the structure learning algorithms. Figures 7.4-7.9 show the different model structures generated for the Ohio stream data from Qian and Miltner [2015], using different discretization methods. We note that the data used to learn the structure was limited to 109 cases, which is relatively small when the discretization at each node is fixed to three levels. Given the large differences in structure, it is expected that predictions and the inference gained by these different models will significantly differ. Nojavan A. et al. [2017] reported significant differences in model predictions for their simple chlorophyll-a BN model even when the model structure was fixed and only the number of bins and/or the method of discretization was varied. Ultimately, these discrepancies in predictions and inference are a result of differing CPTs, as CPTs define the underlying relations among variables post discretization.

Continuous BN

There have been several attempts to allow for the inclusion of continuous variables within the BN modeling framework. Some efforts have attempted to include continuous nodes as part of a BN model that is dominated by discrete nodes. Others have attempted to develop a framework that completely overcomes the need for discretization. Each of these methods has their advantages and limitations as summarized below.

Implementation in Hugin

Hugin allows for the partial inclusion of continuous random variables in

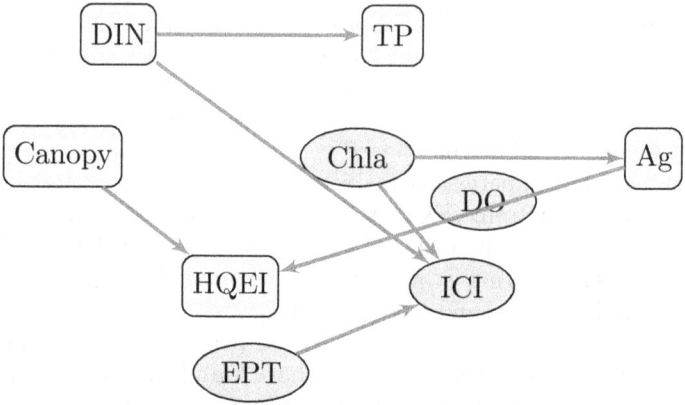

FIGURE 7.4: Impact of structure learning and binning on the structure of the BN model for the Ohio stream data – PC algorithm and equal interval.

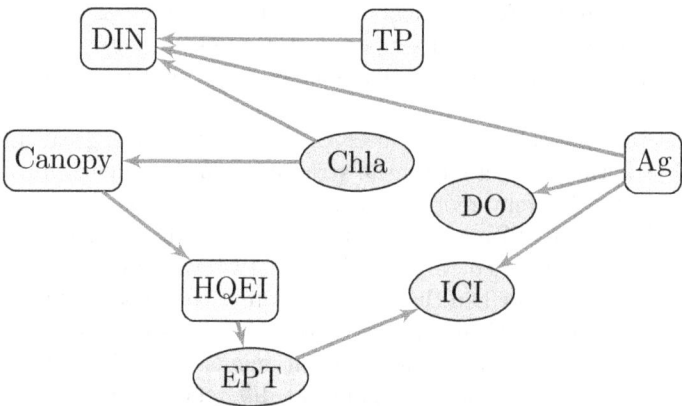

FIGURE 7.5: Impact of structure learning and binning on the structure of the BN model for the Ohio stream data – PC algorithm and equal frequency.

the BN model if they are normally distributed. Yet, the inclusion of these Gaussian continuous nodes is restricted by a set of rules. For example, discrete variables in a BN model are not allowed to have continuous parents; yet continuous variables can have discrete or continuous Gaussian parents. Moreover, creating the CPT for a continuous node is a demanding task. Given that continuous variables are limited to be Gaussian, Hugin requires only the specification of the sufficient statistics for that node, namely its mean and variance. While this is a trivial task for parent nodes, it is challenging when the parents of the continuous node are discrete. In that case, a mean and variance must be assigned to each unique combination of the states of the discrete parents. In the event that the continuous Gaussian mode is a child

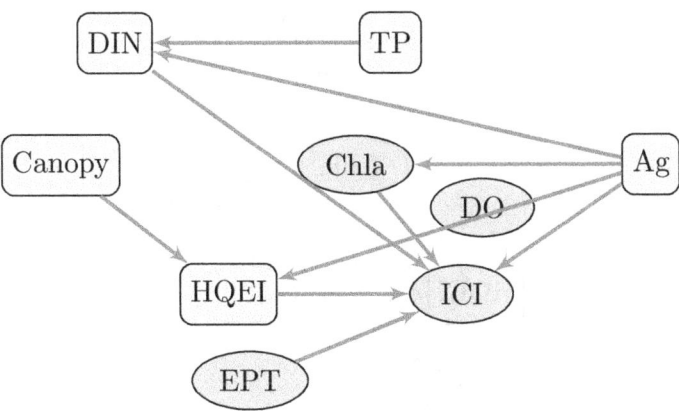

FIGURE 7.6: Impact of structure learning and binning on the structure of the BN model for the Ohio stream data – NPC algorithm and equal interval.

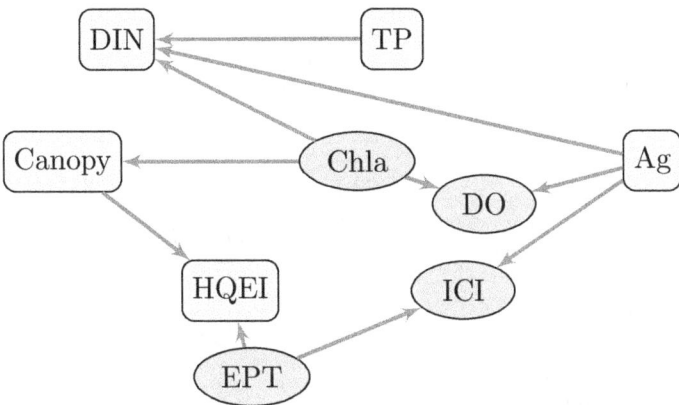

FIGURE 7.7: Impact of structure learning and binning on the structure of the BN model for the Ohio stream data – NPC algorithm and equal frequency.

node to a mixed parent (some are Gaussian and other are discrete) then a regression coefficient for each continuous parent for each configuration of the states of the discrete parents will need to be defined. Thus the distribution for a continuous variable Y that has a discrete parent X and a continuous parent Z is a (one-dimensional) Gaussian distribution conditional on the values of the parents [Hugin Expert, 2021]. This is congruent to specifying a separate regression model for each unique combination of the discrete parents. The regression models can thus have separate intercepts, slopes, and errors; yet they must share the same functional form. Only the mean of the continuous Gaussian child node depends linearly on the continuous parent nodes, while the variance is assumed to be constant for each state of the discrete parent(s).

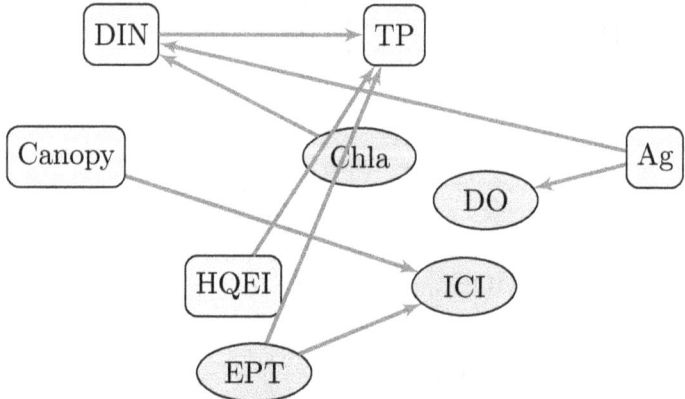

FIGURE 7.8: Impact of structure learning and binning on the structure of the BN model for the Ohio stream data – PC algorithm and equal interval with log transformation.

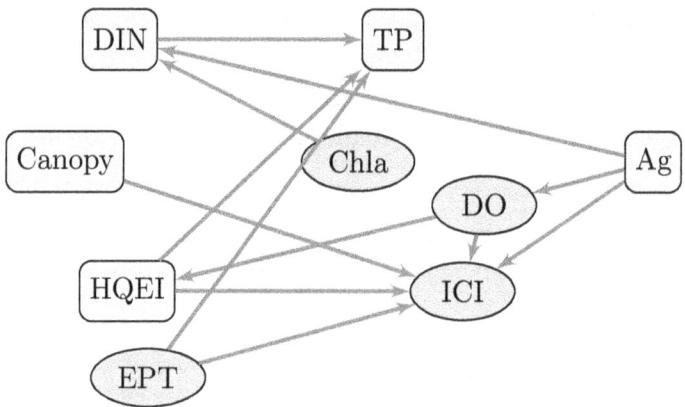

FIGURE 7.9: Impact of structure learning and binning on the structure of the BN model for the Ohio stream data – NPC algorithm and equal interval with log transformations.

Finally, if a continuous node has one or more continuous parents, then the means of each of its states will be linearly dependent on the states of these continuous parents.

$$\Pr\left(Y \mid X = x, Z = z\right) = N\left(\alpha_i + \beta(x)^T z; \sigma(x)^2\right)$$

Implementation in R and Stan; Gibbs Sampling

Several attempts have been made to build continuous variable BN models using Monte Carlo simulation, Gibbs sampler or more generally Markov chain Monte Carlo simulations [Borsuk et al., 2004, Qian and Miltner, 2015]. These methods replace the need to define conditional probability distributions needed for the model's CPT tables with specifying marginal distributions on parents and conditional distributions on children. Figure 7.10 shows the conceptual model structure for the Ohio Stream data as defined by Qian and Miltner [2015].

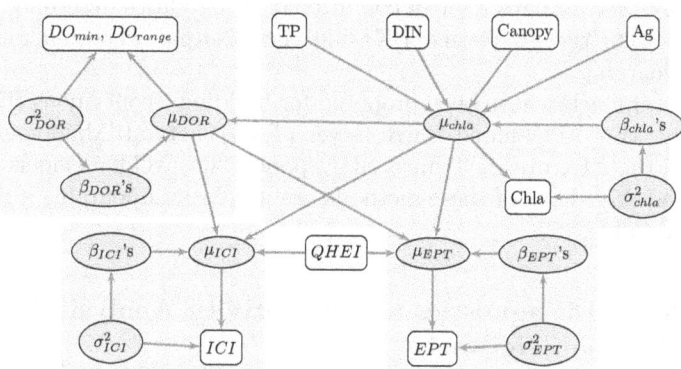

FIGURE 7.10: Continuous BN for the Ohio stream water quality data developed by Qian and Miltner [2015] (Figure 4).

The structure implies a set of regression equation as shown below:

$$
\begin{aligned}
\log(chla) &\sim N(\mu_{chla}, \sigma^2_{chla}) \\
\mu_{chla} &= \beta^{chla}_0 + \beta^{chla}_1 \log(DIN) + \beta^{chla}_2 \log(TP) + \beta^{chla}_3 \text{logit}(Ag) \\
&\quad + \beta^{chla}_4 \log(Canopy) \\
\log\left(\frac{DO_{\min}}{DO_{\max}}\right) &\sim N(\mu_{DOR}, \sigma^2_{DOR}) \\
\mu_{DOR} &= \beta^{DO}_0 + \beta^{DO}_1 I(\log(Chla) - \phi) \times (\log(Chla) - \phi) \\
\log(EPT) &\sim N(\mu_{EPT}, \sigma^2_{EPT}) \\
\mu_{EPT} &= \beta^{EPT}_0 + \beta^{EPT}_1 \mu_{Chla} + \beta^{EPT}_2 \mu_{DOR} + \beta^{EPT}_3 QHEI \\
ICI &\sim N(\mu_{ICI}, \sigma^2_{ICI}) \\
\mu_{ICI} &= \beta^{ICI}_0 + \beta^{ICI}_1 \mu_{Chla} + \beta^{ICI}_2 \mu_{DOR} + \beta^{ICI}_3 QHEI.
\end{aligned}
$$

One of the main advantages of this approach is that it does not require the discretization of the variables in the model. Variables are connected through a series of linear and non-linear models, whose parameters are simultaneously estimated using the Gibbs sampler. Furthermore, continuous and categorical variables can be mixed in the model [Qian et al., 2021a, e.g.]. Once the joint distribution is quantified, statistical inference can be conducted through Monte Carlo simulations. The structure of these continuous BN models allows them to be updated seamlessly over time as new data becomes available.

While these models have the potential to have an attractive directed acyclic diagram associated with them, computational overhead limits their ability to be used effectively as decision making tools by non-modelers. Moreover, these approaches require that the structural form of the model is predefined and parameterized, often as a linear model and less commonly as a non-linear model.

In an effort to showcase differences between the discretized and the continuous BN, we compare a set of conditional probabilities determined by the continuous BN, the discretized BN, and the BN that were generated from structure learning.

Other approaches have been proposed for building a continuous BN. These include the Tree Augmented Naive Bayes (TAN) method [Maldonado et al., 2016] and the Mixture of Truncated Exponentials (MTE) models [Ropero et al., 2014]. Yet, both of these methods are not easily updatable if new data become available.

7.1.2   Model Diagnostics and Sensitivity Analysis for Bayesian Networks

Like all models, BNs require model diagnostics to assess the sensitivity of the models to findings and to quantify their predictive performance. Typically, a BN model's sensitivity and performance should be evaluated both quantitatively and qualitatively including the sensitivity to findings (how the posterior probability distributions (PPDs) change under different conditions) and the sensitivity to parameters (which measures how PPDs change, when input variables are modified) [Chen and Pollino, 2012, Moe et al., 2016, Pollino et al., 2007, Radl et al., 2018].

7.1.2.1   Sensitivity to Findings

The sensitivity to findings assesses the relative influence of collecting evidence in one node on the outcome of another node(s). This is possible given the d-separation properties associated with BN models. The influence of the nodes on the outcome is often described relatively and aims to provide guidance to help prioritize future data collection, check on whether the model reflects the domain experts' intuitions, and identify the main driver nodes in the model. Sensitivity to findings is quantified using two types of measures, entropy and mutual information.

The entropy of a node $(H(X) - \sum_x \Pr(X) \log(\Pr(X)))$ is commonly used to evaluate the uncertainty, or randomness, of a given probability distribution. It measures how much of the probability mass is scattered around the states of a given node. Maximum entropy is achieved when the probability mass function is distributed uniformly across all states. Under such conditions, entropy will reach a value of $\log(n)$. On the other end, when all the mass is within one state, entropy is 0.

We are often interested in assessing the entropy at a node, given a set of observations we have witnessed in the other nodes. The entropy of a variable X given introducing evidence at variable Y is given by:

$$H(X|Y) = H(X) - I(X|Y)$$

and

$$I(X \mid Y) = \sum_Y \Pr(Y) \sum_X \Pr(X|Y) \times \log\left(\frac{\Pr(X,Y)}{\Pr(X) \times \Pr(Y)}\right)$$

where $I(X \mid Y)$ is the mutual information (MI) of X and Y, representing the information shared by X and Y. It represents a way to measure the value of observing Y when it comes to reducing the uncertainty in X. MI can thus be used to identify the input nodes that are associated with the most informative connections regarding the set of target nodes in a given BN. Nodes with larger MI values between them have a stronger link between their variables. As such, it is common to rank the MI values for a specified set of target nodes of interest, given a set of evidence introduced to a set of observed nodes. This assessment is often referred to as assessing the sensitivity to findings by quantifying the value of information (VOI) [Marcot, 2012, Pollino et al., 2007, Radl et al., 2018]. The VOI will thus identify the variables with the highest MI with respect to a selected target node. The VOI ranges between 0 and 1, with lower values associated with mutually independent variables and higher values associated with more informative variables [Pollino et al., 2007]. The VOI analysis is often implemented on the main model endpoint node. As Woodberry et al. [2005] indicated, the MI can be used by the domain experts to assess if a given endpoint in the model is either too sensitive or insensitive to other nodes and thus it can help identify errors in the defined model structure or in the generated CPTs.

Implementing the concept of entropy on the equal frequency discretized version of the Qian and Miltner [2015] model, the entropy for ICI and EPT were both equal to 1.09. The MI between the three immediate parent nodes for ICI and EPT (CHLA, QHEI, and DOR) ranged between 0.03 and 0.08, indicating that information collected on chlorophyll-a, QHEI, and DOR provide little information on the final states of the response variables (Table 7.2). This is to be expected, as most of these links were not proposed by the two structure learning algorithms.

Sensitivity to Parameters

The sensitivity to parameters (also known as influence analysis) can be evaluated either by quantifying changes in the posterior probability distributions of the target nodes when the parent nodes are altered [Marcot, 2012, Nojavan A. et al., 2014, Pollino et al., 2007] or by computing the posterior probability certainty index (PPCI) that was proposed by Marcot [2012]. For example if we compare the changes in the posterior probability of having high ICI (>50) or high EPT (>19) values as a function of changes made to the

TABLE 7.2: Entropy and mutual information of the Ohio stream equal frequency BN.

Parameter	ICI	EPT
Entropy	1.09	1.09
Mutual information		
CHLA	0.04	0.04
QHEI	0.07	0.08
DOR	0.06	0.03

states of their parents (Figure 7.11), it becomes apparent that the high ICI state is largely equally sensitive to the three parents. Meanwhile, the high EPT state appears to be sensitive mostly to changes in QHEI and DOR and least to CHLA. The one-sample Kolmogorov-Smirnov (KS) non-parametric test can also be used on the PPDs to determine if introducing evidence in one of the parent nodes results in a statistically significant change in the PPD of the target node as compared to the normative case [Marcot, 2012]. Conducting the KS test on the PPDs of the ICI and EPT nodes after changing the states of one of their three parents indicated that providing evidence through the parents did not statistically change the PPDs of the two target nodes. This is a further indication of the weak sensitivity between EPT and ICI on one hand and their parents on the other.

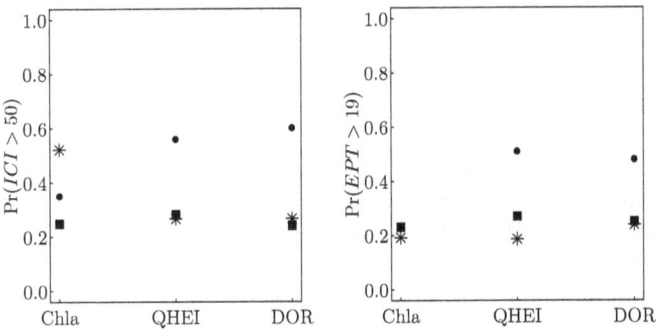

FIGURE 7.11: Probability of ICI and EPT to be in the high interval as a function of the states of their parents. Squares represent the probability associated with the evidence being in the highest interval for the parent; the circle is when the evidence is in the medium range of the parent; the star is when the evidence is at the lowest interval of the parent.

The PPCI metric was first proposed by Marcot [2012]. PPCI quantifies the entropy level for a given node. It can be used to evaluate the uncertainty of model outcomes through indexing the degree of dispersion of their posterior probability values among the outcome states after normalization with the number of states and possible minimum and maximum values. The PPCI is calculated as shown in Equation (7.6). The PPCI values range between 0 and 1; higher values suggest greater certainty in outcome predictions and more concentrated posteriors. Given that the PPCI is normalized in terms of the numbers of outcome states in a node, it can be used to compare the sensitivity to parameters across different models. Figure 7.12 represents the different PPCI values for the Ohio stream equal frequency BN that was based on the Qian and Miltner [2015] proposed model structure. In the absence of any evidence, the PPCIs for both ICI and EPT are close to 0, indicating high uncertainty in the predictions. Entering evidence in any of the parent nodes improves the PPCI marginally; yet the PPCI remains below 0.2. Only when evidence is provided in all three parent nodes does the PPCI significantly increase. It reaches one when the chlorophyll-a is set to low while QHEI and DOR are set to high. Under that combination, the model's prediction is to expect high ICI and EPT with 100% certainty.

$$
\begin{aligned}
PPCI &= 1 - \frac{H'}{H'_{max}} \\
H' &= -\sum_{i=1}^{N} p_i \times L \\
H'_{max} &= \log(N)
\end{aligned}
\tag{7.6}
$$

where $L = \begin{cases} \log(p_i); & p_i > 0 \\ 0; & p_i = 0 \end{cases}$.

7.1.2.2 Model Validation

The validation of BNs remains to date a major challenge and shortcoming of most environmental BN models, largely due to data scarcity and the dependence of the model (or parts of it) on expert judgment. Validation is thus often restricted to rigorous peer review and model reconciliation through a qualitative assessment of model resilience against changes of inputs [Moe et al., 2016]. Other studies have attempted to validate models through assessing their hindcast skills [Marcot, 2012]. Even when data are available, the ability to conduct cross-validation is often limited given the increase in model size and the associated data needed to fully parameterize the CPTs. As such and while several validation approaches have been proposed (e.g., error rates and confusion tables, area under (ROC) curve, k-fold cross validation, spherical payoff, Schwartz's Bayesian Information Criterion, Cohen's Cappa) and some have even been successfully implemented in several of the major BN commercial software [Marcot, 2012], model validation remains infrequent [Aguilera et al., 2011, Barton et al., 2008, Moe et al., 2016].

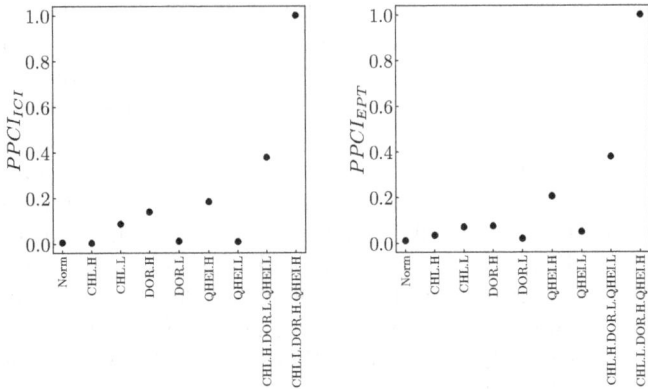

FIGURE 7.12: The posterior probability certainty index (PPCI; 1 = full certainty, 0 = full uncertainty) for the posterior probability distributions of *ICI and EPT*, under normative (Norm) and under selected influence analysis scenarios. CHL is chlorophyll-a; DOR is dissolved oxygen ratio; QHEI is the habitat quality index; H corresponds to setting the parent to its highest state in the BN; L corresponds to setting the parent node to its lowest state in the BN.

7.1.3   Spatio-temporal BN

In environmental and ecological applications, accounting for space and time are often critical steps in any modeling framework [Carpenter et al., 2009]. Most BN applications do not explicitly account for space or time correlations in their models. As a matter of fact, the geographical and temporal scale(s) are often specified implicitly [Barton et al., 2008]. Thus, one has to ensure that the adopted spatio-temporal domain aligns with the identified core management problem(s) it is trying to address [Marcot, 2012, Pollino and Henderson, 2010]. Recent advances in BNs have allowed for a better integration of spatial, temporal, or even spatio-temporal data in the BN models; yet their full integration is still limited. Many of these advances became possible due to the advancement of Object-Oriented Bayesian Networks (OOBN) that expanded the capabilities of traditional BN by allowing them to connect to other networks [Molina et al., 2013].

The seamless integration of time in BNs remains an active research topic and its advancement will certainly increase the penetration of BNs in the environmental field, given that most environmental variables experience significant changes over time and have temporal autocorrelations. The integration of time in BNs is relatively new as most BNs are developed as static models [Uusitalo, 2007]. Several methods have been proposed to allow for the integration of time within a BN model. For example, dynamic BNs (DBNs) have been proposed and successfully used to model time series data. Rachid et al.

[2021] recently used the concept of the DBN to model saltwater intrusion and its expected socioeconomic impacts in a coastal aquifer over 20 years, while accounting for the variabilities and uncertainties of climate change, urbanization, demand and supply management, and population growth. DBNs are now implemented across several BN software, including Hugin [Hugin Expert, 2021]. They work by implementing the concept of "time-slicing." In DBNs, some links in the network are considered to represent the effect of time for the variables they connect [Das and Ghosh, 2020]. DBNs create individual BN models for each time slice and allow for the realization of selected variables at a given time to be dependent on their previous state, while maintaining the same DAG and node relationships throughout the time slices [Marcot and Penman, 2019, Hugin Expert, 2021]. The variables that are connected across the time slices are known as temporal clones; they represent the interface between two successive time slices in the model [Rachid et al., 2021, Hugin Expert, 2021]. These connections across time slices allow for updating the probabilities of the states for all nodes including the clone nodes once information is introduced to any time slice. Clone nodes can thus transmit their updated states to their clone in the next time slice so that the BN of the next time slice will estimate the updated probabilities of all nodes accounting for the carried input from the previous time slice [Rachid et al., 2021]. One of the main limitations of the DBN methodology is the large number of entries needed to fill the CPTs. This often causes the models to run slowly. As such, this method is largely suitable when the time steps are coarse and limited.

Another method that incorporates temporal dependency in a BN model is the use of the Bayesian Network with Residual Correction (BNRC) method. The BNRC method has shown to be useful when the number of influencing variables is reasonably small. The BNRC trains individual BN models for each time step and generates the needed CPTs. Predictions and the associated marginal and conditional probabilities are then made through temporally weighted predictions from each of the fitted BN models. Weights are determined in terms of how far away the prediction is from each specific BN for a given year. This approach adopts temporal autocorrelation, whereby it assumes that inter-variable relationships in the prediction year are expected to be more similar to those closer in time [Das and Ghosh, 2020].

The inclusion of space in BNs is challenging. Most environmental and ecological applications do not explicitly incorporate space and disregard neighborhood effects and spatial interactions. Some environmental BNs attempted to account for space indirectly by incorporating parent nodes that hold relevant information to describe the space being modeled. Yet, the introduction of representative nodes corresponding to each spatial location within the model will result in a complicated causal dependency graphical structure that consists of a large number of nodes and edges. These structures will require a large set of data to fill their resulting CPTs [Das and Ghosh, 2020].

Other methods have been proposed to deal more efficiently with space within the context of a BN. Many of these methods are restricted to raster data, whereby inference in the BN model is implemented at the pixel level [Stritih et al., 2020]. Das and Ghosh [2020] proposed the SpaBN to model spatial data. A SpaBN model is made of a combination of typical BN nodes as well as a set of composite nodes. The latter are a set of nodes that represent the same variable but at different spatial locations. The size of the composite node is as large as the spatial domain of the model. These composite nodes can help diminish the learning time and space complexity of the spatial Bayesian network model [Das and Ghosh, 2020]. As such, the SpaBN models are ill-constructed to work with raster data. Their framework is composed of three sequential steps that start with calculating spatial weights/importance, then that is followed by parameter learning, and finally inference generation. For the determination of the spatial weight of the ith neighboring location with regard to a given prediction location, both the spatial distance separating the prediction location to the neighboring location as well as the correlation between the time series associated with the two locations are estimated. The spatial weights are eventually normalized across all neighbors [Das and Ghosh, 2019, 2020]. This is followed by calculating the marginal and conditional probabilities of the composite and regular nodes. Note that the marginal probabilities of the composite nodes are calculated as a weighted average of the probabilities of the sub-nodes based on the determined spatial weights. Similarly, conditional probabilities are calculated by accounting for the spatial importance of the nearby locations [Das and Ghosh, 2020]. Once the marginal and conditional probabilities are determined, inference is generated.

Recently, Stritih et al. [2020] developed a BN environment that is able to integrate space and time with some simplifying assumptions. Their platform is called gBay (`gbay.ethz.ch`), which is currently operated as an online modeling platform that allows users to couple their BN to spatial data and implement the geo-processing calculations needed to account for spatial interactions. The gBay platform also allows users to run the network iteratively and to incorporate dynamics and feedbacks between the nodes [Stritih et al., 2020]. The model is able to incorporate both vector and raster spatial data and takes into account spatial interactions and cross-scale effects. The platform allows for incorporating local, focal, and zonal processes although the focal and zonal processes have to be introduced through Python scripts.

7.2   Bayesian Change Point and Threshold Models

In statistics, a change point model or a change point identification problem refers to the type of model or inference about the location of one or more points along a sequence of data at which the underlying model or parameters changed. A change point model aims at estimating both model parameters and the change point. The predictor in many applications is time. For example,

Figure 7.13 show the monthly average total phosphorus (TP) concentrations monitored at a location in the upper Neuse River near Raleigh, North Carolina, USA, from 1971 to 2001. The TP concentration distribution appears to have two distinct periods. Before 1988, the distribution has a high mean and a large variance. The distribution changed abruptly after 1988 to a distribution with a lower mean and lower variance. The change is largely due to the state of North Carolina's ban on phosphate detergent effective statewide in January 1988 (the vertical line). The monthly average TP concentrations decreased rapidly in 1988. By the end of 1989, the TP concentration distribution reached a new stable distribution with a lower mean and a lower variance. This is an example of a step change, where the distribution parameters (mean and variance) change abruptly from one set of values to another when crossing the change point.

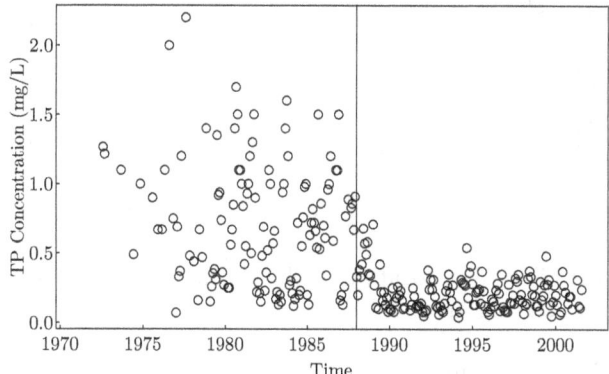

FIGURE 7.13: TP concentration distribution in the Neuse River near Raleigh, NC, USA, changed abruptly shortly after the ban on phosphate detergent was enacted in January 1988.

While the cause of the change in Neuse River TP concentration distribution is known, the timing of change in this example is after the date when the law took effect (January 1988), as unknown amounts of phosphate detergent in homes across the region were being used. The timing of the change is often a quantity of interest. In this case, we can use the time of the abrupt change to estimate the lag time between the legislation being enacted and the improved water quality. In other cases, we know the cause of the change but the timing is largely unknown. Qian [2016] showed the change in the first bloom date of flowering lilac trees (*Syringa vulgaris*) in several Pacific Northwest U.S. locations in response to climate change. Warmer weather prompted many trees to bloom earlier. In Qian [2016], a change point model in the form of a piecewise linear model was used:

$$y_i = \beta_0 + (\beta_1 + \delta \cdot I(x - \phi))(x_i - \phi) + \epsilon_i$$

where y_i is the observed first bloom date (ordinal date), x_i is the year when the ith observation was made, and ϕ is the change point when the change in first bloom date can be detected by the change point model. The model residual is assumed to be a normal random variable with mean 0 and a constant variance. In this model, the intercept (β_0) is the mean response variable value at the change point, similar to the piecewise linear model in Qian and Richardson [1997] (equation (2.8) on page 47). Before the change point, the average first bloom date is β_0 (because $\beta_1 \approx 0$); after the change point, the average first bloom date changed by δ (in days) per year (Figure 7.14).

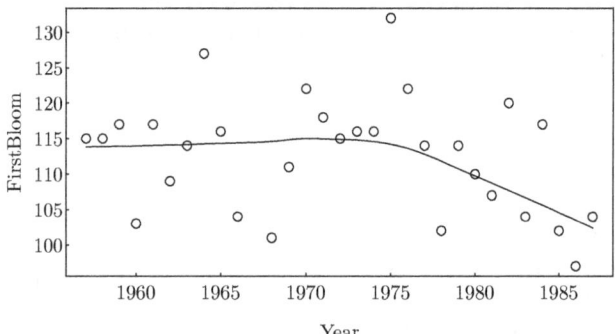

FIGURE 7.14: Lilacs at a location in the Pacific Northwest of the U.S. are blooming earlier starting around 1975.

Figure 7.13 is an example of a step function:

$$y_i \sim N(\mu_0 + I(x_i - \phi)\delta_\mu, \sigma_0^2 + I(x_i - \phi)\delta_\sigma) \tag{7.7}$$

and Figure 7.14 is an example of the piecewise linear (or hockey stick) model. It can be presented as a normal regression model when assuming a common standard deviation for the two segments (equation (7.8)):

$$y_i \sim N(\beta_0 + (\beta_1 + I(x_i - \phi)\delta)(x_i - \phi), \sigma^2). \tag{7.8}$$

Although many applications of change point models are focused on detecting changes over time, we can use change point models in many ecological applications to model the changes of various aspects of an ecosystem along environmental gradients. As reasoned in Richardson et al. [2007], an ecosystem can withstand a certain level of disturbance (e.g., increased level of pollution) without losing the system's function and service. As the disturbance intensifies, an abrupt change of the ecosystem may occur, often in the form of rapid transition from the previous stable state to an alternative stable state once the disturbance exceeds a threshold. In our Everglades example in Chapter 6, we mentioned that bladderworts (*Utricularia* spp.) are a keystone species of the Everglades wetland. It provides structure support to form the characteristic periphyton mat community of the Everglades wetland ecosystem. We used the stem density in the experimental mesocosm as a measure of the species response to increased phosphorus concentrations. The floating plant uses free CO_2 in the water for photosynthesis. As phosphorus concentration increases, algal photosynthesis uses aqueous CO_2 leading to increased pH level during the day. High pH levels are linked to low levels of free CO_2. Increased algal growth prevents bladderwort photosynthesis during the day. The abrupt change in bladderwort stem count density along a TP gradient is very similar to the abrupt change in Neuse River TP over time (Figure 7.15).

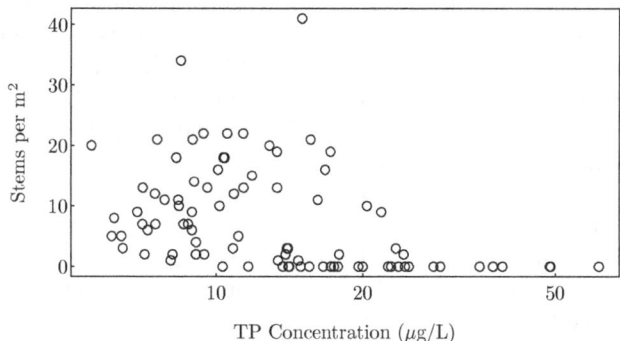

FIGURE 7.15: Density of bladderworts (*Utricularia* spp., stems per square meter) changes abruptly along a phosphorus gradient in a mesocosm experiment in the Everglades. Data from Qian et al. [2003a].

In our Gibbs sampler example of estimating the Everglades wetland's phosphorus retention capacity (Chapter 2), we used a hockey stick model to characterize the long-term phosphorus retention process. The long-term TP retention capacity of the wetland is the change point along the TP gradient.

In these examples, change points have important practical meanings. The change point in the Neuse River TP concentrations time series can be used to measure the temporal lag of a law's effect. The change point in the lilac first bloom date example is an estimate of the time when the effect of climate change can be retrospectively detected. The hockey stick model not only estimates the onset of climate change effect, but also provides a more accurate estimate of the climate change effect (the slope after the change point). The more frequently used linear modeling approach inevitably underestimates the climate change effects. In the two Everglades examples, a change point represents an important ecological threshold separating two states of the ecosystem. The threshold (in TP concentrations) of bladderworts was considered as the basis for setting environmental standards and the threshold in TP loading rate can be used as a reference when designing a constructed wetland for phosphorus retention.

The Gibbs sampler is an effective numerical method for change point models. For the step function model, we can derive Gibbs sampler algorithms for responses with different probability distributions. For example, Qian et al. [2003a] derived algorithms for normal, binomial, and Poisson response variables and Qian et al. [2004a] derived an algorithm for multinomial responses. However, a Gibbs sampling algorithm must be purposely developed for each type of problem. The process of deriving the conditional posterior distributions can be tedious and the process of writing the code is prone to error as we discussed in Chapter 2. The change point model can be implemented in Stan using the step(x) for real-valued x or int_step(x) function for integer-valued x. The two step functions have the opposite value (0 or 1) for x=0: int_step(0) returns 0 whereas step(0) returns 1. The Stan User's Guide warns that these functions "can seriously hinder sampling and optimization efficiency for gradient-based methods (e.g., NUTS, HMC, BFGS) if applied to parameters (including transformed parameters and local variables in the transformed parameters or model block)." With the warning in mind, we start with implementing the hockey stick model.

We first fit the step-function model (equation (7.7)) to the Neuse River total phosphorous data. As concentration variables are typically log-normal, the response variable is the log TP concentration. We use typical weakly informative priors for μ_0, δ_μ and σ_0. For simplicity, we assume a common residual variance for the model (i.e., $\delta_\sigma = 0$). The prior of ϕ is uniform across the range of x.

```
stepchange <- "
data{
    int N;
    real y[N];
    real x[N];
    real minX;
    real maxX;
    real mu0;
}
parameters{
    real beta0;
    real delta;
    real<lower=minX, upper=maxX> phi;
    real<lower=0> sigma;
}
transformed parameters{
    real mu[N];
    for (i in 1:N)
        mu[i] = beta0 + delta*step(x[i]-phi);
}
model{
    beta0 ~ normal(mu0, 10);
```

```
    delta ~ normal(0, 5);
    sigma ~ normal(0, 5);
    y ~ normal(mu, sigma);
}
"
```

For the *Utricularia* spp. stem density data, the response variable is a count variable, and as such, we used a Poisson response model:

```
### Partial Stan Code ###
data{
...
  int y[N];
...
model{
...
  y ~ poisson_log(mu);
}
```

The model was slow and some parameters did not converge after 50,000 iterations when fitting the *Utricularia* spp. stem density data. There was a warning of a large number of divergent transitions after warm-up. Using the `pairs` function, we noticed a strong correlation between β_0 and δ. The fitted model with the Neuse River TP data captured the data pattern well (Figure 7.16, upper panel).

As an alternative, we used the four-parameter logistic function as a smoothed version of the step function (equation (4.14) on page 123), where the parameter x_{mid} can be used to approximate the change point (ϕ). Chiu et al. [2006] noted that statistical methods (e.g., MLE) often cannot distinguish a discontinuous abrupt change (broken stick) from a continuous (smoothed) abrupt change (bent cable). As such, replacing the step function with a four-parameter logistic function is reasonable. The four-parameter logistic function fits the data well (Figure 7.16, lower panel) and the estimated mean of x_{mid} for the Neuse River TP data is 1988.96. That is, the lag of the phosphorus detergent ban effect is nearly one year (Figure 7.16). Because x_{mid} is the x-variable value when the change in the response y is halfway between the two bounds, the estimated x_{mid} suggests that the full effect of the ban was reached after nearly two years.

The use of the four-parameter logistic function reduced the computing time of the Neuse River example from over 1200 seconds (using the step function model) to less than 35 seconds on a Windows PC. Furthermore, the four-parameter logistic function effectively captures the abrupt change. When used on the Everglades (*Utricularia* spp. stem count) example, we see the same computational improvement. The resulting model, however, shows a pattern that is closer to a gradual change than an abrupt change (Figure 7.17). The estimated mean change point (x_{mid}) is 26 μg/L, beyond which the observed

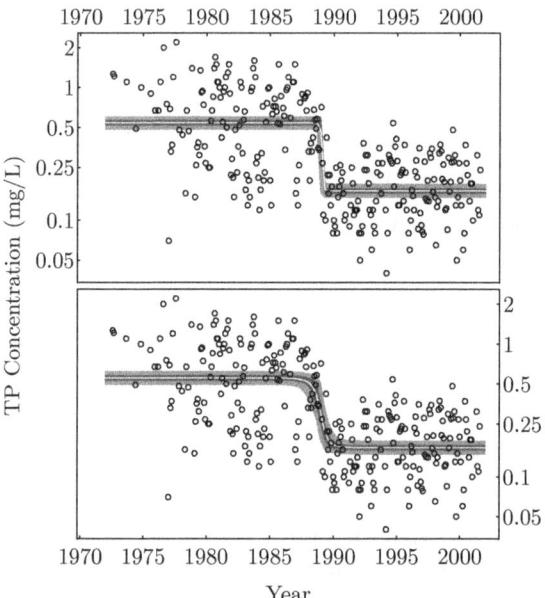

FIGURE 7.16: The Neuse River TP concentration change due to the phosphorus detergent ban is modeled using the step function model (upper panel) and the four-parameter logistic function, a smoothed model for an abrupt change (lower panel). The white lines in the middle of the shaded polygons are the estimated mean TP concentration and the shaded polygons are the 50% and 95% credible intervals of the mean.

stem counts are all 0 (Figure 7.18). Recall that the parameter x_{mid} is the predictor variable value at which the expected response variable value is at the mid-point between the lower and upper bounds. Because the four-parameter logistic function is defined on the logarithmic scale of the total stem count in the model, the resulting midpoint seems to define the point where the bladderwort community collapses. As such, the parameter x_{mid} may not be appropriate as a reference point for setting an environmental standard. Should the four-parameter logistic model be used, the environmental standard should be defined as the TP concentration that results in a certain level of reduction (e.g., 25%) of the stem density from the expected upper bound.

We now fit the hockey stick model of equation (7.8) to the lilac first bloom dates. Priors for model parameters were derived based on our understanding of the first bloom dates. For example, we have no prior knowledge of the change point ϕ and assume that the change point is uniformly distributed within the range of the years for which we have data. When the change point does not

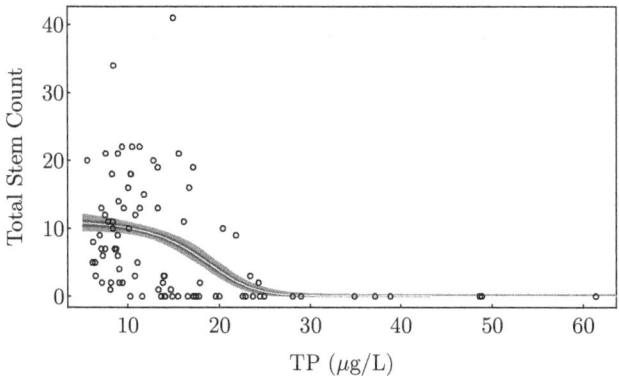

FIGURE 7.17: The total bladderwort (*Utricularia* spp.) stem count change due to changes in phosphorus concentration is modeled using the four-parameter logistic function.

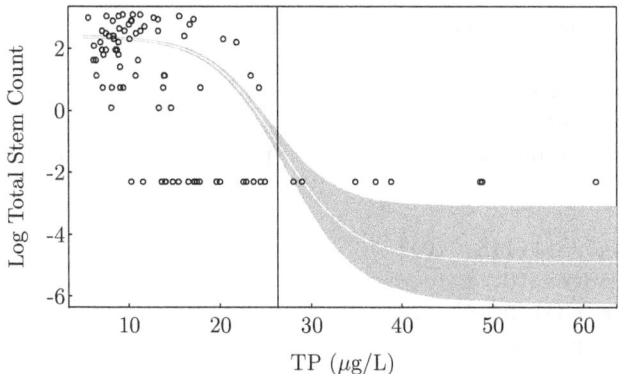

FIGURE 7.18: The four-parameter logistic model estimated mean log total bladderwort (*Utricularia* spp.) stem count as a function of phosphorus concentration (the white line) and the 50% credible interval (gray polygon) show that the estimated midpoint (vertical line) separates TP concentration gradient into one area with all zero counts (shown by the dots near $y = -2$) and the other with positive counts.

exist, the posterior of the change point would be near one of the two ends of the year range. The prior for β_0 (the average first bloom date before the change point) should be centered around mid to late April (92nd–121st day of the year), and as such, $\beta_0 \sim N(115, 10)$ (standard deviation 10) is reasonable. Before the change point, that is, before the effect of climate change on lilac blooming time can be detected, we expect the average first bloom date did not have a persistent temporal trend. In other words, the prior for β_1 should be centered around 0. We initially used $\beta_1 \sim N(0, 5)$.

```
### Stan Code ###
stepchange <- "
data{
  int N;
  real y[N];
  real x[N];
  real minX;
  real maxX;
}
parameters{
  real beta0;
  real beta1;
  real<upper=0> delta;
  real<lower=minX, upper=maxX> phi;
  real<lower=0> sigma;
}
transformed parameters{
  real mu[N];
  for (i in 1:N)
    mu[i] = beta0 +
        (beta1+delta*int_step(x[i]-phi))*(x[i]-phi);
}
model{
  beta0 ~ normal(115, 10);
  beta1 ~ normal(0, 5);
  delta ~ normal(0, 5);
  sigma ~ normal(0, 5);
  y ~ normal(mu, sigma);
}
"
### End ###
```

There were many divergent transitions after warm-up initially when the prior of β_1 was $N(0, 5)$, the usual weakly informative prior. The diagnostic plots show that all divergent transitions appeared in samples with large β_1 values. In other words, the selection of priors in this example can have direct influence on the behavior of the MCMC process. For example, the usual relatively non-informative prior for β_0 (e.g., $N(0, 10)$) would be highly informative suggesting that the first bloom date is most likely less than 20, whereas the typical first bloom dates are in April, or β_0 should be between 92 and 121. Likewise, β_1, the slope before the change point, should have a prior mean of 0 and a very small standard deviation because the average first bloom dates should not change consistently over time before the change point. We then modified the model by using $N(0, 0.5)$ as the prior.

For the hockey stick model, the discontinuity lies in the first derivatives. The first-order derivative of equation (7.8) is a step function:

$$\frac{dy}{dx} = \begin{cases} \beta_1 & \text{if } x \le \phi \\ \beta_1 + \delta & \text{if } x > \phi. \end{cases}$$

As before, the step function can be approximated by a four-parameter logistic function (FPL):

$$\frac{dy}{dx} = \beta_1 + \frac{\delta}{1 + e^{-\frac{x - x_{mid}}{scal}}}. \tag{7.9}$$

The shape parameter *scal* (and the difference δ) controls the maximum rate of change of the derivative curve ($\frac{\delta}{4scal}$). The smaller the shape parameter is, the closer the function in equation (7.9) is to the step function. Integrating the FPL, we have the smooth hockey stick model:

$$y = \beta_0 + \beta_1(x - x_{mid}) + \delta \cdot scal \cdot \log\left(1 + e^{\frac{x - x_{mid}}{scal}}\right). \tag{7.10}$$

Mathematically, the term $\log(1 + e^z)$ approaches 0 as z decreases ($z \to -\infty$). Likewise, the term $\log(1 + e^z)$ approaches z as z increases ($z \to +\infty$). In other words, when $x \ll x_{mid}$, $\log\left(1 + e^{\frac{x - x_{mid}}{scal}}\right)$ approaches 0. The function is approaching a linear model ($y = \beta_0 + \beta_1(x - x_{mid})$). When $x \gg x_{mid}$, $\log\left(1 + e^{\frac{x - x_{mid}}{scal}}\right)$ approaches $\frac{x - x_{mid}}{scal}$ and the function is close to a linear function again ($y = \beta_0 + (\beta_1 + \delta)(x - x_{mid})$). The shape parameter $scal > 0$ when estimated as a free parameter can lead to complicated posterior geometry, especially when *scal* approaches 0 where the bent cable (smooth line) turned into a broken stick. As a result, we often treat *scal* as known (e.g., 0.01 of the predictor variable range). Unlike the step function, using the smoothed hockey stick model in this model did not bring computational gains, although the estimated parameter values are comparable (Table 7.3).

7.2.1   Hierarchical Change Point Model

In the lilac first bloom dates data, we notice the large variation in the first bloom dates from year to year, as shown in Figure 7.14. Such a large variation is very typical in phenology data because of the natural annual variation in weather. Furthermore, the large annual variation also leads to high variability in the estimated model parameters (Table 7.3). In the lilac data, we have observations from multiple locations across the continental U.S. We expect that (1) all locations are affected by the global climate change (hence the hockey stick model applies) and (2) when fitting data from different locations to the hockey stick model the estimated model parameters will vary by location. With the large number of sites, pooling data under a hierarchical

TABLE 7.3: The hockey stick model estimated model parameter posterior distributions (mean, standard deviation, and selected percentiles) are compared to comparable parameters estimated from the smoothed change point model for the lilac first bloom dates data.

Model	Parameter	mean	2.5%	25%	50%	75%	97.5%
	β_0	114.67	110.76	113.38	114.75	115.99	118.445
	β_1	0.019	-0.195	-0.059	0.020	0.092	0.234
Eq. (7.8)	δ	-1.437	-3.668	-1.876	-1.280	-0.800	-0.167
	ϕ	1977.6	1965.2	1975.1	1977.9	1981.1	1984.6
	σ	7.473	5.828	6.796	7.375	8.0592	9.686
	β_0	115.34	110.03	113.69	115.56	117.15	120.14
	β_1	0.118	-0.296	-0.048	0.108	0.264	0.658
Eq. (7.10)	δ	-1.522	-3.722	-1.990	-1.384	-0.896	-0.170
	x_{mid}	1976.76	1962.92	1974.12	1977.09	1980.65	1985.01
	$scal$	0.799	0.0353	0.322	0.678	1.151	2.249
	σ	7.487	5.772	6.770	7.380	8.118	9.781

structure is desirable. That is, we can expand the hockey stick model (equation (7.8)) to:

$$
\begin{aligned}
y_{ij} &\sim N(\beta_{0j} + (\beta_{1j} + I(x_{ij} - \phi_j)\delta_j)(x_{ij} - \phi_j), \sigma^2) \\
\begin{bmatrix} \beta_{0j} \\ \beta_{1j} \\ \phi_j \\ \delta_j \end{bmatrix} &\sim \left[\begin{pmatrix} \mu_{\beta_0} \\ \mu_{\beta_1} \\ \mu_\phi \\ \mu_\delta \end{pmatrix}, \Sigma \right].
\end{aligned}
\tag{7.11}
$$

The multivariate prior for the model parameters is modeled using the same method described in Chapter 6.4.3 (the Chelosky decomposition method was used). The estimated parameter β_1 (the slope before the effect of climate change can be detected) using data from one single site at a time was not statistically different from 0 for all sites we examined (e.g., Table 7.3). As a result, we fit the model in equation (7.11) setting $\beta_1 = 0$ in an effort to compare the generated results to those generated from the single site model shown in Figure 7.14. The estimated model parameters (β_0, δ, and ϕ) using only data from the site shown in Figure 7.14 all have wider 95% credible intervals compared to the same site-specific parameters estimated using the hierarchical model (less so with β_0). These site-specific parameters are closer to the respective hyper-parameters (Figure 7.19).

The amount of shrinkage of site-specific estimates from the hierarchical model depends on the levels of uncertainty. Parameters with a higher level of uncertainty in the model fitted using data from the site alone (i.e., δ, ϕ) are pulled toward their hyper-parameters more than the parameter with a lower level of uncertainty (i.e., β_0). Statistical theories show that shrinkage estimators such as the hierarchical model reduce the overall estimation error,

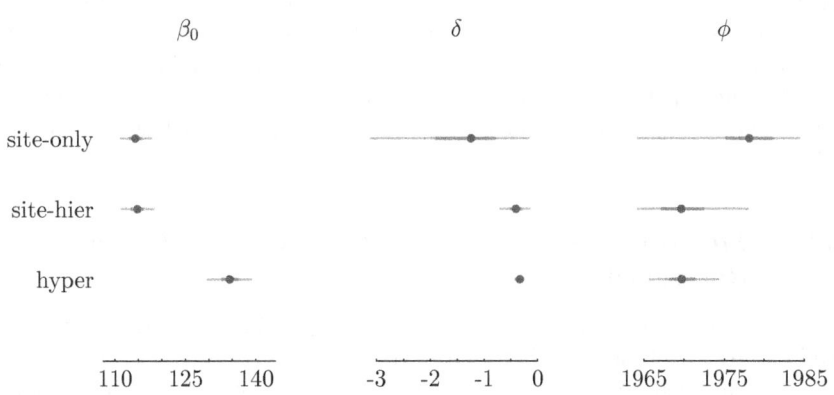

FIGURE 7.19: Selected hockey-stick model parameters are compared: parameters estimated using site data only (site-only), site-specific parameters estimated using the hierarchical model (site-hier), and the hyper-parameters of the hierarchical model (hyper).

although the shrinkage estimated model parameters for a specific site may not be the optimal. The hierarchical model assumption that site-specific model parameters are exchangeable allows us to use a common prior for all locations. When the exchangeable assumption is in question, for example, when we have knowledge to divide the 53 sites in the data into groups of relatively homogeneous locations where lilac phenological changes as a result of climate change are similar within group but differ from locations in other groups, the hierarchical model should be modified to impose the exchangeable assumption only on sites within a group. Just as in the two examples in Section 6.4.3, grouping sites can be theory-driven (e.g., grouping lakes and reservoirs along a natural soil iron gradient) or based on the initial model result (e.g., grouping EUSE regions by antecedent agricultural land use in the watershed). The Bayesian hierarchical model is a versatile tool as part of the iterative process of scientific research.

The use of the hockey-stick model to describe the pattern of change in lilac first bloom date is based on our assumption that the average long-term pattern of the phenological date should resemble the pattern of long-term mean temperature due to climate change. But for plants with a wide range of temperature tolerance such as lilac and Japanese cherry, the hockey-stick pattern can only be part of the story because plant phenological patterns are a result of multiple factors (e.g., daylight hours) that may not be affected by greenhouse gas emission-induced global warming. As such, we can also argue that the better model for phenological pattern change may be the four-parameter logistic function (e.g., Figure 7.16, lower panel). The long-term trend may have three phases: the pre-change stable state, the post-change stable state, and a transition between the two. The hockey stick model approximates the pre-change stable state and the transition phase. As it is unlikely that we have already reached the post-change stable state, analyzing available phenological data using a hockey-stick model seems to be reasonable, at least for the time being.

7.2.2   Modeling Temporal Changes in the Flow-Concentration Relationship

The hockey-stick model can be used to approximate another commonly used empirical relationship between nutrient concentrations and stream flow, especially in locations under the influence of both point and non-point sources of nutrient release. When a stream is predominately under the influence of a major point source, such as a waste water treatment plant, nutrient concentrations in the stream tend to decrease as stream flow increases. Such a negative correlation reflects the dilution effect. When a river receives nutrients from mostly non-point sources, nutrient concentration may increase as flow increases when stream flow is low. The positive relationship is a result of the increased non-point source input. As the stream flow increases further (as a result of, for example, increased precipitation or upstream input), the nutrient concentration may start to decrease reflecting a dilution effect (Figure 7.20). If we define the flow at which the concentration-flow relationship changes from a positive correlation to a negative correlation, we can express the change as in equation (7.10), or

$$\log(Conc_i) = \beta_0 + \beta_1(\log(flow_i) - x_{mid}) + \delta \cdot scal \cdot \log\left(1 + e^{\frac{\log(flow_i) - x_{mid}}{scal}}\right) + \epsilon_i.$$
(7.12)

Alameddine et al. [2011] documented such a change in the concentration-flow relationship in response to nutrient point source loading in the upper Neuse River in North Carolina, USA. They observed that the change of the nitrogen oxide (NO_2+NO_3) concentration and flow relationship after the implementation of a Total Maximum Daily Load (TMDL) program. A TMDL program is mandated by the U.S. Clean Water Act when a water is declared to be impaired. The Neuse River Estuary was designated as a nutrient sensitive water and put on the 303(d) list, which identified nitrogen as the main culprit behind the eutrophication symptoms in the Neuse River estuary. These symptoms include the widely publicized extensive algal blooms, frequent fish kills, and hypoxia and anoxia. As a result, the state of North Carolina adopted in 1997 rules aimed at reducing the amount of nitrogen delivered to the Neuse River Estuary by 30% (based on the average 1991 to 1995 loads). The study reported by Alameddine et al. [2011] was to evaluate whether the TMDL program achieved its stated goal.

Before the implementation of the TMDL, pollution loading to the stretch of the Neuse River was dominated by a point source (wastewater treatment

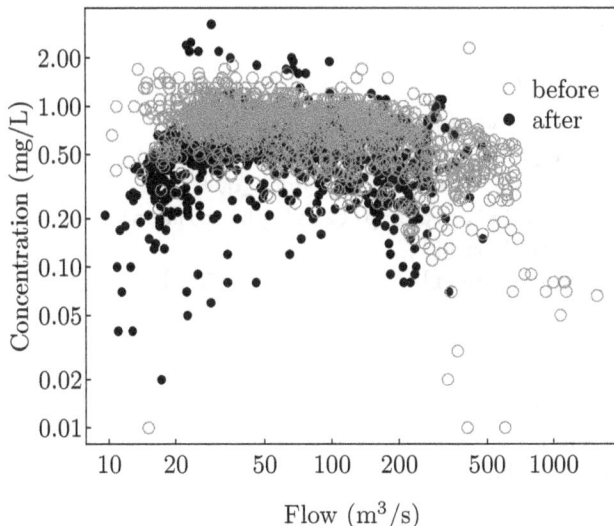

FIGURE 7.20: The nitrogen oxides concentration-flow relationship has two distinct patterns, before and after the implementation of a nutrient loading reduction program (TMDL). Before the implementation (shaded open circles), the correlation is largely negative. After the TMDL program (black dots), the correlation is positive when the flow is low and negative when the flow is high.

plant of the City of Raleigh, North Carolina, USA). As a result, the nitrogen oxide-flow relationship was approximately log-log linear with a negative slope. After the TMDL program (including installing a tertiary treatment process at the wastewater treatment plant), release of nutrients from the wastewater treatment plant was greatly reduced. Using the `step` function in WinBUGS, Alameddine et al. [2011] estimated the flow threshold (x_{mid} in equation (7.12)) and the time change point (when did the change in the concentration-flow relationship occurred) simultaneously. In their WinBUGS program, a categorical distribution was used to model the change point in time (in years), as well as the threshold in the concentration-flow relationship. Stan does not support categorical random variables. We modify the model to use the `step` function only once to model the temporal change point and use equation (7.12) to model the concentration-flow relationship after the temporal change point.

In the Stan code, we used two mean functions to describe the mean function before and after the change point:

```
### Partial Stan code ###
transformed parameters{
    real mu_hat[N];
    real phiYR[N];
```

```
    real phiQ[N];
    real mu1[N];
    real mu2[N];
    for (i in 1:N){
      phiYR[i] = 1-step(yr[i]-phi_yr);
      mu1[i] = alpha0+betaT*wtrTemp[i]+alpha1*x[i];
      mu2[i] = beta0 + beta1*(x[i]-phi_q)+
          delta*scal*log1p_exp((x[i]-phi_q)/scal)+
          betaT*wtrTemp[i];
      mu_hat[i] = phiYR[i]*mu1[i]+(1-phiYR[i])*mu2[i];
    }
}
model{
    scal ~ normal(0,1);
    sigma ~ cauchy(0, 2.5);
    y ~ normal (mu_hat, sigma);
}
### End ###
```

We centered the two predictor variables (water temperature and log flow) to avoid the correlation between regression slopes and intercept. The model identified the temporal change point precisely (from 1999.01, the 1st percentile, to 1999.99, the 99th percentile). The pre-change-point model (a log-log linear model) is as expected, while the post-change-point model caused a large number of divergent transitions. Scatter plots of posterior samples of selected parameters show strong correlations among ϕ_q, δ, and β_1 (Figure 7.21), suggesting that these three parameters cannot be uniquely identified.

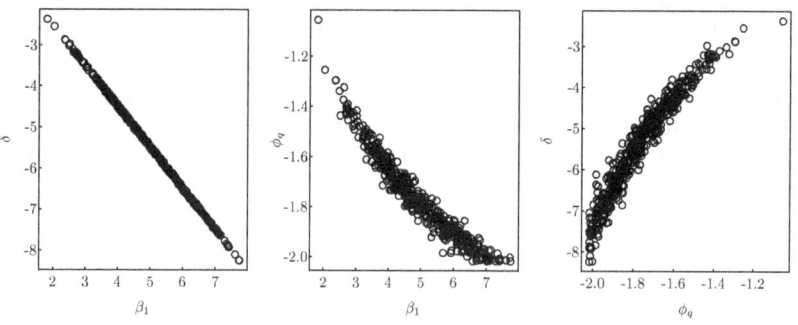

FIGURE 7.21: Scatter plots of posterior samples from β_1, δ, and ϕ_q show strong correlations among these parameters.

To understand the potential cause of the non-identifiable problem, we used posterior simulation to see how well the model fits the data. Using the posterior samples of the model parameters, we predicted the nitrogen concentrations when temperature is at the observed mean value (Figure 7.22). Although the mean models for the pre- and post-change-point periods are well matched with the observed data, the estimated flow threshold is very close to the low end of the flow range. As a result, the parameter β_1 is highly dependent on the location of ϕ_q, which, in turn, influences the change in slope (δ).

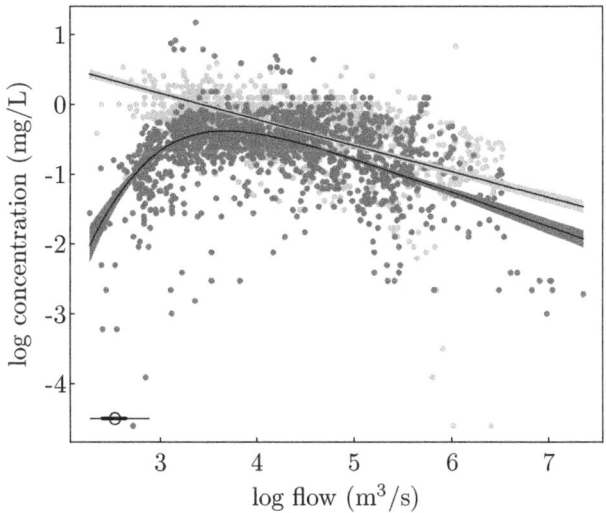

FIGURE 7.22: The posterior model predicted concentration-flow relationship. Although the two main model lines are well matched with the data, the flow threshold (near the lower left corner) is very close to the low end of the flow range.

The fitted curve seems to suggest that the smoothed hockey stick model formulation is problematic – not all parameters can be uniquely identified with this particular data set. A more informative prior of ϕ is needed.

The objective of the original study was to show that the concentration-flow relationship is not static. A static concentration-flow model is often assumed when estimating nutrient loadings from streams to receiving waters (e.g., lakes and coastal waters). The resulting model is often used to "estimate" daily mean concentrations using daily flow measurements. The estimated concentrations are often used to estimate the daily nutrient loads and the total annual loads. This allows for assessing the effectiveness of the implemented measures in the river basin towards achieving the TMDL set goal of reducing loading by 30%. Additionally, the model was able to highlight the shift in the source of pollution loading in the Neuse Estuary. While the TMDL appears to have been able to reduce the load across the entire flow range, the largest gains were at low flows, where nitrogen discharges from point sources used to dominate the system.

Chapter 8

Concluding Remarks

Because statistics is a tool for inductive reasoning, statistical inference is, therefore, subject to the particularities of applications in different science disciplines. The unique features in a discipline are often reflected in the specific sub-branch of statistics. As with most of our readers, we received our statistical lessons in graduate school with a branch of statistics designed for biological data analysis (biostatistics), including topics such as experimental design (data collection), analysis of data from these experiments, and interpretation of the results. In universities around the world, ecology and environmental science graduate students may be required to take at least one statistics course that is largely based on biostatistics designed along the line of Galton and Pearson (summary statistics and correlation), Fisher (randomized experiments, ANOVA, and the maximum likelihood estimator), and Neyman-Pearson (confidence intervals and hypothesis testing).

The development of biostatistics started from individual studies, for example, Pierre C.A. Louis's numerical analysis of the cause of child-bed fever and the effects of bloodletting (who can forget his exasperated response to his critics "Quels faits! Quelle logique!"). These studies, which shared common features within the disciplines and data, led to case studies, new theories, and development of common methods. The process is exemplified in Fisher's examination of agriculture experimental data that led to randomized experiments and ANOVA. Ultimately, the statistical theories and methods become part of life science disciplines. For example, the concept of the randomized experiment is part of many biological studies and the modern clinical trials underpinning the development of all new medicines and treatments. Modern medicine and biology cannot be separated from biostatistics.

In analyzing environmental and ecological data, we similarly must define the features of environmental and ecological data through summarizing individual studies and developing case studies. However, rather than following a linear process, we advocate for an iterative modeling process that intertwines the model formulation, parameter estimation, and model evaluation components. In many applications of Bayesian statistics, the focus is on the use of the Bayes' theorem to replace the parameter estimation step in biostatistics. Such an approach fails to take full advantage of the Bayesian analysis, even when the MCMC-based computation methods were used.

We find that using Stan helped us to integrate these three components. The strong diagnostic capabilities of the Hamiltonian Markov chain method implemented in Stan can alert us to computational difficulties and help us propose alternative models. In a way, the new computational tool combines the estimation and model evaluation steps with the model formulation problem, thereby integrating the three statistical problems in a coherent process. As a result, a Bayesian analysis is characterized by the iterative interactions among the three components, rather than the linear process of moving from model formulation to parameter estimation to model evaluation. In this chapter, we summarize some of the examples used in this book in terms of developing a coherent procedure of model formulation, parameter estimation, and model evaluation in the context of analyzing environmental and ecological data.

8.1   Model Formulation

A typical application of biostatistics includes data from an experiment designed for a specific question along with a statistical model for analyzing the data. In a way, model formulation was decided before data were collected. As a result, statistical analysis can often be standardized. When taking statistical classes, we learn how to fit these standard models and how to verify statistical assumptions, such as the normality and independence assumptions of model residuals. There are limited remedial options when assumptions are not met. For example, when the normality assumption is violated, we often try the log transformation; when residuals are not random, we may try to include one or more additional predictor variables. Typically, such exercises are straightforward because the data were generated based on the intended models.

Analyzing data from environmental and ecological studies, however, can be far more complicated because the data are most likely observational. Many factors can affect the outcome and we have a limited capacity to know or to measure all these factors. As a result, the task of model formulation is often the most important part of a data analysis project, although it is often neglected in our statistical education. Model formulation should be an iterative process, including identifying questions related to data collection (e.g., why and how the data were collected) and subject matter knowledge (e.g., what do we know about factors influencing the response variable). We often start with an initial model, which can be a standard model in a statistics textbook or the simplest model that we can easily fit. In the snake fungal disease example, we should ask, for example, whether the snakes were collected in one small area (to make sure that the snakes represent the target population, rather than, perhaps, from the same family), whether the false positive and false negative probabilities of the testing method are consistent from test to test. When we have satisfactory answers, we may start from the binomial model assuming the fungal disease detection method is perfect (i.e., $f_p = f_n = 0$). We started with the binomial model because we know the analytical form of the posterior distribution and the computation process is very simple, which gives us a starting point. The estimated probability of observing a positive result can be used as a default estimate of the disease's prevalence in the population. We can also use the posterior distribution as the prior of the prevalence for the next study. In our next iteration, we can expand the binomial model by incorporating probabilities of false positive and false negative. When assuming f_p and f_n as known, we specify the probability of a positive result as a function of the prevalence θ (equation (5.13)). The new model can be used to derive the posterior distribution of the parameter of interest (θ), but is computationally more complicated. We used the numerical method applied to the posterior distribution in equation (1.4) (on page 9) and the Metropolis-Hastings method in Section 2.4.1 (see Figure 2.6 on page 45).

As in most statistical models, increased complexity is inevitably associated with a higher computation demand. For the snake fungal disease example, this increased demand does not impede us from learning about the model. In other cases (e.g., the Crypto in drinking water example in Section 6.4.5.3 on page 278), simplifying the model is necessary to ease the computation burden. The model of equation (1.4) (with known f_p and f_n) is unsatisfactory because we do not know f_p and f_n. We learned later that the model can be further expanded by treating these two parameters as unknown and estimated using the Metropolis-Hastings algorithm in a Gibbs sampler (Section 2.5.1, page 55), or using Stan (Section 4.1.1, page 85). The complexity of this model, however, is problematic because the likelihood function (and the posterior distribution) cannot uniquely separate the three model parameters. We discussed this issue and suggested that the model is non-identifiable because the observed count data provide information on the probability of a positive response only.

An identifiability issue is not necessarily easy to recognize. Fortunately, Stan is quite capable of indicating when a model has an identity crisis. We mentioned that Stan shows a warning message regarding divergent transitions after warm-up in many examples. These messages are often an indication that Stan cannot effectively explore the complex posterior distribution to produce reliable estimate of it. These complexities are an indication of a model formulation problem, either the model is wrong for the data or the data are not informative enough for the model (e.g., sample size is too small, observation error is large). In the snake fungal model fit using Stan (Section 4.1.1), we have warnings that nearly half of posterior MCMC samples were from divergent transitions. The warning is a cry for help and should not be ignored. We used pairwise scatter plots of posterior MCMC samples to explore the posterior joint posterior distribution. The plots from the example with typical data of this kind (5 infected out of 20 snakes) did not reveal anything specific except a weak correlation between θ and f_p and the divergent transitions appeared in no particular pattern (Figure 8.1).

As we know that these three parameters (θ, f_p, and f_n) cannot be separated based on the observed number of infected snakes alone, we attempted

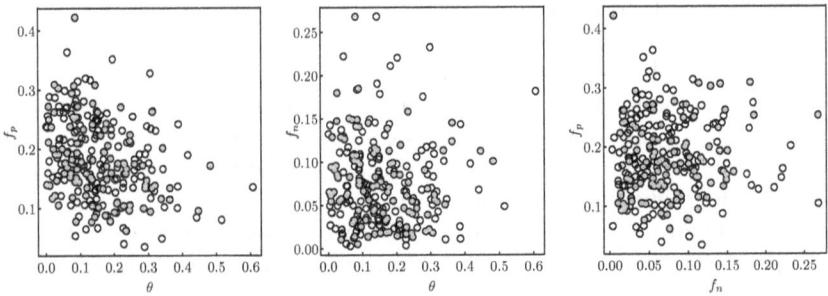

FIGURE 8.1: Pairwise scatter plots of the posterior samples (open circles) from the snake fungal model do not show a particular pattern with divergent transitions marked by the shaded dots.

another model run using data with 500 infected snakes from 2000 snakes. The increased sample size does not change the non-identifiable nature of the model, but we hope that increased sample size (hence reduced estimation uncertainty) would better help us identify the likely problems. In this case, the pairwise scatter plots show that θ and f_p are highly correlated (Figure 8.2).

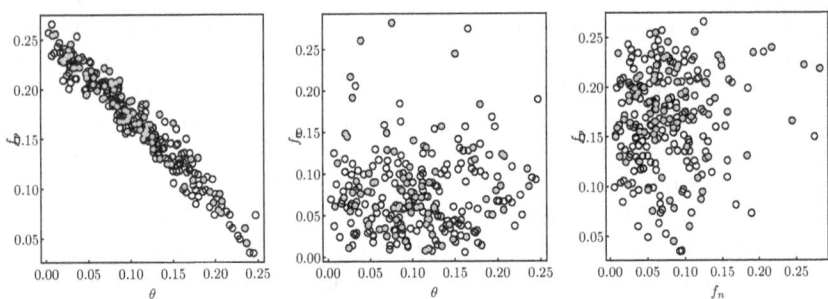

FIGURE 8.2: Pairwise scatter plots of the posterior samples (open circles) from the snake fungal model fit with increased sample size show a strong correlation between θ and f_p. Divergent transitions are marked by the shaded dots.

Figure 8.1 is a result of the estimation process. The warning about divergent transitions indicates a problem that is not obvious from the diagnostic plots. Figure 8.2 is a result of model evaluation. Based on these figures, we simplified the model by assuming that f_p is known (e.g., $f_p = 0$) and noticed yet another problem. The posterior marginal distribution of f_n is now strongly correlated with θ (Figure 8.3, left panel). These figures show that a stable estimate of θ is only possible when f_n is restricted in a narrow range (Figure 8.3, right panel), although the relationship between θ and f_n is still defined through the probability of observing a positive response $(\theta(1 - f_n))$. The observed number of positive results can only provide information of the product. To decouple the two parameters, we need to know (or have a strong prior of) one of them.

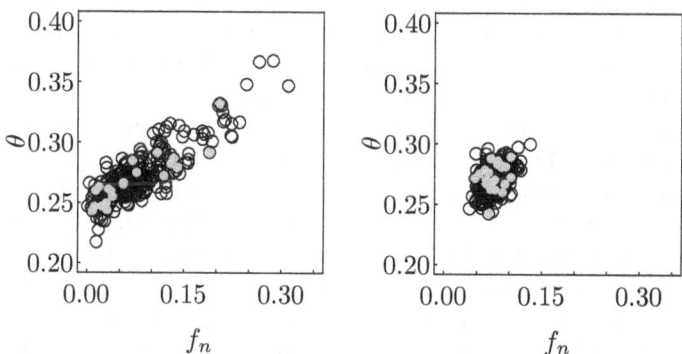

FIGURE 8.3: Scatter plots of the posterior samples (open circles) from the snake fungal model with f_p set to be 0 shows a strong correlation between θ and f_n (left panel). The correlation is reduced only when the prior of f_n is strongly informative ($f_n \sim beta(20, 250)$ shown in the right panel). Divergent transitions are marked by the shaded dots.

From the exploration, we learned that if we are collecting data to learn about the prevalence of the disease, we must first characterize the testing method better. Without reasonably informative priors on the two error probabilities, we are unable to accurately estimate the prevalence. However, if the precise value of prevalence is not of interest, rather we are concerned with the change in prevalence over time or space, then we can simplify the model to estimate the probability of a positive result, which is a linear function of the two error probabilities. This assumes we are reasonably confident that the performance of the detection method is consistent, that is, both f_p and f_n are stable. In either case, a standard experimental and sampling protocol implemented to ensure stable error probabilities would benefit both approaches.

The lessons learned from the snake fungal disease example were applied in two recent studies. Both studies are related to the effort of controlling the spread of grass carp (*Ctenopharyngodon idella*), an invasive fish species, in Lake Erie.

Grass carp were imported to the U.S. from China in the 1960s to help control nuisance aquatic vegetation. Over time, these fish escaped to surrounding rivers and lakes, first in the Mississippi River basin [Guillory and Gasaway, 1978]. Grass carp is a species of concern because it grows fast and can quickly reach a size that is too big for many Great Lakes native predator fish species. It can consume a large amount of aquatic vegetation that may lead to habitat destruction [Cudmore et al., 2017]. Grass carp have been found in Lake Erie since the 1980s. In 2015, grass carp spawning were confirmed in Sandusky River, a tributary of Lake Erie near Sandusky, Ohio [Embke et al., 2016]. A regular grass carp egg monitoring program was established, and annual sampling during the likely spawning season has been occurring since then. In addition to the egg monitoring program, regional and federal agencies also started a joint targeted removal program for adult grass carp [Herbst et al., 2021]. Data from both the egg sampling and adult fish removal programs are counts: counts of eggs and counts of fish captured.

Jaffe [2021] used grass carp egg sampling data to understand the conditions that are favorable for spawning. The egg sampling program recorded whether eggs were captured during each sampling event, along with the flow and temperature on the day the river was sampled. The data are binary. Jaffe [2021] divided the data into bins with relatively homogeneous flow and temperature conditions. Within each bin, the data are the number of times the river was sampled (n) and the number of times eggs were collected (x). The data can be modeled using the snake fungal disease model. In this case, a false positive would be misidentifying a non-grass carp egg as a grass carp egg. A false negative is a result of failure to capture an egg when grass carp spawned. The probability of spawning is similar to the prevalence in the snake fungal disease example. Because grass carp eggs are mophologically distinct from other pelagophilic spawners in the region and temporal spatial overlap is uncommon, mis-identification is virtually impossible. As a result, we can set $f_p = 0$. In fisheries literature, we often use detection probability instead of false negative probability ($p_d = 1 - f_n$). Figure 8.3 indicates that we cannot separate θ and f_n. However, if we know that f_n (hence p_d) is a constant, we can directly estimate the probability of a positive result (θp_d) as a quantity proportional to the probability of spawning. In this case, the actual value of θ is of no particular value as we already know that grass carp spawning occurred in the river. We are interested in the flow-temperature conditions that are favorable for spawning. We can either reduce the model to a simple binomial model or estimate θ using a reasonable value of p_d. This was possible because the same sampling protocol was used throughout the study, thus detection probability was assumed constant and data were pooled together. However, if a new sampling protocol were used in the future, the assumption of a constant p_d and model structure would have to be re-evaluated.

In analyzing data from the grass carp removal project, we are interested in estimating the total number of fish in the river. Because the number of grass carp captured in a given removal event is mostly 0 with occasional captures of one or two fish, we treated the data as binary, as we did in the Crypto example (Section 6.4.5.3, specifically, equations (6.18) and (6.19) on page 284). Similar to the grass carp egg problem, misidentification of a grass carp is highly unlikely (hence $f_p = 0$). In Gouveia et al. [2022], the parameter λ (equation (6.19)) is defined as the average density of grass carp measured in number of fish per kilometer because the removal operations used a fixed length of river. As a result, equation (6.19) was modified to be $p0 = 1 - e^{-f\lambda}$, were f is the length (in kilometers) of the removal operation segment. Because we are interested in estimating the density λ, a reasonable estimate of the detection probability (r in equation (6.18)) is necessary (as shown in Figure 8.3). As a result, a separate study was carried out to estimate the detection probability [Gouveia et al., 2022].

8.2 Estimation

Estimation is more than the process of applying the Bayes' theorem for acquiring the posterior distributions of model parameters. It is part of the iterative process of model formulation, as we illustrated in the snake fungal disease example in the previous section. Estimation using Stan can reveal weaknesses in the model and suggest potential improvements. For example, an ill-formulated model often has a high demand on computational resources leading to a slow MCMC process and divergent transitions. The Hamiltonian Monte Carlo algorithm used in Stan is highly capable of detecting posterior distributions that are widely spread or overly complex (often led to the estimated posterior distributions being unreliable). When we encounter this issue, we should examine the model for defects and solutions by graphically exploring the estimated posterior distributions. A widely spread posterior distribution is often indication of model formulation problems.

In the mixture of two normal distributions example (Section 4.5 on page 131), the iterative estimation process pointed to the necessary constraints we must impose on the model through prior distributions in order to obtain an identifiable joint posterior distribution. In other words, model formulation includes the formulation of prior distributions. The constraint that the soil lead concentration mean in a contaminated area must be larger than the mean in a reference area is reasonable physically and necessary statistically to avoid the problem of interchangeable components. In many models, we have subject matter knowledge on what may be reasonable parameter values. For example, the prior distribution for β_0 in equation (7.8) for the lilac first bloom example (page 328) should not be the usual weakly informative prior (e.g., $N(0, 10)$) because the parameter represents the first bloom date of lilacs in the Pacific Northwest, which is typically in April (i.e., β_0 should be between 92 and 121). A prior of $N(0, 10)$ would put the typical bloom date beyond 10 prior standard deviations away from the prior mean, which is highly (and wrongly) informative.

Estimation must be repeatedly performed each time a model is revised. As a result, computation efficiency is often a concern when using MCMC-based methods. In the Crypto in drinking water example, we modified the binomial-Poisson mixture model (equation (6.14) on page 281) to a mixture of two Bernoulli distributions (equations (6.18) and (6.19)). In doing so, we changed the meaning of the detection probability. In the binomial-Poisson mixture, the detection probability r is the probability of detecting a crypto oocyst when it is present. In the mixture of two Bernoulli distributions, the detection probability is the probability of capturing at least one oocyst when an unknown number of oocysts are present. The two models would be the same if a water sample contains only one oocyst at most. When the number of oocysts captured in a water sample is mostly low, the Bernoulli-Bernoulli model is an approximation of the binomial-Poisson model. In the grass carp study in Gouveia et al. [2022], this approximation is reasonable as grass carp are rare in Lake Erie and no more than two fish were captured in any of the removal events. The approximation makes the computation manageable.

In many of our examples, we started the iterative process in Figure 1.5 with a classical model with fast estimation algorithms. In the EUSE example as shown in Qian et al. [2010], the iterative steps started from fitting independent simple linear regression models for each of the nine regions. The differences in these models led to the use of a multilevel model to partially pool the data from all regions (still using classical multilevel model implemented in R function lmer). The results raised more questions, which led to the use of region-level predictors such as the antecedent agriculture land cover and regional average temperature and precipitation. This is a more typical example as we often start our model exploration by using a simple model that can be easily and quickly fit using MLE in R without using a Bayesian method. As the complexity of the model gradually increases, we may need to move the model to Stan for better parameter estimation in some cases and for formulating a more realistic model. In the EUSE example, the lmer-fit model in Qian [2016, Figure 10.10] showed that the MLE-estimated standard deviations of the region-level intercepts are nearly zero (along with a convergence failure warning). Implementing MLE-estimation in R (using functions such as lmer) yields point estimates of the variance parameters. A variance parameter is often difficult to estimate, especially when the sample size is small or the model is complicated. In this case, the number of levels in the model is small (3 regions with high antecedent agriculture) and we allowed both the intercept and slope to vary by region, such that, the lmer estimated variances are not reliable. Once we have reached a reasonable model with the fast lmer function, we should refit the model in Stan to better quantify the variances in the model (Figure 6.6). The nested group multilevel model in Tang et al. [2019] is another example. In this study, the authors designed the data collection with the intention of fitting a multilevel model similar to the model used in our EUSE example (Section 6.4.3 on page 250). Once the lmer-based non-nested model is fit, we have a good understanding of the model. The implementation of the nested version of the same model in Stan allowed confirmation of the results using a more accurate estimation method, especially for variance parameters.

This iterative process can be hidden in published papers. In Section 6.4.4, we used a multilevel model to explore the regional differences in gill-net catchability of walleye in Lake Erie and how to understand the regional differences. Our example was largely based on the use of R function `lmer` as an exploratory tool. However, the published paper reported the results from models fit using MCMC only because these models are more accurate, especially in the estimation uncertainty. This practice of reporting the final model is common because of the limited space in a journal paper.

The final model in the species-length relationship example followed this process. We began with a simple logistic regression that would appropriately quantify the transition in species composition with size. From that point, we recognized that this relationship may vary across the survey and we used exploratory data analysis to examine spatial patterns in the environmental conditions. Based on these results and what we know regarding the association between walleye and turbidity [Nieman and Gray, 2019, e.g.], we included turbidity as a grid-level predictor in the model. We fit this initial model using maximum likelihood methods in R:

```
wly.glmer<-glmer(walleye~len.c+Turb+Turb:len.c+
                    (1+len.c|Grid),
             data=data, family="binomial")
```

which confirmed that intercepts and slopes were positively correlated with turbidity. Additionally, we knew that other environmental conditions varied across the survey area, but it was not clear how these variables may influence the species composition. Therefore, we included an upper-level set of region-specific hyper-parameters which shared information among grids within regions, further improving grid-specific parameter estimates. The final model came together over time, beginning with a simple logistic regression which grew in complexity as additional information became available. At each step, estimation procedures remained robust. At each step, we monitored estimation performance before moving on to the next model formulation.

8.3   Model Evaluation

Model evaluation can be done on two levels. One is the assessment of how well a model fits the data, often based on the estimated variance parameters. The use of figures similar to an ANOVA table (e.g., Figures 5.2, 5.4, 5.5, and 5.9) gives us a familiar way to understand the "amount of variance explained" by the model. The other level is using fake data simulation to understand the model's predictive performance on important aspects of the data. In the snake fungal disease example, we used simulation (Figure 8.2) to understand how the estimated parameter posterior distribution would change if we increased the sample size. We can also directly use the MCMC samples from the joint posterior distribution to "predict" the observed number of positives to see how well the model can replicate the observed data (a form of posterior simulation). This approach was used in Qian [2016] to replicate the proportion of zeros in several examples. In the snake fungal disease example, the simulation can simply derive the posterior distribution of the probability of positive results, followed by drawing n binomial random numbers:

```
### R Code ###
firstrun <- extract(fit2keep)
p_posit <- firstrun$theta*(1-firstrun$fn)+
           (1-firstrun$theta)*firstrun$fp,
post_sim <- rbinom(length(p_posit), size=20, p_posit)
postsims <- table(post_sim)
barplot(postsims)
### End ###
```

The simulated data have a widespread distribution (Figure 8.4), with a 95% credible interval of (1, 11), an indication that the model (with the estimated parameters) cannot properly replicate the observed data.

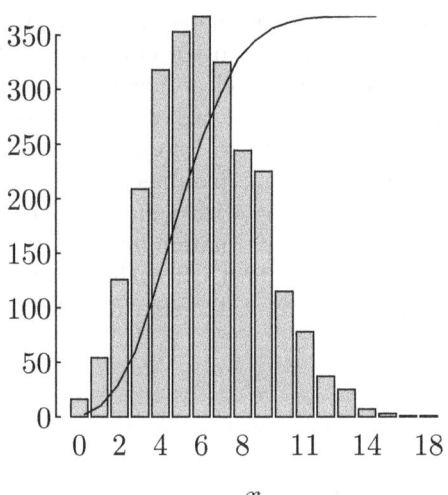

FIGURE 8.4: Random samples of number of infected snakes in a sample of 20 snakes were drawn using the joint posterior distribution of the three model parameters shown in Figure 8.1. The solid line is the cumulative distribution of the simulated data distribution.

In more complicated examples, posterior simulation can be used to summarize key statistics of interest and compare the distribution of the statistics to the corresponding observed value. For example, in the Gulf of Mexico example (Section 4.2.2, page 100), we can use posterior simulation to replicate the observed mean differences among the three zones. Because the original model could not estimate the hyper-parameters properly and the first alternative model does not have parameters representing zone means, we use the second alternative model to replicate the observed data.

To simulate the observed data, we start from random samples of α_k and β_j (equation (4.7) on page 107), which leads to a sample for each core mean (μ_i). For each core, we draw three random variates from the data distribution ($N(\mu_i, \sigma_y^2)$) to calculate the replicated zone averages and differences among the three zones.

```
### R Code ###
rich_stan3 <- rvsims(as.matrix(as.data.frame(extract(fit2keep))))

## the GOM model was fit to standardized response variable
input_sd <- input.to.stan$y_spd
input_mu <- input.to.stan$y_cen

nms3 <- names(rich_stan3)
## 1. core means
muK <- rich_stan3[substring(nms3, 1, 3)=="muK"]
## zone 1
tmp <- unique(input.to.stan$data$core[input.to.stan$data$zone==1])
zn1_core <- rich_stan3[nms3=="mu0"]+muK[tmp]+
            rich_stan3[nms3=="muZ.1"]
zn1_rep <- rvnorm(3, zn1_core, rich_stan3[nms3=="sigmaY"])
zn1_mean <- input_mu+input_sd*mean(zn1_rep)

## zone 2
tmp <- unique(input.to.stan$data$core[input.to.stan$data$zone==2])
zn2_core <- rich_stan3[nms3=="mu0"]+muK[tmp]+
            rich_stan3[nms3=="muZ.2"]
zn2_rep <- rvnorm(3, zn2_core, rich_stan3[nms3=="sigmaY"])
zn2_mean <- input_mu+input_sd*mean(zn2_rep)
## zone 3
tmp <- unique(input.to.stan$data$core[input.to.stan$data$zone==3])
zn3_core <- rich_stan3[nms3=="mu0"]+muK[tmp]+
            rich_stan3[nms3=="muZ.3"]
zn3_rep <- rvnorm(3, zn3_core, rich_stan3[nms3=="sigmaY"])
zn3_mean <- input_mu+input_sd*mean(zn3_rep)

## simulated differences
delta1 <- zn2_mean-zn1_mean
delta2 <- zn2_mean-zn3_mean
delta3 <- zn1_mean-zn3_mean
### End ###
```

The estimated zone means and zone mean differences are very close to the observed means and mean differences (Figure 8.5).

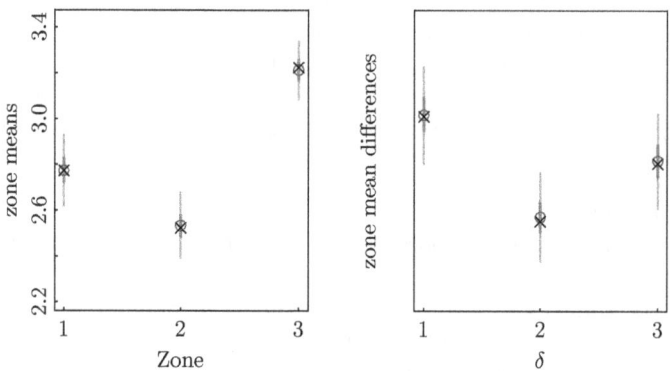

FIGURE 8.5: Replicated observations were repeatedly drawn from the alternative model 2 to replicate the mean log richness for each zone (left panel) and the zone mean differences (right panel). The observed means and mean differences are represented by crosses ($\times$).

In addition to the zone means, we use the replicated data to estimate the range of core means within each zone to see if the model captures the within-zone variances. The simulated ranges tend to be somewhat smaller than the observed ones (Figure 8.6).

The posterior simulation results provided assurance that the estimated differences among the three zones from the two alternative models are consistent with the observed data. As a result, the estimated effects of hypoxia on benthic macroinvertebrates (Figures 4.10 and 4.11) are likely reliable.

We evaluated model fit in the fishery catchability example by comparing observed mean log CPUE overall and by region to the model estimated values. We initially used linear regression in R (`lm(y~x)`) to quantify the relationship between CPUE and N, pooling together the region-specific data. However, additional information suggested the transition in lake conditions from west to east may influence catchability, and model parameter estimates, so we also fit individual region-specific models. Further, we assumed that paired samples within regions were independent of one another, and similarly, without further information on the region-level parameters, we assumed the regions themselves were exchangeable. As a result, we explored three region levels within the model using maximum likelihood methods in R (`lmer(y~x+(1+x|region))`), and this model structure documented the varying relationship between CPUE and N across the survey area. Finally, we translated the maximum likelihood model code to Stan, and used MCMC methods to estimate parameters and uncertainty. One of the challenges with this study was that data were sparse

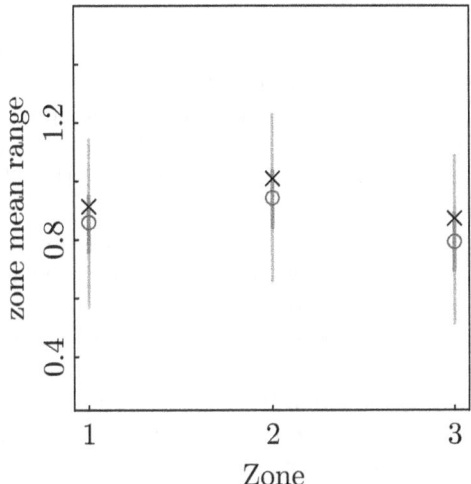

FIGURE 8.6: Replicated core mean log richness ranges within each zone. The observed ranges are represented by the cross ($\times$).

and variable, which may cause a region-specific difference to be driven by random variation. Using the hierarchical model, we shared information across regions, which led to reduction in model uncertainty and shrunk estimates toward the overall mean. When using the hierarchical modeling approach, we can properly organize the model to represent what we know and what we do not know, to help improve estimates from sparse and variable data.

8.4 Statistical Significance and Bayesian Posterior Distribution

The Gulf of Mexico hypoxia example was initially presented in Baustian et al. [2009]. Although the data were observational in nature, the initial analysis used ANOVA to evaluate the effect of hypoxia on benthic macroinvertebrate community using a significance test. Significance tests are widely used in ecological and environmental studies. However, the relevance of a significance test in ecological studies such as the one in the Gulf of Mexico hypoxia example is often debated. Reckhow [1990] observed that the meaning of a p-value (a long-run frequency-based probability value) is questionable in ecological studies where repeated observations are rare. As a result, using a significance test can be confusing. A more consistent approach is the Bayesian approach under which we directly estimate the probability of a hypothesis being true.

The vast majority of ecologists and environmental scientists are trained in classical statistics (most likely biostatistics) and the concept of significance testing is often the most familiar one. In addition, significance testing can be a useful tool in many problems where decision making is relevant. For example, environmental standard compliance assessment under the Clean Water Act is a repeated decision-making process. Even though a given water body would be only assessed once in a given time period, the concept of long-run frequency is still relevant from the perspective of the regulatory agency. The agency is responsible for evaluating all waters in their jurisdiction. Even in the Gulf of Mexico hypoxia example, where the sampling was not repeated, showing that hypoxia did have a measurable effect on the two important measures of benthic macroinvertebrate community is necessary to justify further research on the problem. Using the error probability concept in classical statistics, we can measure the uncertainty about a decision or inference using a familiar number. Whether we interpret the error probability as a long-run frequency or a degree of belief is usually irrelevant. What we need is a high degree of assurance that the inference or decision has passed rigorous testing and the likelihood of making a mistake is low.

The controversy of null hypothesis testing in scientific research is nearly always associated with the idea of reproducible results. A key misunderstanding in this discussion may be the measure of "reproducibility." Some may interpret that a reproducible study is one that can be replicated to produce the same level of statistical significance as the original one, or a similar p-value in a replicated null hypothesis test. But the p-value is a random variable, a conditional probability of observing data more extreme than the one observed if the null hypothesis is true. The variability of the p-value is a function of many factors, including sample size, population variance, and, more importantly, the magnitude of the underlying effect. Simply reporting whether a study is "significant" or not does not capture what roles these factors play. In some cases, a significant result is reported as the sole indication of a large (but undefined) difference between the null and the alternative means [Wasserstein and Lazar, 2016]. The undefined difference is another level of controversy: the lack of a specific alternative hypothesis when the null is rejected. A statistically significant result can come from an observed difference ranging from small values that are scientifically negligible to large ones that are physically impossible, making the "reproducible crisis" inevitable.

In nearly all applications of a null hypothesis testing, the null hypothesis is a target to be rejected. In the Gulf of Mexico hypoxia example, we know that hypoxia does impact benthic macroinvertebrates. What we do not know is the magnitude of the impact. As a result, an estimation-oriented approach (e.g., the Bayesian modeling we used) is more suited for the problem. Action may be warranted if, for example, the impact of hypoxia is severe. The hypothesis testing approach seems to meet such a need when declaring that the result is "highly significant." The question is how to reconcile the estimation-oriented Bayesian approach with the decision-oriented hypothesis testing. The answer lies in the logic of statistical hypothesis testing. This logic is reflected in the difference between how we explain the performance of a hypothesis test before and after observing data.

Before observing data, we want a test to be able to reject a false null hypothesis with a high probability and accept a true null hypothesis most of the time (not necessarily with a high probability). As a result, pre-data criteria for assessing a test are its probabilities of making the type I and type II errors. If we step away from the long-run frequency description of these error probabilities, we can see that the low type I error probability is designed to ensure that we do not make the most relevant type of error easily. Only when the data showed overwhelming evidence against the null could we conclude that the null should be rejected. Once we have observed the data and rejected the null hypothesis, simply stating that the result is significant seems to be unsatisfactory at best. We want to propose a specific alternative hypothesis and subject it to the same level of scrutiny. In other words, the existing hypothesis testing process explicitly defines a rigorous pre-data procedure that would reject the null hypothesis based on overwhelming evidence. Once we have the data, we need the same post-data procedure to defend any specific alternative hypothesis with strong evidence. This is the topic of "severe testing" of Mayo [2018].

We use a one sample t-test problem to illustrate the severe testing concept. In a t-test contrasting the null hypothesis of $H_0 : \mu \leq \mu_0$ against the alternative hypothesis $H_a : \mu > \mu_0$, we decide which one is supported by the data $y_1, \cdots, y_n$ by first assuming that H_0 is true. Under H_0, the t-test assumption is that the observed data follows a normal distribution with mean μ_0 (i.e., $y_i \sim N(\mu_0, \sigma^2)$), which implies that the test statistic $t = \frac{\bar{y} - \mu_0}{s/\sqrt{y}} \sim t(df = n-1)$, where $\bar{y}$ is the sample average and s is the sample standard deviation. The t-distribution has a range of $(-\infty, +\infty)$. Although any value of the test statistic is possible under the null hypothesis, the likelihood of observing a value of the t-statistic decreases under H_0 and increases under H_a as the observed value increases. Statistical hypothesis testing is, then, a means to weigh the evidence for and against H_0. The evidence is in the form of the p-value.

The Neyman-Pearson lemma defines a procedure of dividing the space of $\bar{Y}$ into a rejection region and an acceptance region. Specifically for the one-sided t-test, the rejection region is derived to ensure that the probability of making a type I error is limited to α, which is $\bar{Y} > \bar{y}_{threshold} = \mu_0 + t_{n-1}(1-\alpha)s/\sqrt{n}$, where $t_{n-1}(1 - \alpha)$ is the $1 - \alpha$ quantile of the t-distribution with degrees of freedom of $n - 1$. The Neyman-Pearson lemma shows that the process also minimizes the chance of making a type II error (failing to reject the null when the alternative is true). The long-run frequency interpretation of the process is obvious: should the process be repeated and the null is true, we would wrongly reject the null 5% of the time (when $\alpha = 0.05$) ; if the alternative is true, we will reject the null most of the time. The long-run frequency interpretation explains what will happen if using a t-test repeatedly, a pre-data explanation. Long-run frequency is the most intuitive explanation that can be easily demonstrated via Monte Carlo simulation in a classroom. It is by no means the only explanation. A small probability of error indicates the procedure of rejecting the null is based on strong evidence.

In practice, rejecting the null allows us to propose a more specific alternative hypothesis based on the data we have (post-data). As such, interpretation of test results must consider the post-data feature. When observing a sample average much larger than $\bar{y}_{threshold}$ (e.g., a sample average associated with $p = 0.0001$), we know that the observed data are more contradictory to the null than $\bar{y}_{threshold}$ is. If observing $\bar{y} = \bar{y}_{threshold}$ is evidence to conclude that $\mu > \mu_0$, observing a more contradictory sample average ($\bar{y} > \bar{y}_{threshold}$) requires us rejecting the null more severely. That is, to conclude that the true mean is not merely larger than μ_0, but also larger than $\mu_0 + \delta$ (for a specific $\delta > 0$).

We can present the hypothesis testing procedure as a logic statement of "if A (p-value is small), then B (the null is false)." For the statement to be true, its logic contrapositive of the statement, "if not B (the alternative is false) then not A (p-value is large)," must also be true. The post-data logic statement is then: if the probability of observing a sample mean more contradictory (larger) than the observed sample average under the null hypothesis (i.e., the p-value) is small (much smaller than 0.05), then we conclude $\mu > \mu_0 + \delta$. The logic contrapositive statement is: if our conclusion is wrong (i.e., $\mu \leq \mu_0 + \delta$), the probability of observing a sample average more in agreement with the null (less than the observed mean, or $\Pr(\bar{Y} < \bar{y}; \mu = \mu_0 + \delta)$) should be large (e.g., > 0.95). The value δ represents the magnitude of the difference between the sample average and the null hypothesis mean, and the probability $\pi(\delta) = \Pr(\bar{Y} < \bar{y}; \mu_0 + \delta)$ represents the levels of scrutiny we imposed on the declared difference. We can call δ the severity and the probability $\pi(\delta)$ the severity score. The data allow us to reject the null hypothesis more severely, that is, concluding that the mean is larger than $\mu_0 + \delta$, with strong evidence. For a t-test (or any given test) problem, the severity score is readily available when $\bar{y}$ and δ are known. It is the cumulative probability of $\frac{\bar{y}-(\mu_0+\delta)}{s/\sqrt{n}}$ of the t-distribution with degrees of freedom of $n - 1$. As such, the severity δ with a severity score of $\pi(\delta) = 1 - \alpha$ can be derived by

$$\frac{\bar{y} - (\mu_0 + \delta)}{s/\sqrt{n}} = t_{n-1}(1 - \alpha).$$

That is, the minimum alternative mean is $\mu_0 + \delta = \bar{y} - t_{n-1}(1 - \alpha) \times s/\sqrt{n}$, which is the lower bound of the $(1 - \alpha/2)100$ confidence interval of the sample average. The question is now whether the difference (δ), with strong evidence from the data, is large enough to be practically and scientifically meaningful and yet not too large as to be physically impossible.

The value $\mu_0 + \delta$ with a severity score of 0.975 coincides with the lower bound of the 95% confidence interval of the mean when the null hypothesis

($H_0 : \mu \leq \mu_0$) is rejected ($p < 0.05$). Likewise, when the null hypothesis is not rejected ($p > 0.05$), the value $\mu_0 + \delta$ with a severity score of 0.975 is the upper bound of the 95% confidence interval of the mean. That is, when we accept the null, we conclude that we have evidence to show that the mean is at most $\mu_0 + \delta$. If we are to believe that the null is true, we should be able to show that the difference δ is practically/scientifically negligible. Otherwise, the test result may suggest the need of further study. The sampling distribution of the sample average coincides with the Bayesian posterior distribution of the population mean. As a result, we can use the Bayesian estimated posterior distribution to carry out a hypothesis test – comparing the 2.5 or 97.5 percentile of the posterior distribution of the parameter of interest to the null hypothesis value. If the difference is practically meaningful, we conclude that the mean is at least as large as the 2.5 percentile of the posterior distribution. By presenting the magnitude of the minimum difference, we can use subject matter knowledge to decide whether the difference is scientifically meaningful/important or likely due to noise/error (either too small to be meaningful or too large to be physically justifiable).

The practical implication of the severe testing concept is that we can expand the realm of hypothesis testing beyond the limited number of tests in the classical statistics repertoire. Furthermore, we can use more realistic models for better estimating the parameters of interest. The Gulf of Mexico hypoxia example is a case in point. Using ANOVA, we are forcing a simplified model to suit the data. The resulting large estimation uncertainty makes the F-test of a low statistical power. As a result, a much larger difference in the test statistics between the observed and the null hypothesis is needed in order to reject the null hypothesis. The reduced estimation uncertainty in the three Bayesian models allowed us to conclude that the observed differences among the three zones are "significant," especially when we use the second alternative model. Using the second alternative model, the estimated log-differences between the hypoxia zone and inshore zone are -0.24 for richness and -0.64 for abundance, or the ratios of richness and abundance between the two zones are 0.79 and 0.53. Likewise, the ratios of richness and abundance between the hypoxia zone and offshore zone are 0.51 and 0.76 (Table 8.1). The estimated differences in abundance and richness between the inshore and offshore zones are quite large. As the hypoxia zone lies between the two zones, we can approximate the expected richness and abundance (without hypoxia) using the mean of the two zones. The ratios of hypoxia richness over the expected are labeled as "H/Exp" in Table 8.1. The estimated expected ratio of abundance and richness are 0.64 and 0.63, respectively. This is a near 40% decrease. Using the severe test, the data showed that the decline in abundance (0.82) is at least 18% and the decline in richness (0.72) is at least 28%. Ecologically speaking, such levels of decline are practically important.

TABLE 8.1: Posterior distributions of hypoxia effects (mean, standard deviation, and selected percentiles) are expressed as the estimated ratios of richness and abundance between the hypoxia zone (H) and the inshore (I) and offshore zones (O).

Ratio	mean	sd	2.5%	25%	50%	75%	97.5%
			Abundance				
H/I	0.53	0.087	0.39	0.48	0.53	0.58	0.73
H/O	0.76	0.103	0.59	0.69	0.75	0.82	0.99
H/Exp	0.64	0.083	0.49	0.58	0.63	0.69	0.82
			Richness				
H/I	0.79	0.061	0.68	0.74	0.78	0.83	0.92
H/O	0.51	0.035	0.44	0.48	0.50	0.53	0.58
H/Exp	0.63	0.04	0.56	0.6	0.63	0.66	0.72

8.5 Formulating a Prior Distribution Based on Hyper-distribution

In Section 3.3, we recommended that we can use a conjugate family of priors, especially the relevant physical interpretation of the conjugate prior parameter(s), to develop a proper prior distribution that reflects our knowledge. When discussing the Bayesian hierarchical modeling approach in Chapter 6, we nearly always used non-informative priors for hyper-parameters. Gelman and Hill [2007] discussed the hyper-distribution in the context of the Bayesian hierarchical modeling as the vehicle for partially pooling information across local scale data. At the same time, the hyper-distribution serves as the prior for local-level parameter estimation. In the two water quality standard assessment related examples (Neuse River Estuary in Section 4.4 and the water quality standard compliance assessment example in Section 6.4.2), we discussed the idea of using the hyper-distribution of the hierarchical model to serve as the prior distribution of the mean parameters of individual groups. In the Neuse River Estuary example, an individual group is represented by data collected in summer of a calendar year and we used a sequential updating process to incrementally update the hyper-distribution over time. The sequential-updating estimated annual mean distributions are comparable to the annual mean distributions estimated jointly using the hierarchical model (Figure 4.16 on page 130). The computation of the sequential updating was initiated by the hierarchical model. When updating the annual mean using data from a specific year, the hierarchical model is reduced to a Bayesian estimator of a normal distribution with informative prior for the mean and variance. The empirical Bayes interpretation of the hierarchical model (e.g., equations (4.15) and (4.16)) suggests that the hyper-distribution (equation (4.16)) is the prior distribution for individual annual means. In the hierarchical model, we justified the use of a common prior for all years based on two facts: (1) annual means are likely different from each other and (2) we are ignorant about the nature of the differences. The same argument was used in the water quality standard compliance assessment example (Section 6.4.2), where we argued that nutrient concentration means from different streams are likely different from each other, but we have no specific information to indicate how the means will be different among streams. As a result, a hierarchical model imposing a common prior for all streams is the only logical choice.

If we assume that μ and τ^2 in equation (4.16) are known, the posterior distribution of θ_j is

$$
\begin{aligned}
\theta_j \mid \mu, \tau^2, y &\sim N(\mu_j, \tau^2) \\
\mu_j &= \frac{\frac{n_j}{\sigma^2}\bar{y}_j + \frac{1}{\tau^2}\mu}{\frac{n_j}{\sigma^2} + \frac{1}{\tau^2}}
\end{aligned}
\tag{8.1}
$$

which shows that the hierarchically estimated group-level mean (μ_j) is a weighted average between the overall mean and the group-level sample average. As a result, μ_j is always closer to the overall mean than $\bar{y}_j$ is, which is why the hierarchical model is a shrinkage estimator. Efron [1975] compared sample averages $\bar{y}_j$ to the true underlying means μ_j and showed that when y_j's are from a multivariate normal distribution with an overall mean μ, the following relationship holds:

$$
\Pr\left[\sum_j (\bar{y}_j - \mu)^2 > \sum_j (\mu_j - \mu)^2\right] > 0.5.
\tag{8.2}
$$

In other words, the maximum likelihood estimator (sample average) is more likely to result in estimates farther away from the overall mean μ than the true means θ_j are. The theorem (equation (8.2)) implies that shrinking sample averages toward the overall mean can reduce the overall estimation error. Furthermore, when a proper prior for the mean is available, the Bayes estimator as shown in equation (8.1) has the smallest "Bayes risk" among all estimators [Lehmann and Casella, 1998].

Not only is the use of a shrinkage estimator, such as the Bayesian estimator, justified by mathematical theories in terms of Bayes risk, the Bayesian estimator as presented in equation (8.1) is also operationally and intuitively appealing. Using the Bayesian estimator, the level of shrinkage depends on the two variance parameters (σ^2/n_j and τ^2). A large among-group variance (τ^2) suggests that group means are not close to each other. The value of the overall mean as a reference is small (hence the low weight of μ in equation (8.1)). A small within-group variance (σ^2) or a large sample size (n_j), on the other hand, suggests that we are quite sure that the group-level sample average is a reliable estimate of the group mean. As a result, the weight on the sample average is large.

The sequential updating process for estimating annual means in the Neuse River Estuary example showed that hyper-distribution estimated based on data from previous years can be used as the prior for the current year. The comparison of the sequentially estimated annual means and the hierarchical (jointly) estimated annual means (Figure 4.16 on page 130) suggests that using hyper-distribution as prior is appropriate. In that example, the updated sequence of annual mean distributions is comparable to the hierarchically estimated annual mean distributions.

The hyper-distribution is the distribution of exchangeable means from different groups. As a result, we expect that deriving an informative prior for a mean parameter can be guided by identifying whether we have information on similar systems from existing studies. If we call these similar systems "exchangeable units," a practical approach for deriving an informative prior may be the empirical distribution of the quantity of interest among exchangeable units. We explored the potential of this idea in the water quality compliance assessment example (Section 6.4.2), where total phosphorus concentration data from streams in Ohio within one eco-region in the Lake Erie watershed were used to fit a Bayesian hierarchical model. The fitted hyper-distribution was used as the prior for the mean total phosphorus concentration in another river in the same eco-region in Upstate New York. The use of an informative prior for the mean parameter made the assessment process more stable, overcoming the effect of the fickle p-value when using hypothesis testing.

The above discussion led to the proposal of revising the currently used hypothesis-testing based methods to an estimation-based approach in water quality standard compliance assessment. Because water quality standard compliance assessment is water-body-specific, the current practice evaluates the compliance one water body at a time. When the sample size of the target water body is small, the hypothesis-testing based method will always be unsatisfactory due to the low power of the statistical test. However, water quality standard compliance assessment is the responsibility of a state. The state agency responsible for the assessment must evaluate all water-bodies in the state. There are many types of water in a state and we can group them based on their ecological and hydrologic characteristics. In the example in Section 6.4.2, we grouped small wadable streams by eco-region in the Lake Erie watershed. Likewise, we can group lakes by their size and trophic levels. Once water-bodies of similar characteristics are identified, we can pool existing data to fit a hierarchical model to estimate annual means of individual water-bodies. After the initial hierarchical model of multiple similar (or exchangeable) water-bodies, we can start the sequential updating process for each water body separately. Computationally, this process can be automated, and the assessment decision can be based on the comparison of a pre-selected upper percentile (e.g., 80-percentile) of the estimated mean concentration distribution to the water quality standard.

In our formulation of the sequential updating algorithm, we approximated the estimated posterior distributions of the mean parameters as normal-inverse-gamma distributions and the posterior distributions of variance parameters as inverse-gamma distributions. The normal-inverse-gamma and inverse gamma distributions are conjugate priors for the normal distribution mean and variances. Although intended to simplify the computation of the sequential updating process, the approximation process is applicable in many modeling situations because the posterior distributions of most regression estimated model parameters are conditionally normal. For example, in the EUSE example, we fit a Bayesian hierarchical (linear) model using data from nine metropolitan regions. When data are available for the tenth region, we can summarize the posterior hyper-distributions of all model coefficients to derive informative priors for the tenth regional model coefficients. The hyper-distribution serves as a record of information from the existing nine regions. When fitting the model for the tenth region, we do not need to carry the existing data forward, thereby simplifying the computation by avoiding repeating the models for the existing nine regions. The updated hyper-distribution of model parameters summarizes information from all ten regions. A comparison of the updated hyper-distribution to the hyper-distribution estimated based on data from the previous nine regions can inform us about the changes of the updated hyper-distribution from the previously estimated hyper-distribution.

8.5.1 Example: Forecasting the Likelihood of High Cyanobacterial Toxin Concentration Events in Western Lake Erie

As an example of using the exchangeable unit concept to derive informative prior distributions, we summarize a short-term risk assessment model based on the sequentially updated empirical relationship between the cyanobacterial toxin (microcystin) concentration and the chlorophyll a concentration (a measure of lake phytoplankton density). The study is part of National Oceanic and Atmospheric Administrations's (NOAA) effort to forecast harmful algal blooms in Western basin of Lake Erie. Currently NOAA makes annual predictions of the size of the bloom based on observed spring total phosphorus loading from the Maumee River, the largest source of phosphorus to Lake Erie. The short-term forecast of the likelihood of high toxicity events can be used to supplement the annual size predictions to help local public and private entities to develop and deploy remedial plans in a timely fashion [Qian et al., 2021b]. A notable remedial strategy is to strengthen the carbon filtration treatment in many drinking water treatment plants.

The empirical relationship between microcystin (MC) concentration and chlorophyll a (Chla) concentration in Western Lake Erie was characterized by a hockey-stick model because of the high level of uncertainty in the measured MC concentration, as demonstrated by Qian et al. [2015a]. The measurement uncertainty is related to the calibration curve method discussed in Section 4.3.2.1 and detailed in Qian [2016, Chapters 6 and 10]. When Chla concentrations were low (likely occurred in spring/early summer or early full), the phytoplankton community in Western basin of Lake Erie was likely dominated by non-cyanobacteria species. Therefore, MC concentrations should be low. The high level of measurement uncertainty, however, often obscures the typical log-log linear relationship between MC and Chla concentrations, leading to a random pattern at the low end of the Chla concentration spectrum. When plotted on the log-log scale, the MC-Chla data cloud resembles a hockey stick. If a log-log linear regression is used, the high level of uncertainty in the lower end of the Chla range may result in underestimation of the slope, and thereby underestimating the risk of high MC concentration probability when Chla is high. As a result, the smoothed change point model (equation (7.10), with $\beta_0 = 0$) was used.

The relationship between MC and Chla cannot be viewed as a causal relationship. Although the presence of phytoplankton is a necessary condition for MC production, only a few cyanobacteria are known to produce these toxins. Furthermore, most toxin-producing cyanobacteria do not produce toxin all the time. At the same time, we are unclear about what triggers the production of MC. As a result, the predictor (Chla) represents only the necessary condition, not the sufficient condition, for MC production. Over a large spatiotemporal scale, we observe a log-log relationship between MC and Chla. However, the apparent correlation between MC and Chla is likely a result of some unknown factors that influence both MC and Chla. If these unknown factors are stable over time, the correlation between MC and Chla can be used to predict how MC changes as a function of Chla. But we do not know what these factors are and data show that the MC-Chla relationship varies over time. If we use data from multiple years to fit the MC-Chla regression model, the model would be of no near-term predictive value as the MC-Chla model fit with long-term data reflects the average pattern. This is another manifestation of Simpson's paradox – the average correlation estimated based on data from multiple years is likely different from the correlation estimated based on data from a short time period (e.g., one or two weeks).

The modeling approach used in Qian et al. [2021b] used a two-tier sequential updating process. These two tiers represent two temporal scales: annual and prediction periods within a sampling season (each period is between one to two weeks). At the annual temporal scale, a hierarchical model was initially fit to data from the first nine years of the monitoring program (2008-2016). The goal of this annual hierarchical model is to derive the hyper-distributions of model coefficients to be used as priors for subsequent years. The first-tier models represent annual mean patterns of the MC-Chla relationship. The sequential updating process is used with hyper-distributions of model parameters from the initial hierarchical model as the initial informative priors for models fit in subsequent years. The hyper-distribution is then updated, along with the annual model using new data each year. For short-term (one to two

weeks) prediction, second-tier sequential updating is used. At the beginning
of a sampling season, the most recently updated hyper-distributions of the
annual model parameters are used as the prior for the first short-term model
fit with the data from the first one to two weeks of the sampling season. The
resulting model is then used as a predictive model for the next prediction
period. The predicted MC concentration distribution is a function of Chla
concentration. Because automated monitoring platforms have been installed
in many important locations in Lake Erie, we can use these real-time reporting data streams to predict the probability of MC concentration exceeding a
certain threshold. Once data from the next sampling period are available, the
model is updated. At the end of each sampling season, the annual model is
updated (Figure 8.7).

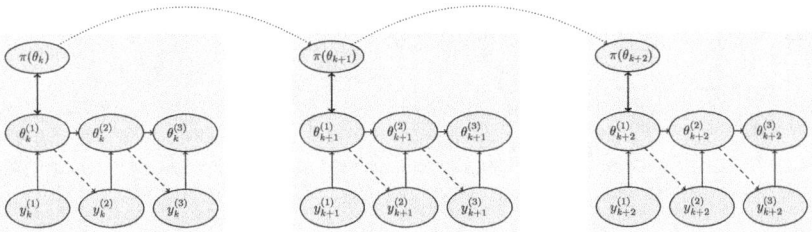

FIGURE 8.7: A schematic representation of the sequential updating and
short-term risk assessment of high microcystin concentration events in Western Lake Erie using weekly harmful algal bloom monitoring data. The dotted
lines represent the annual updating to derive annual prior distributions of
model parameters (θ_k) and the shaded blocks represent within-year sequential updating-forecasting using data from individual sampling periods to derive
sampling-period posterior distributions ($\theta_k^i, i = 1, \cdots, n_k$) for predicting MC
concentration distribution for the next sampling period. Within each year, the
initial priors ($\pi(\theta_k)$) are based on data from the previous year.

At the annual scale, model parameters represent the annual mean relationship between log MC and log Chla. As such, prior distributions for parameters
of an annual model can be derived from the hyper-distributions of a hierarchical model fit to data from previous years. The sequential updating process
eases the computation burden. As the MC-Chla relationship changes within
a year, the annual mean model is ill-suited for short-term prediction. At the
same time, we do not have enough data to fit the MC-Chla model for each
sampling period. Using the hyper-distribution updated from the previous year
as the priors for model coefficients, the regression model becomes more relevant to the current sampling period.

Bibliography

S. Acid, L.M. de Campos, J.M. Fernández-Luna, S. Rodrıguez, J.M. Rodrıguez, and J.L. Salcedo. A comparison of learning algorithms for Bayesian networks: A case study based on data from an emergency medical service. *Artificial Intelligence in Medicine*, 30(3):215–232, 2004.

A. Agresti. *Analysis of Ordinal Categorical Data*. John Wiley & Sons, Ltd., Hoboken, NJ, 2nd edition, 2010.

P. Aguilera, A. Fernández, Fernández R., R. Rumí, and A. Salmerón. Bayesian networks in environmental modelling. *Environmental Modelling and Software*, 26:1376–1388, 2011.

I. Alameddine, Y.K. Cha, and K.H. Reckhow. An evaluation of automated structure learning with Bayesian networks: An application to estuarine chlorophyll dynamics. *Environmental Modelling and Software*, 26(2):163–172, 2011.

B.J. Alder and T.E. Wainwright. Studies in molecular dynamics. I. General method. *The Journal of Chemical Physics*, 31(2):459–466, 1959.

P.J. Allen, Z.A. Mitchell, R.J. DeVries, D.L. Aboagye, M.A. Ciaramella, S.W. Ramee, H.A. Steward, and R.B. Shartau. Salinity effects on Atlantic sturgeon (*Acipenser oxyrinchus oxyrinchus Mitchell, 1815*) growth and osmoregulation. *Journal of Applied Ichthyology*, 30(6):1229–1236, 2014.

M.C. Allender, D.B. Raudabaugh, F.H. Gleason, and A.N. Miller. The natural history, ecology, and epidemiology of *Ophidiomyces ophiodiicola* and its potential impact on free-ranging snake populations. *Fungal Ecology*, 17:187–196, 2015.

M.J. Alvarez-Martínez, J.M. Miró, M.E. Valls, A. Moreno, P.V. Rivas, M. Solé, N. Benito, P. Domingo, C. Muñoz, E. Rivera, H.J. Zar, G. Wissmann, A.R.S. Diehl, J.C. Prolla, M.T.J. de Anta, J.M. Gatell, P.E. Wilson, and S.R. Meshnick. Sensitivity and specificity of nested and real-time PCR for the detection of *Pneumocystis jiroveci* in clinical specimens. *Diagnostic Microbiology and Infectious Disease*, 56(2):153–160, 2006.

D.P. Ames, B.T. Neilson, D.K. Stevens, and U. Lall. Using Bayesian networks to model watershed management decisions: An east Canyon Creek case study. *Journal of Hydroinformatics*, 7(4):267–282, 2005.

ASMFC. Atlantic sturgeon benchmark stock assessment and peer review report. Technical report, Atlantic States Marine Fisheries Commission, Arlington, VA., 2017.

S.G. Baker. The multinomial-Poisson transformation. *The Statistician*, 43(4): 495–504, 1994.

M.T. Barbour and M.J. Paul. Add value to water resource management through biological assessment of rivers. *Hydrobiologia*, 651:17–24, 2010.

M.T. Barbour, J. Gerritsen, B.D. Snyder, and J.B. Stribling. Rapid bioassessment protocols for use in streams and wadeable rivers: Periphyton, benthic macroinvertebrates and fish, 2nd edition, EPA 841-B-99/002. Technical report, U.S. Environmental Protection Agency; Office of Water; Washington D.C., 1999.

J. Barnard, R. McCulloch, and X. Meng. Modeling covariance matrices in terms of standard deviations and correlations, with application of shrinkage. *Statistica Sinica*, 10(4):1281–1311, 2000.

V. Barnett and A. O'Hagan. *Setting Environmental Standards: The Statistical Approach to Handling Uncertainty and Variation*. Chapman and Hall, London, UK., 1997.

D. Barton, T. Saloranta, S. Moe, H. Eggestad, and S. Kuikka. Bayesian belief networks as a meta-modelling tool in integrated river basin management – pros and cons in evaluating nutrient abatement decisions under uncertainty in a Norwegian river basin. *Ecological Economics*, 66(1):91–104, 2008.

D.M. Bates. *lme4: Mixed-effects Modeling with R*. Springer, 2010. URL `http://lme4.r-forge.r-project.org/book/`.

M.M. Baustian, J.K. Craig, and N.N. Rabalais. Effects of summer 2003 hypoxia on macrobenthos and Atlantic croaker foraging selectivity in the northern Gulf of Mexico. *Journal of Experimental Marine Biology and Ecology*, 381:531–537, 2009.

P.M. Berthouex and L.C. Brown. *Statistics for Environmental Engineers*. Lewis Publishers, Boca Raton, 1994.

J. Besag, J. York, and A. Mollie. Bayesian image restoration, with two applications in spatial statistics (with discussion). *Annals of the Institute of Statistical Mathematics*, 43:1–59, 1991.

T. Beuzen, L. Marshall, and K.D. Splinter. A comparison of methods for discretizing continuous variables in Bayesian networks. *Environmental Modelling and Software*, 108:61–66, 2018.

P.J. Bickel, E.A. Hammel, and J.W. O'Connell. Sex bias in graduate admissions: Data from Berkeley. *Science*, 187:398–404, 1975.

A.A. Binsaeed, A.A. Al-Khedhairy, A.M. Mandil, S.A. Shaikh, R. Qureshi, A.S. Al-Khattaf, H.A. Habib, A.A. Alam, L.A. Al-Ansary, and M. Al-Omran. A validation study comparing the sensitivity and specificity of the new Dr. KSU H1N1 RT-PCR kit with real-time RT-PCR for diagnosing influenza A (H1N1). *Annals of Saudi Medicine*, 31(4):351–355, 2011.

J. A. Bishop. An experimental study of the cline of industrial melanism in Biston Betularia (L.) (Lepidoptera) between urban Liverpool and rural North Wales. *The Journal of Animal Ecology*, 41(1):209–243, 1972.

M. E. Borsuk, C. A. Stow, and K. H. Reckhow. A Bayesian network of eutrophication models for synthesis, prediction, and uncertainty analysis. *Ecological Modelling*, 173(2-3):219–239, 2004.

G.E.P. Box. Science and statistics. *Journal of the American Statistical Association*, 71(356):791–799, 1976.

G.E.P. Box and G.C. Tiao. *Bayesian Inference in Statistical Analysis*. Addison-Wesley, Reading, MA, 1973.

J. Bromley, N.A. Jackson, O.J. Clymer, A.M. Giacomello, and F.V. Jensen. The use of Hugin to develop Bayesian networks as an aid to integrated water resource planning. *Environmental Modelling and Software*, 20(2):231–242, 2005.

L.R. Brown, T.F. Cuffney, J.F. Coles, F. Fitzpatrick, G. McMahon, J. Steuer, A.H. Bell, and J.T. May. Urban streams across the USA: Lessons learned from studies in 9 metropolitan areas. *Journal of the North American Benthological Society*, 28(4):1051–1069, 2009.

J. N. Carleton and H. J. Montas. A modeling approach for mixing and reaction in wetlands with continuously varying flow. *Ecological Engineering*, 29(1): 33–44, 2007.

B. Carpenter, A. Gelman, M.D. Hoffman, D. Lee, B. Goodrich, M. Betancourt, M. Brubaker, J. Guo, P. Li, and Al. Riddell. Stan: A probabilistic programming language. *Journal of Statistical Software*, 76(1):1–32, 2017.

S.R. Carpenter, H.A. Mooney, J. Agard, D. Capistrano, R.S. DeFries, S. Díaz, T. Dietz, A.K. Duraiappah, A. Oteng-Yeboah, H.M. Pereira, C. Perrings, W.V. Reid, J. Sarukhan, R.J. Scholes, and A Whyte. Science for managing ecosystem services: Beyond the millennium ecosystem assessment. *Proceedings of the National Academy of Sciences*, 106(5):1305–1312, 2009. ISSN 0027-8424. doi: 10.1073/pnas.0808772106. URL https://www.pnas.org/content/106/5/1305.

G. Casella and E.I. George. Explaining the Gibbs sampler. *The American Statistician*, 46(3):167–174, 1992. doi: 10.1080/00031305.1992.10475878.

T. C. Chamberlin. The method of multiple working hypotheses. *Science*, 15 (old series):92, 1890.

Y.E. Chee, L. Wilkinson, A.E. Nicholson, P.F. Quintana-Ascencio, J.E. Fauth, D. Hall, K.J. Ponzio, and L. Rumpff. Modelling spatial and temporal changes with GIS and spatial and dynamic Bayesian networks. *Environmental Modelling and Software*, 82:108–120, 2016.

S.H. Chen and C.A. Pollino. Good practice in Bayesian network modelling. *Environmental Modelling and Software*, 37:134–145, 2012.

F.Y. Cheng and N.B. Basu. Biogeochemical hotspots: Role of small water bodies in landscape nutrient processing. *Water Resources Research*, 53(6): 5038–5056, 2017.

K.S. Chin, D.W. Tang, J.B. Yang, S.Y. Wong, and H. Wang. Assessing new product development project risk by Bayesian network with a systematic probability generation methodology. *Expert Systems with Applications*, 36 (6):9879–9890, 2009.

G. Chiu, R. Lockhart, and R. Routledge. Bent-cable regression theory and applications. *Journal of the American Statistical Association*, 101(474): 542–553, 2006.

D.G. Clayton. Generalized linear mixed models. In W.R. Gilks, S. Richardson, and D.J. Spielelhalter, editors, *Markov Chain Monte Carlo in Practice*, pages 275–301. Chapman and Hall, London, 1996.

R.T. Clemen. *Making Bard Decisions: An Introduction to Decision Analysis*. Brooks/Cole Publishing Company, 1996.

R.T. Clemen and R.L. Winkler. Combining probability distributions from experts in risk analysis. *Risk Analysis*, 19(2):187–203, 1999.

J.F. Coles, T.F. Cuffney, and G. McMahon. The effects of urbanization on the biological, physical, and chemical characteristics of coastal New England streams. Technical report, U.S. Geological Survey Professional Paper 1695, Reston, Virginia, USA, 2004.

Norsys Software Company. *Netica User's Manual*. Vancouver, Canada, 2010.

S. Cooper, M. Goman, and Richardson C.J. Historical changes in waster quality and vegetation in WCA2A determined by paleoecological analyses. In C.J. Richardson, editor, *The Everglades Experiments: Lessons for Ecosystem Restoration*, pages 321–350, New York, 2008. Springer-Verlag.

S.R. Cooper, J. Huvane, P. Vaithiyanathan, and C.J. Richardson. Calibration of diatoms along a nutrient gradient in Florida Everglades Water Conservation Area-2A, USA. *Journal of Paleolimnology*, 22:413–437, 1999.

R.M. Couture, S.J. Moe, Y. Lin, Ø. Kaste, S. Haande, and A.L. Solheim. Simulating water quality and ecological status of Lake Vansjø, Norway, under land-use and climate change by linking process-oriented models with a Bayesian network. *Science of the Total Environment*, 621:713–724, 2018.

R.G. Cowell. *Probabilistic Networks and Expert Systems*. Springer-Verlag, New York, NY, 1999.

C.B. Craft and C.J. Richardson. Peat accretion and nitrogen, phosphorus andoganic carbon accumulation in nutrient-enriched and unenriched Everglades peatlands. *Ecological Applications*, 3:446–458, 1993.

B. Cudmore, L.A. Jones, N.E. Mandrak, J.M. Dettmers, Chapman, D.C., C.S. Kolar, and G. Conover. Ecological risk assessment of grass carp (*Ctenopharyngodon idella*) for the Great Lakes Basin, 2017.

T.F. Cuffney and J.A. Falcone. Derivation of nationally consistent indices representing urban intensity within and across nine metropolitan areas of the conterminous United States. Technical report, U.S. Geological Survey, Scientific Investigations Report 2008-5095, 36 pp., 2008.

T.F. Cuffney and S.S. Qian. A critique of the use of indicator species scores for identifying thresholds in species responses. *Freshwater Science*, 32(2): 471–488, 2013.

T.F. Cuffney, H. Zappia, E.M.P. Giddings, and J.F. Coles. Effects of urbanization on benthic macroinvertebrate assemblages in contrasting environmental settings: Boston, Massachusetts; Birmingham, Alabama; and Salt Lake City, Utah. *American Fisheries Society Symposium*, 47:361–407, 2005.

T.F. Cuffney, G. McMahon, J.A. May, and I.A. Waite. Responses of benthic macroinvertebrates to environmental changes associated with urbanization in nine metropolitan areas of the conterminous United States. In R.M.T. Webb and D.J. Semmens, editors, *Planning for an Uncertain Future—Monitoring, Integration, and Adaptation. Proceedings of the Third Interagency Conference on Research in the Watersheds*, pages 187–194. U.S. Geological Survey Scientific Investigations Report 2009-5049, 2009.

T.F. Cuffney, R.A. Brightbill, J.T. May, and I.R. Waite. Responses of benthic macroinvertebrates to environmental changes associated with urbanization in nine metropolitan areas. *Ecological Applications*, 20:1384–1401, 2010.

M. Das and S.K. Ghosh. FB-STEP: A fuzzy Bayesian network based data-driven framework for spatio-temporal prediction of climatological time series data. *Expert Systems with Applications*, 117:211–227, 2019.

M. Das and S.K. Ghosh. Spatial Bayesian network. In *Enhanced Bayesian Network Models for Spatial Time Series Prediction*, volume 858 of *Studies in Computational Intelligence*. Springer, 2020.

S.P. Davies and S.K. Jackson. The biological condition gradient: A descriptive model for interpreting change in aquatic ecosystems. *Ecological Applications*, 16(4):1251–1266, 2006.

J.H. Davis. The natural features of southern Florida, especially the vegetation, and the Everglades. Technical report, Florida Geological Survey Bulletin, No. 25, 1943.

L.M. de Campos and J.G. Castellano. Bayesian network learning algorithms using structural restrictions. *International Journal of Approximate Reasoning*, 45(2):233–254, 2007.

R.G. Death, F. Death, R. Stubbington, M.K. Joy, and M. van den Belt. How good are Bayesian belief networks for environmental management? A test with data from an agricultural river catchment. *Freshwater Biology*, 60(11): 2297–2309, 2015.

A.P. Dempster, N.M. Laird, and D.B. Rubin. Maximum likelihood from incomplete data via the EM algorithm. *Journal of the Royal Statistical Society: Series B (Methodological)*, 39(1):1–22, 1977.

P. J. Dillon and F. H. Rigler. Phosphorus-chlorophyll relationship in lakes. *Limnology and Oceanography*, 19:767–773, 1974.

W.M. Dlamini. A Bayesian belief network analysis of factors influencing wildfire occurrence in Swaziland. *Environmental Modelling and Software*, 25(2): 199–208, 2010.

M.R. DuFour, S.S. Qian, C.M. Mayer, and C.S. Vandergoot. Evaluating catchability in a large-scale gillnet survey using hydroacoustics: Making the case for coupled surveys. *Fisheries Research*, 211:309–318, 2019.

M.R. DuFour, Qian S.S., C.M. Mayer, and C.S. Vandergoot. Embracing uncertainty to reduce bias in hydroacoustic species apportionment. *Fisheries Research*, 233:105750, 2021.

M.F. D'Angelo, R.M. Palhares, L.B. Cosme, L.A. Aguiar, F.S. Fonseca, and W.M. Caminhas. Fault detection in dynamic systems by a Fuzzy/Bayesian network formulation. *Applied Soft Computing*, 21:647–653, 2014.

B Efron. Biased versus unbiased estimation. *Advances in Mathematics*, 16: 259–277, 1975.

B. Efron. Controversies in the foundations of statistics. *The American Mathematical Monthly*, 85(4):231–246, 1978.

B. Efron and C. Morris. Stein's paradox in statistics. *Scientific American*, 236:119–127, 1977.

H.S. Embke, P.M. Kocovsky, C.A. Richter, J.J. Pritt, C.M. Mayer, and S.S. Qian. First direct confirmation of grass carp spawning in a Great Lakes tributary. *Journal of Great Lakes Research*, 42(4):899–903, 2016.

U. M. Fayyad and K. B. Irani. Multi-interval discretization of continuous valued attributes for classification learning. In *Proceedings of the 13th International Joint Conference on Artificial Intelligence*, pages 1022–1029, Chambery, France, 1993. Morgan-Kaufmann.

FDEP. Overview of approaches for numeric nutrient criteria development in marine waters. Technical report, Florida Department of Environmental Protection, Division of Environmental Assessment and Restoration, Standards and Assessment Section, Tallahassee, FL 32399, 2011.

T.S. Ferguson. A Bayesian analysis of some nonparametric problems. *Annals of Statistics*, 1:209–230, 1973.

M.N. Fienen, J.P. Masterson, N.G. Plant, B.T. Gutierrez, and E.R. Thieler. Bridging groundwater models and decision support with a Bayesian network. *Water Resources Research*, 49(10):6459–6473, 2013.

R. A. Fisher, A. S. Corbet, and C. B. Williams. The relation between the number of species and the number of individuals in a random sample of an animal community. *Journal of Animal Ecology*, 12:42–58, 1943.

R.A. Fisher. On the mathematical foundations of theoretical statistics. *Philosophical Transactions of the Royal Society of London, Series A*, 222:309–368, 1922.

R.A. Fisher. *Statistical Methods and Scientific Inference*. Hafner Publishing Co., Oxford, England, 1956.

M.D. Flora, D.R. Walker, D.J. Scheidt, R.G. Rice, and D.H. Landers. The response of the Everglades marsh to increased nitrogen and phosphorus loading. Part I: Nutrient dosing, water chemistry and periphyton productivity. Technical report, Everglades National Park, Report to the Superintendent, Homestead, FL, USA, 1988.

M.A.E. Forio, D. Landuyt, E. Bennetsen, K. Lock, T.H.T. Nguyen, M.N.D. Ambarita, P.L.S. Musonge, P. Boets, G. Everaert, and L. Dominguez-Granda. Bayesian belief network models to analyse and predict ecological water quality in rivers. *Ecological Modelling*, 312:222–238, 2015.

Jr. Gauch, H. G. and R. H. Whittaker. Coenocline simulation. *Ecology*, 53 (3):446–451, 1972.

A.E. Gelfand and A.F.M. Smith. Sampling-based approaches to calculating marginal densities. *Journal of American Statistical Association*, 85:398–409, 1990.

A. Gelman. Analysis of variance – why it is more important than ever (with discussions). *The Annals of Statistics*, 33(1):1–53, 2005.

A. Gelman. Prior distributions for variance parameters in hierarchical models (comment on an article by Browne and Draper). *Bayesian Analysis*, 1(3): 515–533, 2006.

A. Gelman. *Red State, Blue State, Rich State, Poor State: Why Americans Vote the Way They Do*. Princeton University Press, 2009.

A. Gelman and J. Hill. *Data Analysis Using Regression and Multi-level/Hierarchical Models*. Cambridge University Press, New York, 2007.

A. Gelman, A. Jakulin, M.G. Pittau, and Y.S. Su. A weakly informative default prior distribution for logistic and other regression models. *The Annals of Applied Statistics*, 2(4):1360–1383, 2008.

A. Gelman, J. Hill, and M. Yajima. Why we (usually) don't have to worry about multiple comparisons. *Journal of Research on Educational Effectiveness*, 5:189–211, 2012.

S. Geman and D. Geman. Stochastic relaxation, Gibbs distributions, and the Bayesian restoration of images. *IEEE Transactions on Pattern Analysis and Machine Intelligence*, PAMI-6(6):721–741, Nov 1984. ISSN 0162-8828. doi: 10.1109/TPAMI.1984.4767596.

R. Giné-Garriga, D. Requejo, J.L. Molina, and A. Pérez-Foguet. A novel planning approach for the water, sanitation and hygiene (WaSH) sector: The use of object-oriented Bayesian networks. *Environmental Modelling and Software*, 103:1–15, 2018.

A. Gleit. Estimation of small normal data sets with detection limits. *Environmental Science and Technology*, 19:1201–1206, 1985.

J. Gonzalez-Redin, S. Luque, L. Poggio, R. Smith, and A. Gimona. Spatial Bayesian belief networks as a planning decision tool for mapping ecosystem services trade-offs on forested landscapes. *Environmental Research*, 144: 15–26, 2016.

A.R. Gouveia, S.S. Qian, C. Mayer, J. Smith, J. Bossenbroek, W.D. Hintz, R. Mapes, J. Navarro, P. Kocovsky, J.M. Dettmers, R. Young, and J.T. Buszkiewicz. A Bayesian approach to estimate abundance of a rare and invasive fish. *Biological Invasions*, In Review, 2022.

V. Guillory and R.D. Gasaway. Zoogeography of the grass carp in the United States. *Transactions of the American Fisheries Society*, 107:105–112, 1978.

P. Guttorp. Setting environmental standards: A statistician's perspective. *Environmental Geosciences*, 13(4):261–266, 2006.

S. Hansson and L.G. Rudstam. Gillnet catches as an estimate of fish abundance: A comparison between vertical gillnet catches and hydroacoustic abundances of Baltic Sea herring (*Clupea harengus*) and sprat (*Sprattus sprattus*). *Canadian Journal of Fisheries and Aquatic Sciences*, 52:75–83, 1995.

S.J. Harley, R.A. Myers, and A. Dunn. Is catch-per-unit-effort proportional to abundance? *Canadian Journal of Fisheries and Aquatic Sciences*, 58: 1760–1772, 2001.

W. K. Hastings. Monte Carlo sampling methods using Markov chains and their applications. *Biometrika*, 57:97–109, 1970.

J. Hejzlar, K. Samalova, P. Boers, and B. Kronvang. Modelling phosphorus retention in lakes and reservoirs. In B. Kronvang, J. Faganeli, and N. Ogrinc, editors, *The Interactions between Sediments and Water*, page 123–130, Dordrecht, Netherlands, 2007. Springer.

S.J. Herbst, L.R. Nathan, T.J. Newcomb, M.R. DuFour, J. Tyson, E. Weimer, J. Buszkiewicz, and J.M. Dettmers. An adaptive management approach for implementing multi-jurisdictional response to grass carp in lake erie. *Journal of Great Lakes Research*, 47(1):96–107, 2021.

R. Hilborn and M. Mangel. *The Ecological Detective: Confronting Models with Data*. Princeton University Press, Princeton, New Jersey, 1997.

E.T. Hileman, M.C. Allender, D.R. Bradke, L.J. Faust, J.A. Moore, M.J. Ravesi, and S.J. Tetzlaff. Estimation of *Ophidiomyces* prevalence to evaluate snake fungal disease risk. *The Journal of Wildlife Management*, page doi:10.1002/jwmg.21345, 2017.

M.D. Hoffman and A. Gelman. The no-U-turn sampler: Adaptively setting path lengths in Hamiltonian Monte Carlo. *Journal of Machine Learning Research*, 15:1351–1381, 2014.

K. Hornik, C. Buchta, and A. Zeileis. Open-source machine learning: R meets Weka. *Computational Statistics*, 24(2):225–232, 2009.

Hugin Expert. *Hugin GUI Manual 9.0*. Aalborg, Denmark, 2021.

J. Huisman, H. Olff, and L. F. M. Fresco. A hierarchical set of models for species response analysis. *Journal of Vegetation Science*, 4(1):37–46, 1993.

S. Jaffe. Assessing the risk of grass carp spawning in Lake Erie tributaries using discharge and water temperature. Master's thesis, The University of Toledo, Toledo, Ohio, USA, 2021.

W. James and Charles Stein. Estimation with quadratic loss. In *Proceedings of the 4th Berkeley Symposium Mathematics, Statistics and Probability*, volume 1, pages 361–379. University of California Press, Berkeley, California, 1961.

H. Jeffreys. An invariant form for the prior probability in estimation problems. *Proceedings of the Royal Society of London. Series A, Mathematical and Physical Sciences*, 186(1007):453–461, 1946.

H. Jeffreys. *Theory of Probability*. Oxford Univ Press, Oxford, 3rd edition, 1961.

J. Jensen, S. Cooper, and C. Richardson. Calibration of modern pollen along a nutrient gradient in Everglades Water Conservation Area-2A. *Wetlands*, 19:675–688, 1999.

X. Jin, B.P. Carlin, and S. Banerjee. Generalized hierarchical multivariate CAR models for areal data. *Biometrics*, 61(4):950–961, 2005.

S. Johnson, F. Fielding, G. Hamilton, and K. Mengersen. An integrated Bayesian network approach to *Lyngbya majuscula* bloom initiation. *Marine Environmental Research*, 69(1):27–37, 2010.

J.R. Jones and R.W. Bachmann. Prediction of phosphorus and chlorophyll levels in lakes. *Journal of Water Pollution Control Federation*, 48(9):2176–2182, 1976.

R.O. Kashuba. *Bayesian Methods to Characterize Uncertainty in Predictive Modeling of the Effect of Urbanization on Aquatic Ecosystems*, 2010. PhD dissertation.

A.A. Keller and L. Cavallaro. Assessing the US Clean Water Act 303(d) listing process for determining impairment of a waterbody. *Journal of Environmental Management*, 86:699–711, 2008.

J.G. Kennen and M.A. Ayers. Relation of environmental characteristics to the composition of aquatic assemblages along a gradient of urban land use in New Jersey, 1996-98. Technical report, U.S. Geological Survey Water-Resources Investigations Report 02-4069, West Trenton, New Jersey, USA, 2002.

M. Kéry, J.A. Royle, and H. Schmid. Modeling avian abundance from replicated counts using binomial mixture models. *Ecological Applications*, 15: 1450–1461, 2005.

A. Keshtkar, A. Salajegheh, A. Sadoddin, and M.G. Allan. Application of Bayesian networks for sustainability assessment in catchment modeling and management (Case study: The Hablehrood River catchment). *Ecological Modelling*, 268:48–54, 2013.

H.J. Kim. *Discretization: Data Preprocessing, Discretization for Classification*, 2012. URL https://CRAN.R-project.org/package=discretization. R package version 1.0-1.

U.B. Kjaerulff and A.L. Madsen. *Bayesian Networks and Influence Diagrams.* Springer Science & Business Media, New York, NY, 2008.

I. Kononenko. On biases in estimating multi-valued attributes. In *Proceedings IJCAI95, Montreal, Que.*, pages 1034–1040, Los Altos, CA, 1995. Morgan Kaufmann.

K.B. Korb and A.E. Nicholson. *Bayesian Artificial Intelligence.* CRC Press, 2010.

D. Lambert. Zero-inflated Poisson regression, with an application to defects in manufacturing. *Technometrics*, 34(1):1–14, 1992.

M. Lavine. An approach to evaluating sensitivity in Bayesian regression analysis. *Journal of Statistical Planning and Inference*, 40:233–244, 1994.

E.L. Lehmann and G. Casella. *Theory of Point Estimation.* Springer, New York, 2nd edition, 1998.

D. Lewandowski, D. Kurowicka, and H. Joe. Generating random correlation matrices based on vines and extended onion method. *Journal of Multivariate Analysis*, 100(9):1989–2001, 2009. ISSN 0047-259X. doi: https://doi.org/10.1016/j.jmva.2009.04.008.

C.S. Li. Identifiability of zero-inflated Poisson models. *Brazilian Journal of Probability and Statistics*, 26(3):306–312, 2012.

Z. Liang, F. Dong, S.S. Qian, Y. Liu, H. Chen, and W. Lu. Ecoregional or site-specific lake nutrient criteria? Evidence from ecological fallacy. *Ecological Indicators*, 111:105989, 2020.

S.S. Light and J.W. Dineen. Water control in the Everglades: A historical perspective. In S.M. Davis and J.C. Ogden, editors, *Everglades: The Ecosystem and Its Restoration*, pages 47–84. St. Lucie Press, Delray Beach, FL, 1994.

D.V. Lindley and M.R. Novick. The role of exchangeability in inference. *The Annals of Statistics*, 9(1):45–58, 1981.

R.J.A. Little and D.B. Rubin. *Statistical Analysis with Missing Data, 3rd Edition.* Wiley, New York, 2019.

J.M. Lorch, S. Knowles, J.S. Lankton, K. Michell, J.L. Edwards, J.M. Kapfer, R.A. Staffen, E.R. Wild, K.Z. Schmidt, A.E. Ballmann, and D. Blodgett. Snake fungal disease: An emerging threat to wild snakes. *Philosophical Transactions of the Royal Society B*, 371(1709):20150457, 2016.

R.H. Love. Dorsal-aspect target strength of an individual fish. *The Journal of the Acoustical Society of America*, 49(3B):816–823, 1971.

378   *Bibliography*

D. Lunn, D. Spiegelhalter, A. Thomas, and N. Best. The BUGS project: Evolution, critique and future directions. *Statistics in Medicine*, 28(25): 3049–3067, 2009.

D.J. Lunn, A. Thomas, N. Best, and D. Spiegelhalter. WinBUGS - a Bayesian modelling framework: Concepts, structure, and extensibility. *Statistics and Computing*, 10(4):325 – 337, 2000.

C.P. Madenjian, R.J. Hesselberg, T.J. Desorcie, L.J. Schmidt, Stedman. R.M., L.J. Begnoche, and D.R. Passino-Reader. Estimate of net trophic transfer efficiency of PCBs to Lake Michigan lake trout from their prey. *Environmental Science and Technology*, 32:886–891, 1998.

A.L. Madsen, M. Lang, U.B. Kjærulff, and F. Jensen. The Hugin tool for learning Bayesian networks. In T.D. Nielsen and N.L. Zhang, editors, *Symbolic and Quantitative Approaches to Reasoning with Uncertainty*, pages 594–605, Berlin, Heidelberg, 2003. Springer Berlin Heidelberg. ISBN 978-3-540-45062-7.

D. Malakoff. Bayes offers a "new" way to make sense of numbers. *Science*, 286(5444):1460–1464, 1999.

A.D. Maldonado, P.A. Aguilera, and A. Salmeron. Continuous Bayesian networks for probabilistic environmental risk mapping. *Stochastic Environmental Research and Risk Assessment*, 30(5):1441–1455, 2016.

O. Malve and S.S. Qian. Estimating nutrients and chlorophyll a relationships in Finnish lakes. *Environmental Science and Technology*, 40(24):7848–7853, 2006.

B.G. Marcot. Metrics for evaluating performance and uncertainty of Bayesian network models. *Ecological Modelling*, 230:50–62, 2012.

B.G. Marcot and T.D. Penman. Advances in Bayesian network modelling: Integration of modelling technologies. *Environmental Modelling and Software*, 111:386–393, 2019.

B.G. Marcot, J.D. Steventon, G.D. Sutherland, and R.K. McCann. Guidelines for developing and updating Bayesian belief networks applied to ecological modeling and conservation. *Canadian Journal of Forest Research*, 36(12): 3063–3074, 2006.

D.G. Mayo. *Statistical Inference as Severe Testing*. Cambridge University Press, New York, NY, 2018.

G. McMahon and T.F. Cuffney. Quantifying urban intensity in drainage basins for assessing stream ecological conditions. *Journal of the American Water Resources Association*, 36(6):1247–1261, 2000.

G. McMahon, R. Alexander, and S. Qian. Support of total maximum daily load programs using spatially referenced regression models. *Journal of Water Resources Planning and Management*, 129(4):315–329, 2003.

R.S. McNay, B.G. Marcot, V. Brumovsky, and R. Ellis. A Bayesian approach to evaluating habitat for woodland caribou in north-central British Columbia (1). *Canadian Journal of Forest Research*, 36(12):3117–3133, 2006.

N. Metropolis and S. Ulam. The Monte Carlo method. *Journal of the American Statistical Association*, 44(247):335–341, 1949. ISSN 01621459.

N. Metropolis, A.W. Rosenbluth, M.N. Rosenbluth, A.H. Teller, and E. Teller. Equation of state calculations by fast computing machines. *The Journal of Chemical Physics*, 21(6):1087–1092, 1953. doi: 10.1063/1.1699114.

S.J. Moe, S. Haande, and R.M. Couture. Climate change, cyanobacteria blooms and ecological status of lakes: a Bayesian network approach. *Ecological Modelling*, 337:330–347, 2016.

J.-L. Molina, D. Pulido-Velázquez, J.L. García-Aróstegui, and M. Pulido-Velázquez. Dynamic Bayesian networks as a decision support tool for assessing climate change impacts on highly stressed groundwater systems. *Journal of Hydrology*, 479:113–129, 2013.

M.G. Morgan, M. Henrion, and M. Small. *Uncertainty: A Guide to Dealing with Uncertainty in Quantitative Risk and Policy Analysis*. Cambridge University Press, Cambridge, UK, 1990.

S. Morita, A. Namikoshi, T. Hirata, K. Oguma, H. Katayama, S. Ohgaki, N. Motoyama, and M. Fujiwara. Efficacy of UV irradiation in inactivating Cryptosporidiumparvum oocysts. *Applied and Environmental Microbiology*, 68(11), 2002.

P. Müller. A generic approach to posterior integration and Gibbs sampling. Technical Report 91-09, Purdue University, 1991.

S. Nadkarni and P.P. Shenoy. A causal mapping approach to constructing Bayesian networks. *Decision Support Systems*, 38(2):259–281, 2004.

R.M. Neal. Slice sampling. *Annals of Statistics*, 31(3):705–767, 2003.

R.M. Neal. MCMC using Hamiltonian dynamics. In S. Brooks, A. Gelman, G.L. Jones, and X.L. Meng, editors, *Handbook of Markov Chain Monte Carlo*, pages 113–142. Chapman & Hall/CRC Press, 2011.

M. Neil, M. Tailor, and D. Marquez. Inference in hybrid Bayesian networks using dynamic discretization. *Statistics and Computing*, 17(3):219–233, 2007.

S. Newcomb. A generalized theory of the combination of observations so as to obtain the best result. *American Journal of Mathematics*, 8(4):343–366, 1880.

J. Neyman and E.S. Pearson. On the problem of the most efficient tests of statistical hypotheses. *Philosophical Transactions of the Royal Society A*, CCXXXL(702):289–337, 1933.

T.D. Nielsen and F.V. Jensen. *Bayesian Networks and Decision Graphs*. Springer Science and Business Media, 2009.

C.L. Nieman and S.M. Gray. Visual performance impaired by elevated sedimentary and algal turbidity in walleye sander vitreus and emerald shiner *Notropis atherinoides*. *Journal of Fish Biology*, 95(1):186–199, 2019.

E.J. Niklitscheck and D.H. Secor. Dissolved oxygen, temperature and salinity effects on the ecophysiology and survival of juvenile Atlantic sturgeon in estuarine waters: II. Model development and testing. *Journal of Experimental Marine Biology and Ecology*, 381:S161–S172, 2009.

F. Nojavan A., S.S. Qian, H.W. Paerl, K.H. Reckhow, and E.A. Albright. A study of anthropogenic and climatic disturbance of the New River Estuary using a Bayesian belief network. *Marine Pollution Bulletin*, 83:107–115, 2014.

F. Nojavan A., S.S. Qian, and C.A. Stow. Comparative analysis of discretization methods in Bayesian networks. *Environmental Modelling and Software*, 87:64–71, 2017.

S.A. Nummer, S.S. Qian, and R.D. Harmel. A meta-analysis on the effect of agricultural conservation practices on nutrient loss. *Journal of Environmental Quality*, 47(5):1172–1178, 2018.

E.P. Odum, J.T. Finn, and E.H. Franz. Perturbation theory and the subsidy-stress gradient. *BioScience*, 29(6):349–352, 1979.

J. Oksanen and P.R. Minchin. Continuum theory revisited: What shape are species responses along ecological gradients? *Ecological Modelling*, 157(2-3): 119–129, 2002.

J.M. Omernik. Ecoregion of the conterminous United States, map (scale 1:7,500,000). *Annals of the Association of American Geographers*, 77(1): 118–125, 1987.

C. Osborne. Statistical calibration: A review. *International Statistical Review*, 59(3):309–336, 1991.

W.R. Ott. *Environmental Statistics and Data Analysis*. Lewis Publishers, Boca Raton, 1995.

J.E. Painter, M.C. Hlavsa, S.A. Collier, L. Xiao, and J.S. Yoder. Cryptosporidiosis surveillance – United States, 2011–2012. *Morbidity Mortality Weekly Report*, 64(3):1–14, 2015.

J.E. Painter, J.W. Gargano, J.S. Yoderm, S.A. Collierm, and M.C. Hlavsa. Evolving epidemiology of reported cryptosporidiosis cases in the United States 1995-2012. *Epidemiology and Infection*, 144(8):1792–1802, 2016.

Y. Pan, R.J. Stevenson, P. Vaithiyanathan, J. Slate, and C.J. Richardson. Changes in algal assemblages along observed and experimental phosphorus gradients in a subtropical wetland, USA. *Freshwater Biology*, 44:339–353, 2000.

J. Pearl. Reverend Bayes on inference engines: A distributed hierarchical approach. In *Proceedings of AAAI National Conference on AI*, pages 133–136, Pittsburgh, PA., 1982.

J. Pearl. *Causality: Models, Reasoning and Inference*. Cambridge University Press, Cambridge, MA, USA, 2000.

J Pearl, M. Glymour, and N.P. Jewell. *Causal Inference in Statistics*. Wiley, Chichester, UK, 2016.

K. Pearson. Contribution to the mathematical theory of evolution. *Philosophical Transactions of the Royal Society of London A*, 185, 1894.

K. Pearson. *The Grammar of Science*. A. and C. Black, 2nd edition, 1900.

R.H. Peters. *A Critique for Ecology*. Cambridge University Press, 1991.

T.D. Phan, J.C. Smart, S.J. Capon, W.L. Hadwen, and O. Sahin. Applications of Bayesian belief networks in water resource management: A systematic review. *Environmental Modelling and Software*, 85:98–111, 2016.

A.I. Pollard, S.E. Hampton, and D.M. Leech. The promise and potential of continental-scale limnology using the U.S. Environmental Protection Agency's National Lake Assessment. *Limnology and Oceanography Bulletin*, May:36–41, 2018.

C.A. Pollino and C. Henderson. Bayesian networks: A guide for their application in natural resource management and policy. Technical report, Department of the Environment, Water, Heritage, and the Arts, Australia, 2010.

C.A. Pollino, O. Woodberry, A. Nicholson, K. Korb, and B.T. Hart. Parameterisation and evaluation of a Bayesian network for use in an ecological risk assessment. *Environmental Modelling and Software*, 22(8):1140–1152, 2007.

S.S. Qian. Estimating the area affected by phosphorus runoff in an Everglades wetland: A comparison of universal kriging and Bayesian kriging. *Environmental and Ecological Statistics*, 4(1):1–29, 1997.

S.S. Qian. *Environmental and Ecological Statistics with R.* Chapman and Hall/CRC Press, 2010.

S.S. Qian. On model coefficient estimation using Markov chain Monte Carlo simulations: A potential problem and the solution. *Ecological Modelling*, 247:302–306, 2012.

S.S. Qian. The frequency component of water quality criterion compliance assessment should be data driven. *Environmental Management*, 56(1):24–33, 2015.

S.S. Qian. *Environmental and Ecological Statistics with R.* Chapman and Hall/CRC Press, 2nd edition, 2016.

S.S. Qian and T. F. Cuffney. To threshold or not to threshold? That's the question. *Ecological Indicators*, 15(1):1–9, 2012.

S.S. Qian and T.F. Cuffney. A hierarchical zero-inflated model for species compositional data – from individual taxon responses to community response. *Limnology and Oceanography: Methods*, 12:498–506, 2014.

S.S. Qian and T.F. Cuffney. The multiple-comparison trap and the Raven's paradox – perils of using null hypothesis testing in environmental assessment. *Environmental Monitoring and Assessment*, 190(409), 2018.

S.S. Qian and M. Lavine. Setting standards for water quality in the Everglades. *Chance*, 16(3):10–16, 2003.

S.S. Qian and R.E. Lyons. Characterization of background concentrations of contaminants using mixture of normal distributions. *Environmental Science and Technology*, 40:6021–6025, 2006.

S.S. Qian and R.J. Miltner. A continuous variable Bayesian networks model for water quality modeling: A case study of setting nitrogen criterion for small rivers and streams in Ohio, USA. *Environmental Modelling and Software*, 69:14–22, 2015.

S.S. Qian and R.J. Miltner. On abandoning hypothesis testing in environmental standard compliance assessment. *Environmental Management*, 2018. doi: 10.1007/s00267-018-1037-2. URL https://doi.org/10.1007/s00267-018-1037-2.

S.S. Qian and Y. Pan. Historical soil total phosphorus concentration in the Everglades. In A.R. Burk, editor, *Focus on Ecological Research*, pages 131–150. Nova Science, 2006.

S.S. Qian and K. H. Reckhow. Combining model results and monitoring data for water quality assessment. *Environmental Science and Technology*, 41(14):5008–5013, 2007.

S.S. Qian and C.J. Richardson. Estimating the long-term phosphorus accretion rate in the Everglades: A Bayesian approach with risk assessment. *Water Resources Research*, 33(7):1681–1688, 1997.

S.S. Qian and Z. Shen. Ecological applications of multilevel analysis of variance. *Ecology*, 88(10):2489–2495, 2007.

S.S. Qian, M.E. Borsuk, and C. A. Stow. Seasonal and long-term nutrient trend decomposition along a spatial gradient in the Neuse River watershed. *Environmental Science and Technology*, 34:4474–4482, 2000a.

S.S. Qian, M. Lavine, and C.A. Stow. Univariate Bayesian nonparametric binary regression with application in environmental management. *Environmental and Ecological Statistics*, 7:77–91, 2000b.

S.S. Qian, R.S. King, and C.J. Richardson. Two statistical methods for the detection of environmental thresholds. *Ecological Modelling*, 166:87–97, 2003a.

S.S. Qian, C.A. Stow, and M.E. Borsuk. On Monte Carlo methods for Bayesian inference. *Ecological Modelling*, 159:269–277, 2003b.

S.S. Qian, Y. Pan, and R.S. King. Soil total phosphorus threshold in the Everglades: A Bayesian changepoint analysis for multinomial response data. *Ecological Indicators*, 4(1):29–37, 2004a.

S.S. Qian, A. Schulman, J. Koplos, A. Kotros, and P. Kellar. A hierarchical modeling approach for estimating national distributions of chemicals in public drinking water systems. *Environmental Science and Technology*, 38 (4):1176–1182, 2004b.

S.S. Qian, K.H. Reckhow, J. Zhai, and G. McMahon. Nonlinear regression modeling of nutrient loads in streams: A Bayesian approach. *Water Resources Research*, 41:W07012, 2005.

S.S. Qian, J.K. Craig, M.M. Baustian, and N.N. Rabalais. A Bayesian hierarchical modeling approach for analyzing observational data from marine ecological studies. *Marine Pollution Bulletin*, 58(12):1916–1921, 2009.

S.S. Qian, T.F. Cuffney, I. Alameddine, G. McMahon, and K.H. Reckhow. On the application of multilevel modeling in environmental and ecological studies. *Ecology*, 91.355–361, 2010.

S.S. Qian, T.F. Cuffney, and G. McMahon. Multinomial regression for analyzing macroinvertebrate assemblage composition data. *Freshwater Sciences*, 31(3):681–694, 2012.

S.S. Qian, J.D. Chaffin, M.R. DuFour, J.J. Sherman, P.C. Golnick, C.D. Collier, S.A. Nummer, and M.G. Margida. Quantifying and reducing uncertainty in estimated microcystin concentrations from the ELISA method. *Environmental Science and Technology*, 49(24):14221–14229, 2015a.

S.S. Qian, C.A. Stow, and Y.K. Cha. Implications of Stein's Paradox for environmental standard compliance assessment. *Environmental Science and Technology*, 49(10):5913–5920, 2015b.

S.S. Qian, C.A. Stow, Farnaz. Nojavan A., J. Stachelek, Y. Cha, I. Alameddine, and P. Soranno. The implications of Simpson's paradox for cross-scale inference among lakes. *Water Research*, 163:114855, 2019.

S.S. Qian, J.M. Refsnider, J.A. Moore, G.R. Kramer, and H.M. Streby. All tests are imperfect: Accounting for false positives and false negatives using Bayesian statistics. *Heliyon*, 6(3):e03571, 2020.

S.S. Qian, J.G. Kennen, J. May, M.C. Freeman, and T.F. Cuffney. Evaluating the impact of watershed development and climate change on stream ecosystems: A Bayesian network modeling approach. *Water Research*, 205: 117685, 2021a.

S.S. Qian, C.A. Stow, F.E. Rowland, Q. Liu, M.D. Rowe, E.J. Anderson, R.P. Stumpf, and T.H. Johengen. Chlorophyll *a* as an indicator of microcystin: Short-term forecasting and risk assessment in Lake Erie. *Ecological Indicators*, 130:108055, 2021b.

G. Rachid, I. Alameddine, M.A. Najm, S. Qian, and M. El-Fadel. Dynamic Bayesian networks to assess anthropogenic and climatic drivers of saltwater intrusion: A decision support tool toward improved management. *Integrated Environmental Assessment and Management*, 17(1):202–220, 2021.

A. Radl, M.J. Lexer, and H. Vacik. A Bayesian Belief Network approach to predict damages caused by disturbance agents. *Forests*, 9(1):15, 2018.

T.H. Rainer, P.K.S. Chan, M. Ip, N. Lee, D.S. Hui, D. Smit, A. Wu, A.T. Ahuja, J.S. Tam, J.J.Y. Sung, and P. Cameron. The spectrum of severe acute respiratory syndrome–associated coronavirus infection. *Annals of Internal Medicine*, 140(8):614–619, 2004.

F. Ramsey and D. Schafer. *The Statistical Sleuth: A Course in Methods of Data Analysis*. Cengage Learning, 2012.

K.H. Reckhow. Robust Bayes models of fish response to lake acidification. In M.B. Beck, editor, *Systems Analysis in Water Quality Management*, pages 61–72, Oxford, UK, 1987. Pergamon Press.

K.H. Reckhow. A comparison of robust Bayes and classical estimators for regional lake models of fish response to acidification. *Water Resource Research*, 24:1061–1068, 1988.

K.H. Reckhow. Bayesian inference in non-replicated ecological studies. *Ecology*, 71(6):2053–2059, 1990.

K.H. Reckhow. Water quality prediction and probability network models. *Canadian Journal of Fisheries and Aquatic Sciences*, 56(7):1150–1158, 1999.

K.R. Reddy, R.D. DeLaune, W.F. DeBusk, and M.S. Koch. Long-term nutrient accumulation rates in the everglades. *Soil Science Society of America Journal*, 57:1147–1155, 1993.

C.J. Richardson, S. Qian, C.B. Craft, and R.G. Qualls. Predictive models for phosphorus retention in wetlands. *Wetlands Ecology and Management*, 4, 1997.

C.J. Richardson, R.S. King, S.S. Qian, P. Vaithiyanathan, R.G. Qualls, and C.A. Stow. Estimating ecological thresholds for phosphorus in the Everglades. *Environmental Science and Technology*, 41(23):8084–8091, 2007.

M. Richey. The evolution of Markov chain Monte Carlo methods. *The American Mathematical Monthly*, 117(5):383–413, 2010.

E.Z. Rizo, S. Xu, Q. Tang, R.D.S. Papa, H.J. Dumont, S.S. Qian, and B.P. Han. A global analysis of Cladoceran body size and its variation linking to habitat, distribution and taxonomy. *Zoological Journal of the Linnean Society*, 187(4):1119–1130, 10 2019.

C.P. Robert and G. Casella. *Monte Carlo Statistical Methods*. Springer-Verlag, 1999.

C.P. Robert and G. Casella. *Introducing Monte Carlo Methods with R*. Springer, 2010.

R. Robinson. Counting unlabeled acyclic digraphs. In C. Little, editor, *Combinatorial Mathematics V*, pages 28–43, Berlin, Heidelberg, 1977. Springer.

J. Rohmer. Uncertainties in conditional probability tables of discrete Bayesian belief networks: A comprehensive review. *Engineering Applications of Artificial Intelligence*, 88:103384, 2020.

R.F. Ropero, P.A. Aguilera, A. Fernandez, and R. Rumi. Regression using hybrid Bayesian networks: Modelling landscape-socioeconomy relationships. *Environmental Modelling and Software*, 57:127–137, 2014.

A.H. Roy, A.D. Rosemond, M.J. Paul, D.S. Leigh, and J.B. Wallace. Stream macroinvertebrate response to catchment urbanization (Georgia, U.S.A). *Freshwater Biology*, 48, 2003.

T.L. Saaty. How to make a decision: The analytic hierarchy process. *European Journal of Operational Research*, 48(1):9–26, 1990.

J.W. Seaman III, J.W. Seaman Jr, and J.D. Stamey. Hidden dangers of specifying noninformative priors. *The American Statistician*, 66(2):77–84, 2012.

Z. Shen. A multiscale study on the vegetation–environment relationship of a mountain forest transect (in Chinese with English abstract). *Acta Ecologica Sinica*, 22:461–470, 2002.

Z. Shen, X. Zhang, and Y. Jin. An analysis of the topographical pattern of the chief woody species at Dalaoling Mountain in the Three Gorges (in Chinese with English abstract). *Acta Phytoecologica Sinica*, 24:581–589, 2000.

E.H. Simpson. The interpretation in contingency table. *Journal of Royal Statistical Society (B)*, 13:238–241, 1951.

E.P. Smith, K. Ye, C. Hughes, and L. Shabman. Statistical assessment of violations of water quality standards under Section 303(d) of the Clean Water Act. *Environmental Science and Technology*, 35(3):606–612, 2001.

G.H. Snyder and J.M. Davidson. Everglades agriculture: Past, present, and future. In S.M. Davis and J.C. Ogden, editors, *Everglades: The Ecosystem and Its Restoration*, pages 85–116. St. Lucie Press, Delray Beach, FL,, 1994.

A. Sperotto, J.-L. Molina, S. Torresan, A. Critto, and A. Marcomini. Reviewing Bayesian networks potentials for climate change impacts assessment and management: A multi-risk perspective. *Journal of Environmental Management*, 202:320–331, 2017.

C.S. Spetzler and C.-A.S. Stael von Holstein. Exceptional paper—probability encoding in decision analysis. *Management Science*, 22(3):340–358, 1975.

D.J. Spiegelhalter and R.P. Knill-Jones. Statistical and knowledge-based approaches to clinical decision-support systems, with an application in gastroenterology. *Journal of the Royal Statistical Society: Series A (General)*, 147(1):35–58, 1984.

D.J. Spiegelhalter, A. Thomas, N.G. Best, and W.R. Gilks. BUGS 0.5: Bayesian inference Using Gibbs Sampler (version ii), 1996.

P. Spirtes, C. Glymour, and R. Scheines. *Causation, Prediction and Search*. Springer Verlag, Berlin, Germany, 1993.

C. Stein. Inadmissibility of the usual estimator for the mean of a multivariate normal distribution. In *Proceedings of the Third Berkeley Symposium on Mathematical Statistics and Probability*, volume 1, pages 197–206. University of California Press, 1956.

C.E. Stephan, D.I. Mount, D.J. Hansen, J.R. Gentile, G.A. Chapman, and W.A. Brungs. *Guidelines for Deriving Numerical Water Quality Criteria for the Protection of Aquatic Organisms and Their Uses*. 822R85100. US Environmental Protection Agency, Office of Research and Development, Cincinnati, OH, 1985.

K.K. Steward and W.H. Ornes. Assessing a marsh environment for wastewater renovation. *Journal Water Pollution Control Federation*, 47(7):1880–1891, 1975a.

K.K. Steward and W.H. Ornes. The autecology of sawgrass in the Florida Everglades. *Ecology*, 56(1):162–171, 1975b.

C.A. Stow and S.S. Qian. A size-based probabilistic assessment of PCB exposure from Lake Michigan fish consumption. *Environmental Science and Technology*, 32(15):2325–2330, 1998.

C.A. Stow, K.H. Reckhow, and S.S. Qian. A Bayesian approach to retransformation bias in transformed regression. *Ecology*, 87(6):1472–1477, 2006.

A. Stritih, S.-E. Rabe, O. Robaina, A. Gret-Regamey, and E. Celio. An online platform for spatial and iterative modelling with Bayesian networks. *Environmental Modelling and Software*, 127:104658, 2020.

D.R. Swift and R.B. Nicholas. Periphyton and water quality relationships in the Everglades Water Conservation Areas. Technical report, South Florida Water Management District, Tech. Publ. 87-2, West Palm Beach, FL., 1987.

Q. Tang, L. Peng, Y. Yang, Q. Lin, S.S. Qian, and B.P. Han. Total phosphorus-precipitation and chlorophyll a-phosphorus relationships of lakes and reservoirs mediated by soil iron at regional scale. *Water Research*, 154:136–143, 2019.

M.A. Tanner. *Tools for Statistical Inference: Methods for the Exploration of Posterior Distributions and Likelihood Functions*. Springer-Verlag, New York, 1996.

S. J. Tetzlaff, M. Allender, M. Ravesi, J. Smith, and B. Kingsbury. First report of snake fungal disease from Michigan, USA involving massasaugas, *Sistrurus catenatus* (Rafinesque 1818). *Herpetology Notes*, 8:31–33, 2015.

N. Tham, V.T. Hang, T.H. Khanh, D.C. Viet, T.T. Hien, J. Farrar, N.V Chau, and H.R. van Doorn. Comparison of the Roche real-time ready influenza A/H1N1 detection set with CDC A/H1N1pdm09 RT-PCR on samples from three hospitals in Ho Chi Minh City, Vietnam. *Diagnostic Microbiology and Infectious Disease*, 74(2):131–136, 2012.

D.M. Titterington, A.F.M. Smith, and U.E. Makov. *Statistical Analysis of Finite Mixture Distributions*. Applied section. Wiley, 1985.

N.H. Urban, S.M. Davis, and N.G. Aumen. Fluctuations in sawgrass and cattail densities in everglades water conservation area 2a under varying nutrient, hydrologic and fire regimes. *Aquatic Botany*, 46(3):203–223, 1993.

U.S. EPA. Risk assessment guidance for superfund. I. human health evaluation manual (part a). Technical Report EPA 540-1-89-002, U.S. Environmental Protection Agency, Office of Emergency and Remedial Response, Washington DC, 1989.

U.S. EPA. *Ambient Water Quality Criteria Recommendations – Information Supporting the Developlment of State and Tribal Nutrient Criteria – Rivers and Streams in Nutrient Ecoregion VII*. EPA 822-B-00-018. U.S. EPA Office of Water, Washington, CD.C., 2000.

U.S. EPA. Guidance for comparing background and chemical concentrations in soil for CERCLA sites. Technical Report EPA 540-R-01-003, OSWER9285.7-41, U.S. Environmental Protection Agency, Office of Emergency and Remedial Response, 2002.

U.S. EPA. EPA protocol for the review of existing national primary drinking water regulations. Technical Report EPA 815-R-03-002, United States Environmental Protection Agency, Washington, DC, 2003.

U.S. EPA. Drinking water health advisory for the cyanobacterial microcystin toxins. Office of Water, U.S. Environmental Protection Agency, EPA-820R15100, June 2015.

U.S. EPA. Effects Assessment for Existing Chemical and Radionuclide National Primary Drinking Water Regulations - Summary Report. Technical Report EPA 822-R-16-008, U.S. Environmental Protection Agency, Office of Water, Washington D.C., December 2016a.

U.S. EPA. Six-Year Review 3 Technical Support Document for Long-Term 2 Enhanced Surface Water Treatment Rule. Technical Report EPA 810-R-16-011, U.S. Environmental Protection Agency, Office of Water, Washington D.C., December 2016b.

L. Uusitalo. Advantages and challenges of Bayesian networks in environmental modelling. *Ecological Modelling*, 203(3-4):312–318, 2007.

L. Uusitalo, M.T. Tomczak, B. Müller-Karulis, I. Putnis, N. Trifonova, and A. Tucker. Hidden variables in a Dynamic Bayesian Network identify ecosystem level change. *Ecological Informatics*, 45:9–15, 2018.

O. Varis. Bayesian decision analysis for environmental and resource management. *Environmental Modelling and Software*, 12(2-3):177–185, 1997.

W. N. Venables and B. D. Ripley. *Modern Applied Statistics with S*. Springer, New York, fourth edition, 2002. URL http://www.stats.ox.ac.uk/pub/MASS4. ISBN 0-387-95457-0.

L. Vilizzi, A. Price, L. Beesley, B. Gawne, A.J. King, J.D. Koehn, S.N. Meredith, and D.L. Nielsen. Model development of a Bayesian belief network for managing inundation events for wetland fish. *Environmental Modelling and Software*, 41:1–14, 2013.

C.J. Vink, P. Paquin, and R.H. Cruickchank. Taxonomy and irreproducible biological science. *BioScience*, 62(5):451–452, 2012.

R.A. Vollenweider. Scientific foundations of the eutrophication of lakes and flowing waters, with particular reference to nitrogen and phosphorus as factors in eutrophication. Technical report, Organization for Economic Co-operation and Development, Technical Report DAS/CSI/68.27. 250p., 1968.

R.A. Vollenweider. Input-output models with special reference to phosphorus loading concept in limnology. *Schweizerische Zeitschrift für Hydrologie-Swiss*, 37:53–84, 1975.

T. Wagner, P.A. Soranno, K.E. Webster, and K.S. Cheruvelil. Landscape drivers of regional variation in the relationship between total phosphorus and chlorophyll in lakes. *Freshwater Biology*, 56:1811–1824, 2011.

C.J. Walsh, A.K. Sharpe, P.F. Breen, and J.A. Sonneman. Effects of urbanization on streams of the Melbourne region, Victoria, Australia – I. Benthic macroinvertebrate communities. *Freshwater Biology*, 46:535–551, 2001.

R.L. Wasserstein and N.A. Lazar. The ASA's statement on p-values: context, process, and purpose. *American Statisticians*, 70(2):129–133, 2016.

WDH and WDNR. Important health information for people eating fish from wisconsin waters. Technical report, Wisconsin Division of Health and Wisconsin Department of Natural Resources, PUB No FH824 97, 1997.

R.W.M. Wedderburn. Quasi-likelihood functions, generalized linear models, and the Gauss—Newton method. *Biometrika*, 61(3):439–447, 1974.

Z. Wei and Y. Wei. Fluoridation in China: A clouded future. *Fluoride*, 35(1): 1–4, 2002.

R. H. Whittaker. Vegetation of the Great Smoky Mountains. *Ecological Monographs*, 26(1):1–80, 1956.

R.H. Whittaker. Gradient analysis of vegetation. *Biological Reviews*, 42(2): 207–264, 1967.

R.L. Winkler. *An Introduction to Bayesian Inference and Decision*. Probabilistic Publishing, Gainesville, Fl., 2003.

O. Woodberry, A.E. Nicholson, K.B. Korb, and C. Pollino. Parameterising Bayesian networks. In G.I. Webb and X. Yu, editors, *AI 2004: Advances in Artificial Intelligence*, pages 1101–1107, Berlin, Heidelberg, 2005. Springer.

R. Wu, S.S. Qian, F. Hao, H. Cheng, D. Zhu, and J. Zhang. Modeling contaminant concentration distributions in China's centralized source waters. *Environmental Science and Technology*, 45(14):6041–6048, 2011.

L.L. Yuan and A.I. Pollard. Deriving nutrient targets to prevent excessive cyanobacterial densities in U.S. lakes and reservoirs. *Freshwater Biology*, 60 (9):1901–1916, 2015.

L.L. Yuan and A.I. Pollard. Using national-scale data to develop nutrient-microcystin relationships that guide management decisions. *Environmental Science and Technology*, 433(51):6972–6980, 2017.

L.A. Zadeh. The concept of a linguistic variable and its application to approximate reasoning-I. *Information Sciences*, 8(3):199–249, 1975.

Z. Zawadzki and M. Kosinski. *Rcpp: Implementation of "FSelector" Entropy-Based Feature Selection Algorithms with a Sparse Matrix Support*, 2021. URL https://github.com/mi2-warsaw/FSelectorRcpp. R package version 0.0.3.

L. Zhang, X. Wu, Y. Qin, M.J. Skibniewski, and W. Liu. Towards a fuzzy Bayesian network based approach for safety risk analysis of tunnel-induced pipeline damage. *Risk Analysis*, 36(2):278–301, 2016.

Index

analysis of deviance, 146
analysis of variance, 91
    Bayesian, 147
    nested, 107

background concentration, 218
Bayes theorem, 2, 4, 65
Bayes, Thomas, 1
Bayesian Monte Carlo, 4, 26–28
Bayesian networks, 298–326
    continuous, 315–320
    CPT, 299, 301, 304, 309–312, 315
    discretization, 299, 311–315
    dynamic, 315, 325, 326
    expert elicitation, 298, 301–302
    Markov equivalent, 303
    mutual information, 308, 320, 321
    NPC algorithms, 303, 305, 307, 308, 315
    OOBN, 324
    PC algorithms, 303, 305, 315
    sensitivity, 299, 301, 308, 320, 321, 323
    spatiotemporal, 324
    structure learning, 303, 305
Bernoulli distribution, 176
beta distribution, 4, 281
binomial distribution, 2
binomial-binomial mixture, 285
binomial-Poisson mixture, 281

calibration, 117
catchability, 262
censored data, 271
change point, 47, 50, 238

Clean Water Act, 244
    303(d), 244, 338
    MDF, 244
conditional autoregressive (CAR), 165
confidence interval, 11, 358
conjugate priors, 51, 73, 77, 79, 84, 85, 94, 117, 130, 146
    beta, 78
    Dirichlet, 300
    gamma, 78, 142–144
    inverse gamma, 92, 114, 247
    norma-gamma, 73
    normal-inverse gamma, 92, 113
contraposition, 358
CPUE, 15, 193, 195, 196, 262–264
credible interval, 5, 13, 39, 153, 161, 238, 239, 241, 249, 332, 336, 352

d-separation, 293, 320
data
    experimental, 344
    observational, 344
data augmentation, 170–177
deduction, 1, 7, 9
detection probability, 168, 280, 348
Dirichlet distribution, 52, 53, 300
drinking water safety, 227
    fluoride, 277

empirical Bayes, 234
entropy, 308, 315, 320, 321
environmental standard
    ideal, 250
    realizable, 250
ergodic, 41

examples, 15
  background contaminant
    concentration, 132–138
  combining nonexchangeable
    units, 289–293
  COVID-19 testing, 177–183
  drinking water safety
    China source water survey,
      276–278
    cryptosporidium, 278–287
    six-year review, 273–276
  effects of soil iron on lake
    eutrophication, 258–260
  effects of urbanization on stream
    ecosystems (EUSE), 16–18,
    196–206, 215–217, 250–258
  environmental standard
    compliance assessment,
    21–22, 243–250
  Everglades studies, 18–21
    environmental standard,
      237–243
    Historical soil TP
      concentrations, 217–222
    phosphorus threshold, 47–51
  fishery by-catch, 144–146,
    188–191
  gill-net monitoring data, 15–16
    sampling methods
      catchability, 261–271
    walleye apportionment, 36–40
  Gulf of Mexico hypoxia,
    100–108, 353, 359
  insect oviposition behavior,
    210–214
  Liverpool Moth, 148–156
  microcystin in Western Lake
    Erie, 363–365
  Neuse River eutrophication, 126
    water quality standard
      compliance assessment,
      66–76
  PCB in fish, 52–54, 110
  seaweed grazer, 93–100
  seedling recruitment, 156–168
  snake fungal disease, 6–9, 26–28,
    30, 55–56, 91, 170, 345, 352
  sturgeon population, 191–196
  Toledo water crisis, 119–126
  water quality standard
    compliance assessment, 126
exchangeable, 103, 131, 194, 196,
    202, 225, 228–230, 232, 234,
    236, 240, 249, 251, 257, 259,
    286, 288, 290, 293, 337, 355,
    362, 363

false negative, 7, 168, 178, 280
false positive, 7, 168, 178

gamma model, 197, 218
generalized linear models, 157
  Bayesian, 160
  zip, 186, 193
Gibbs sampler, *see* Monte Carlo
    simulation
grass carp, 347

hierarchical model, 226, 246, 270
  hyper-distribution, 92, 103, 105,
    129, 131, 234, 242, 243, 245,
    248, 249, 280, 292, 361
  hyper-parameters, 92, 103–105,
    197, 202, 204, 231, 236, 237,
    241–243, 246, 251, 283, 287,
    336, 337
  multivariate normal prior, 252,
    253, 255
  nested groups, 260
  shrinkage, 234
  zip, 202–204
hockey stick model, 47, 50
Hugin, 303, 308, 318, 325
Hume, David, 1
hydroacoustic, 36
hypothesis testing, 11, 244
  alternative, 11
  null hypothesis, 11
  power of, 245
hypothetical deduction, 64

i.i.d., 225
identifiable, 135, 169
imperfect detection, 168–206, 271
induction, 1, 8, 9
instrumental distribution, 30
interaction, 161

James-Stein estimator, 234

latent variable, 170
likelihood function, 4, 12, 171, 176,
    185
logistic regression, 149, 270
logit transformation
    multinomial, 209

maximum contaminant level (MCL),
    227, 276
method detection limit (MDL), 227
method of moments, 90, 130
Metropolis-Hastings, *see* Monte
    Carlo simulation
mixture distribution, 131–138
Monte Carlo simulation, 25–56
    acceptance-rejection, 30–32
    inverse-CDF, 28–30
    Markov chain, 25, 41–54
        Gibbs sampler, 45–55, 171
        Metropolis-Hastings, 42–44,
        55
    numerical integration, 33–35
    relationships, 32–33
morph, 148
mountain ecology, 156
multilevel model, 226, 246, 251, 263
multinomial distribution, 171, 206
multinomial regression, 206–222

negative binomial distribution,
    142–144
Neuse River Estuary, 66
Neyman-Pearson lemma, 11
    rule of behavior, 11

objective knowledge, 228
over-dispersion, 142, 162–164

Poisson distribution, 142–144, 157,
    183, 280
posterior
    distribution, 5, 9
    probability, 3
posterior simulation, 146, 163, 190,
    340, 345, 346, 352
prior, 234, 236
    correlation matrix
        Cholesky decomposition, 253
        LKJ prior, 252
    covariance matrix, 251
        quad-form decomposition, 252
    distribution, 4
    non-informative, 6
    probability, 2
prior distribution, 76–80, 360–363
    conjugate family, 77
    informative, 77
    non-informative, 80
    weakly informative, 80

quasi-likelihood, 163

R
    functions
        anova, 148, 155, 157
        apply, 35
        bayes_binom, 3
        beta_mm, 183
        bmc_sfd_post, 27
        cumsum, 27, 106
        curve, 56, 74
        dbeta, 43, 56
        dbinom, 3
        dt, 74
        extract, 95, 152, 352
        fixef, 246
        glm, 154, 157
        glmer, 269, 351
        hist, 56, 74
        length, 74
        lmer, 246, 263
        log1p, 44
        log_lk, 44

matrix, 35
mean, 74
mlplot, 98, 152
multinom, 212
my.rbinom, 32
my.rnorm, 31
NIGpost, 74
pchisq, 156, 158
post, 56
post_impft, 9
posterior, 115
rbeta, 43, 47, 56
rbinom, 47
rbin_imperfect, 173
rbinom, 352
rnorm, 35
runif, 56
rvnorm, 116, 353
rvsims, 90, 95, 98, 106, 152,
    353
sampling, 89, 90, 95, 152, 183
sd, 35
sd.rv, 152
se.fixef, 246
stan, 89
stan_model, 88, 94, 152, 183
sum, 3
zeroinfl, 187
packages
    rjags, 57
    rstan, 58
    rstan, 86
    rv, 86, 106
regression, 108
    calibration, 117
    linear, 109
    nonlinear, 117

Safe Drinking Water Act (SDWA),
    227, 273
    information collection request,
    273
sequential updating, 126, 182
severe testing, 357
shrinkage, 234

Simpson's paradox, 232
spatial autocorrelation, 165–168
ST50, 201, 206
Stan
    functions
        binomial_lpmf, 282
        diag_pre_multiply, 253, 255,
            256, 260
        lkj_corr, 252, 254
        lkj_corr_cholesky, 253, 255,
            256, 260
        log1m, 185
        log_mix, 134
        log_sum_exp, 286
        log_sum_exp, 134, 175, 177,
            185, 282
        multi_normal_prec, 167
        multinomial, 214
        neg_binomial_2_log_lpmf,
            146
        neg_binomial_2_lpmf, 190,
            192
        normal_lpdf, 88, 122, 134
        poisson_log_lpmf, 145
        poisson_lpmf, 185, 282
        quad_form_diag, 252, 254
        rows_dot_product, 255, 256
        softmax, 214
        sparse_car_lpdf, 167
    models
        euse_stan1, 254
        everg_stan, 241
        GNq_cor_cent, 267
        latent_Bern, 182
        mixture1, 135
        moth_var, 150
        multN, 214
        NB_bycatch, 146
        nested groups, 260
        non-nested groups, 256
        occ_stan1, 275
        Pois_bycatch, 145
        seedStan, 160
        seedStanCar1, 167
        sequp_ch6, 247

`stan_aov`, 94
`stan_aov2`, 99
`walleye_id`, 270
`zinb1`, 195
`zip1`, 187
`zip2`, 199
`zip3`, 204
statistical problems, 14, 343
    distribution, 63, 68
    estimation, 63, 68
    specification, 63, 68
statistical significance, 355–359
Stein's paradox, 234
sub-population, 232
subjective ignorance, 228
superfund, 131

threshold, 242

unidentifiable, 135

variance components, 96–98, 100,
    153, 160, 162, 168

wetlands, 47, 289
    nutrient retention, 47, 238, 289

zero-inflation, 183–206, 280
    identifiable, 186